# Hydroxylapatite Coatings in Orthopaedic Surgery

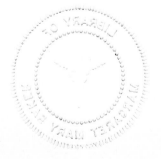

# Hydroxylapatite Coatings in Orthopaedic Surgery

Editors

**Rudolph G. T. Geesink,**
**M.D., Ph.D.**

*State University of Limburg*
*Department of Orthopaedic Surgery*
*University Hospital Maastricht*
*Maastricht, The Netherlands*

**Michael T. Manley, Ph.D.**

*Orthopaedic Bioengineer*
*Franklin Lakes, New Jersey*

Raven Press ⚞ New York

**Raven Press, Ltd., 1185 Avenue of the Americas, New York, New York 10036**

Made in the United States of America

```
Hydroxylapatite coatings in orthopaedic surgery / editors, Rudolph
  G.T. Geesink, Michael T. Manley.
       p.   cm.
    Includes bibliographical references and index.
    ISBN 0-7817-0005-1
    1. Hydroxyapatite coating--Biocompatibility.  2. Orthopedic
  implants.  3. Hydroxyapatite coating--Physiological effect.
  4. Hydroxyapatite coating--Therapeutic use.   I. Geesink, Rudolph G.
  T.  II. Manley, Michael T.
    [DNLM: 1. Hydroxyapatites.  2. Surface Properties.  3. Implants,
  Artificial.  4. Hip Prosthesis.  5. Orthopedics.   WE 172 H995 1993]
  RD755.65.H93   1993
  617.3'0028--dc20
  DNLM/DLC
  for Library of Congress                                 93-24521
                                                             CIP
```

9 8 7 6 5 4 3 2 1

# Foreword

I have followed Dr. Geesink's work on hydroxylapatite (HA) with great, shared interest over the years. It is, therefore, a pleasure to write the foreword to *Hydroxylapatite Coatings in Orthopaedic Surgery.* During our careers in orthopaedic surgery, we have both sought to develop a method that will provide enduring fixation for hip prostheses. We have both come to appreciate that the success of our methods of implant fixation depends on the consistency of our results: consistency achieved not only by joint replacement specialists, but by the general orthopaedists in the community.

Without minimizing the importance that polymethylmethacrylate (PMMA) will always hold in orthopaedic surgery, it must be recognized and accepted that inherent mechanical and biologic drawbacks ultimately limit its successful application. The brittleness, low modulus, low static and fatigue strength of PMMA contributes to mechanical failure of the procedure. Furthermore, the tendency of PMMA to be toxic to tissues, both locally and systemically, invokes inflammatory reactions and osteolytic lesions.

When I began using cementless implants with a sintered metal surface, much of the pioneering work had already been done. In the late 1960s and early 1970s, Judet and Lord had developed and tested hip prostheses with cast rough and porous surfaces. The basics of experimental research on sintered microporous surfaces had also been completed by such pioneers as Bobyn, Cameron, Collier, and Ducheyne. My task was to initiate the clinical trials.

Dr. Geesink's involvement with HA coatings for hip implants began at an earlier stage of development. However, the motivation for Dr. Geesink's work was notably similar to my own. Dr. Geesink had experience using cemented implants. He also had experience with press-fit and porous-surface implants and was not satisfied with the results. The results of his early animal experiments with HA-coated implants were published and presented at numerous international symposia prior to the initiation of the clinical trial phase.

To gain broader acceptance for the use of HA coatings, expanded clinical trials and careful analysis of autopsy-retrieved specimens were conducted. This text reviews the evolution and current application of HA technology and suggests directions for further research.

The clinical trials described in this text are reported by surgeons experienced with press-fit stems for biologic fixation. The impression given by their data is that press-fit stems with HA coatings produce better short-term clinical results than the use of press-fit stems without coating. The reader will note that HA coatings have been applied to a number of different implant designs, including Dr. William Bargar's work with customized implants. I have had the opportunity to examine the postoperative radiographs of Dr. Geesink's HA-coated implants, and there appears to be osseointegration into the HA-coated surface. Long-term follow-up will be needed to assess the durability of this bond.

Thomas Bauer, an internationally recognized orthopaedic pathologist, has performed detailed histologic analysis of autopsy-retrieved material. Acknowledging the biocompatibility and osteoconductive properties of HA, Dr. Bauer maintains that load transfer from implant to bone, implant flexibility, and the state of host bone are the key determinants for bone apposition. Dr. Bauer continues to explore the possible mechanisms for HA loss, including bone remodeling, delamination, dissolution, abrasion, and the consequences of particulate HA.

As it is often stated, any new concept with merit evolves through several stages. First there is a phase of initial enthusiasm; second, a more critical scientific evaluation: and finally, the phase of general acceptance. This text is, to my knowledge, the first comprehensive examination of HA coatings in orthopaedics and will serve as a cornerstone for further research.

*Charles A. Engh, M.D.*
Clinical Assistant Professor of
Orthopaedic Surgery
Georgetown University and
University of Maryland
The Anderson Clinic, Inc.
Arlington, Virginia

# Preface

In the last two decades, major changes have occurred in the practice of reconstructive orthopaedic surgery. Cemented total hip arthroplasty, begun by John Charnley and extended by Maurice Muller, has evolved into a more exacting science with better implant materials, different designs, and improved cement techniques. Demands for hip replacement surgery from a younger and potentially more active patient population stimulated the development of noncemented hip replacement because of the poor mechanical properties and apparent limited lifetime of cement. These demands led, in the United States, to the development of noncemented implants with porous coatings based on the pioneering work of Robert Pilliar in Toronto, Canada. The clinical reporting of Charles Engh with the AML, the PCA group with their implant, and other investigators with various designs have shown that noncemented porous implants can provide good/excellent results in some younger patients. In Europe, where porous ("microbead") implants were never accepted as widely, noncemented implants evolved toward press-fit macrostructured designs such as the Zweimuller and the CLS.

In the hands of their designers, noncemented implants have shown successful clinical outcomes in many patients. Generally, however, success has been mixed, and loose press-fit implants have led to complications such as bead shedding, metal abrasion, pain and revision. The need for a stable initial fit is now accepted as a prerequisite for success. Better and more accurate instrumentation and more rigorous surgical technique have been developed to achieve the requirement of postoperation implant stability.

A little over ten years ago, the editors became aware separately that implant coatings of calcium phosphate ceramics might lead to a predictable bony interface for weight-bearing implants and might be capable of promoting such an interface even if the implant was not completely stable postoperatively. Among the calcium phosphate materials available, hydroxylapatite $[Ca_{10}(PO_4)_6(OH)_2(HA)]$ appeared to be the best candidate because of its natural occurrence in bone, its documented biocompatibility, and because of its apparent predictability in establishing a bony interface *in vivo*. We worked on roughly parallel paths (as did others, some of whom are authors in this book) and became aware of each other in 1987. Since then, we have collaborated in the assessment of HA coatings by experimental and clinical studies and have become convinced that this material can promote favorable bone remodeling at implant interfaces. Further, as clinical follow-up progresses, the data suggest that HA-coated implants retain stability and are associated with a lesser incidence of pain than some contemporary porous designs.

*vii*

In 1992, we decided that a book summarizing the experimental, *in vivo,* and clinical studies on HA coatings would be useful. Rather than writing the book simply about our own experiences, we decided that it would be more interesting to invite independent scientific and clinical investigators in Europe and the United States to write about their own results and their views on HA coatings, whether or not their views coincided with our own.

This book, therefore, contains a compilation of different scientific and clinical studies. The text begins with a review of the available scientific literature on HA in general, follows with papers on scientific *in vivo* studies of HA coatings in animals and in patients, and then describes clinical results with four different types of femoral stems and one knee implant. The impression from all of the data presented is that HA coatings do indeed promote an implant interface with bone rather than fibrous tissue. Autopsy studies have shown a remarkable adaptation of the bone to implant contours. Biological response appears benign, and short- to mid-term clinical follow-up (six years plus) is very favorable.

Some questions yet remain unanswered. It is now known that HA coatings can be digested by osteoclasts and that the coating becomes a part of the remodeling process around the implant. Autopsy specimens suggest that focal digested areas of the coating can be replaced by bone. It is not known whether the entire coating will eventually be remodeled and replaced or, indeed, whether this would have any effect on implant stability. It has yet to be shown conclusively that macrotextured titanium alloy implants are the optimum substrate for the coating. However, it is known that at four, five, and six years postsurgery HA-coated implants are remarkably stable and pain-free. Only time is required to see whether this favorable trend continues into long-term (ten year plus) clinical follow-up.

*Rudolph G. T. Geesink, M.D., Ph.D.*
Maastricht, The Netherlands

*Michael T. Manley, Ph.D.*
Franklin Lakes, New Jersey, U.S.A.

# Contents

*ix*

# Acknowledgments

We thank the authors of the chapters in this book for the time commitment needed to write, finalize, and proofread their manuscripts. The excellent quality of their scientific and clinical work speaks for itself.

Compilation of this volume would have been impossible without the hard work and constant reminders of Terry Zielinski and Joann Gold. Layouts are due to the diligence of Chris Beaudin and Wayne Pollack. Final editing was skillfully completed by Laura Koch. All have our thanks.

Finally, we sincerely acknowledge the support our families have given us. They have tolerated our obsession with this subject and our absences from home with understanding and encouragement.

# Contributors

**William L. Bargar, M.D.**
*The University of California at Davis*
*    School of Medicine*
*Sacramento, California;*
*The Sutter General Hospital*
*Fort Sutter Medical Complex II*
*Suite 450*
*Sacramento, California 95816*

**Thomas W. Bauer, M.D., Ph.D.**
*Department of Pathology and*
*    Orthopedic Surgery*
*The Cleveland Clinic Foundation*
*9500 Euclid Avenue*
*Cleveland, Ohio 44195*

**Clemens A. van Blitterswijk, Ph.D.**
*Laboratory for Otobiology and*
*    Biocompatibility*
*Biomaterials Research Group*
*Leiden, The Netherlands*

**Yvonne P. Bovell, B.Sc.**
*Laboratory for Otobiology and*
*    Biocompatibility*
*Biomaterials Research Group*
*Leiden, The Netherlands*

**Ineke van den Brink, B.Sc.**
*Laboratory for Otobiology and*
*    Biocompatibility*
*Biomaterials Research Group*
*Leiden, The Netherlands*

**Joost D. de Bruijn, B.Sc.**
*Laboratory for Otobiology and*
*    Biocompatibility*
*Biomaterials Research Group*
*Leiden, The Netherlands*

**Cody Bünger, M.D., Ph.D.**
*Biomechanics Laboratory,*
*    Orthopaedic Hospital*
*DK-8200 Aarhus N., Denmark*

**William N. Capello, M.D.**
*Professor of Orthopaedic Surgery*
*Department of Orthopaedic Surgery*
*Indiana University School of Medicine*
*541 Clinical Drive, Rm 600*
*Indianapolis, Indiana 46223*

**Stephen D. Cook, Ph.D.**
*Director, Orthopaedic Research*
*Department of Orthopaedic Surgery*
*Tulane University School of Medicine*
*1430 Tulane Avenue*
*New Orleans, Louisiana 70112*

**James A. D'Antonio, M.D.**
*Clinical Assistant Professor*
*Department of Orthopaedic Surgery*
*University of Pittsburgh;*
*Orthopaedic Surgeon*
*Sewickley Valley Hospital*
*MH & D Orthopaedics*
*1099 Ohio River Boulevard*
*Sewickley, Pennsylvania 15143*

**Lawrence D. Dorr, M.D.**
*Professor and Chief*
*USC Center for Arthritis and Joint*
*    Implant Surgery*
*1510 San Pablo Street*
*Suite 634*
*Los Angeles, California 90033*

**Charles A. Engh, M.D.**
*Clinical Assistant Professor of*
*    Orthopaedic Surgery*
*Georgetown University and University*
*    of Maryland;*
*The Anderson Clinic, Inc.*
*2445 Army-Navy Drive*
*Arlington, Virginia 22206*

**Jean-Alain Epinette, M.D.**
*Clinique Medico-Chirurgicale*
*200 Avenue D'Auverne*
*62700 Bruay en Artois, France*

**Jim S. Flach, M.Sc.**
*Laboratory for Otobiology and*
  *Biocompatibility*
*Biomaterials Research Group*
*Leiden, The Netherlands*

**Michael A. R. Freeman, M.D.,**
  **F.R.C.S.**
*London Hospital Medical College*
*Arthritis and Rheumatism Council Building*
*25-29 Ashfield Street*
*London E1 1AD, United Kingdom*

**Richard J. Friedman, M.D.,**
  **F.R.C.S. (C)**
*Associate Professor*
*Department of Orthopaedic Surgery*
*Medical University of South Carolina*
*171 Ashley Avenue*
*Charleston, South Carolina 29406*

**Ronald Furlong, F.R.C.S.**
*Hon. Consulting Orthopaedic Surgeon*
*St. Thomas Hospital, London;*
*Hon. Consulting Orthopaedic Surgeon*
  *to the Army*
*Lister House*
*11-12 Wimpole Street*
*London W1M 7AB, United Kingdom*

**Rudolph G. T. Geesink, M.D., Ph.D.**
*State University of Limburg*
*Department of Orthopaedic Surgery*
*University Hospital Maastricht*
*P.O. Box 5800 6202 AZ*
*Maastricht, The Netherlands*

**Klaas de Groot, Ph.D.**
*Biomaterials Research Group*
*School of Medicine*
*Leiden University*
*Rijnsburgerweg 10*
*2333 AA Leiden, The Netherlands*

**Ebbe S. Hansen, M.D.**
*Institute of Experimental Clinical*
  *Research*
*Biomechanics Laboratory*
*Orthopaedic Hopital*
*DK-8200 Aarhus N, Denmark*

**Anthony K. Hedley, M.D., F.R.C.S.**
*Chairman, Department of Orthopedics*
*St. Luke's Hospital*
*1800 E. Van Buren Street*
*Phoenix, Arizona 85006*

**Rik Huiskes, Ph.D.**
*Biomechanics Section*
*Department of Orthopaedics*
*University of Nijmegen*
*P.O. Box 9101*
*6500 HB Nijmegen, The Netherlands*

**William L. Jaffe, M.D.**
*Associate Director*
*Department of Orthopaedic Surgery*
*Hospital for Joint Diseases Orthopaedic*
  *Institute*
*New York, New York;*
*Associate Clinical Professor*
*Mt. Sinai School of Medicine*
*1095 Park Avenue*
*New York, New York 10028*

**John A. Jansen, D.D.S., Ph.D.**
*Department of Oral Function*
*Laboratory of Biomaterials*
*Dental School, University of Nijmegen*
*P.O. Box 9101*
*6500 HB Nijmegen, The Netherlands*

**John F. Kay, Ph.D.**
*President/CEO*
*Bio-Interfaces, Inc.*
*11095 Flintkote Avenue*
*San Diego, California 92121*

**Christel P.A.T. Klein, D.V.S., Ph.D.**
*Biomaterials Research Group*
*School of Medicine*
*Leiden University*
*Leiden, The Netherlands*

**Henk Leenders, B.Sc.**
*Laboratory for Otobiology and*
  *Biocompatibility*
*Biomaterials Research Group*
*Leiden, The Netherlands*

**Frank P. Magee, D.V.M.**
*Executive Vice President of Research
and Development
OrthoLogic Corporation
Phoenix, Arizona 85034*

**Michael T. Manley, Ph.D.**
*Orthopaedic Bioengineer
744 Paiute Place
Franklin Lakes, New Jersey 07417*

**Edward J. McPherson, M.D.**
*Associate Professor
USC Center for Arthritis and Joint
Implant Surgery
USC University Hospital
Kerlan-Jobe Orthopaedic Clinic
501 East Hardy Street
Suite 200
Inglewood, California 90301*

**Robert D. Poser, D.V.M.**
*Director of Orthopedic Research
Norian Corporation
1025 Terra Bella Avenue
Mountain View, California 94043*

**Helle B. Rasmussen, M.D.**
*Institute of Pathology at Aarhus
Amtssygehus
DK-8200 Aarhus N, Denmark*

**Gareth Scott, F.R.C.S.**
*London Hospital Medical College
Arthritis and Rheumatism Council
Building
25-29 Ashfield Street
London E1 1AD, United Kingdom*

**Paul Serekian, M.S.**
*Material Scientist
5 Aspen Court
Mahwah, New Jersey 07430*

**Kjeld Søballe, M.D.**
*Biomechanics Laboratory
Orthopaedic Hospital
DK-8200 Aarhus N, Denmark*

**Jeffery K. Taylor, M.D.**
*The Sutter General Hospital
Fort Sutter Medical Complex II
1020 29th Street
Suite 450
Sacramento, California 95816*

**Jan Verhaar, M.D., Ph.D.**
*Department of Orthopaedics
Academic Hospital Maastricht
6202 AZ Maastricht, The Netherlands*

**Harrie Weinans, Ph.D.**
*Biomechanics Section
Department of Orthopaedics
University of Nijmegen
6500 HB Nijmegen, The Netherlands*

**Joop G.C. Wolke, B.Eng.**
*Biomaterials Research Group
School of Medicine
Leiden University
Leiden, The Netherlands*

# Hydroxylapatite Coatings in Orthopaedic Surgery

*Hydroxylapatite Coatings in Orthopaedic Surgery,*
edited by R. G. T. Geesink and M. T. Manley.
Raven Press, Ltd., New York, © 1993.

# Calcium Phosphate Biomaterials: A Review of the Literature

## Michael T. Manley, Ph.D.

In recent years, the calcium phosphate system, and in particular hydroxylapatite (HA), has been the subject of extensive investigation as implant materials and coatings. HA is a naturally occurring mineral and the predominant mineral component of vertebrate bone and tooth enamel. HA has found use as a dietary calcium supplement for pregnant women and nursing mothers, and extensive use as a dental implant material. HA has a calcium -phosphorus ratio (Ca/P) of 1.67.

Synthetic calcium phosphate materials have been prepared and studied extensively *in vitro* and *in vivo*. Although some materials used have been called "hydroxylapatite" by some investigators, they actually vary widely in composition with calcium/phosphorus ratios ranging from 2.0 to as low as 1.3. These materials are rarely well-characterized. Therefore, it can be difficult or misleading to compare and rationalize the results of studies by different investigators with "hydroxylapatite" materials (3, 58).

This chapter is a summation of the extensive literature on calcium phosphate biomaterials, and HA in particular. The review covers the biologic response to the material and its potential degradation *in vivo*. The literature indicates the excellent biocompatibility of HA, the overall lack of inflammatory response to the material, and its favorable biologic profile when used in apposition to living bone. The application of calcium phosphates as coatings to metallic implants in animal studies is summarized also. Finally, a brief review of the emerging clinical data with HA coatings is presented.

## GENERAL BIOLOGICAL CHARACTERIZATION OF CALCIUM PHOSPHATE MATERIALS

### Biocompatibility and Toxicity

In 1981, HA for medical applications was introduced commercially in granular form for alveolar ridge augmentation and periodontal lesion filling. In the decade following, applications have expanded to include blocks and coatings in restorative dental and orthopaedic implants. HA continues to show a highly attractive biologic profile. This profile includes a lack of local or systemic toxicity, a lack of inflammatory or foreign-body response to the material in solid or particulate form, a lack of pyrogenic response, an absence of intervening fibrous tissue between implant and bone, and the ability to become bonded to bone directly (20, 58, 60, 62, 71, 90). Favorable biologic data have been observed with calcium phosphate implant materials of various chemical compositions and material structures. The profile probably is generic to all calcium phosphate implant materials. In addition, when discussing the biocompatibility of HA, Russotti et al., (83), stated, in citing a number of authors, "Repeated studies in animals and humans have shown the substance (HA) to be nontoxic, nonallergenic, and noninflammatory".

Almost all long term investigations of calcium phosphate materials have shown positive results *in vivo*. HA blocks and granules have been studied extensively in orthopaedic and dental animal models, including primates (49), dogs (25, 33), rabbits (35, 78), and rats (2, 5, 33). Results have been uniformly successful with no reported adverse local or systemic response.

An investigation by Hoogendoorn et al. (56) of tissue compatibility and biodegradation of large ceramic porous HA blocks implanted in dog femora for up to three and one-half years did not reveal any signs of inflammation or of adverse tissue reaction. Radiographic and microscopic observations by Gumaer et al. (50) of 22 dog femora implanted with granular and solid ceramic HA for periods of up to eight years revealed normal organs and tissues and no inflammatory response due to the HA material. Gumaer et al. also observed that both granular and solid types of HA implants interfaced directly with dense lamellar bone on all surfaces, with little to no resorption of the ceramic material (50). Jarcho (58) reported that the undesirable migration of an implant from a bony site into adjacent soft tissue did not produce an inflammatory response, because the calcium phosphate materials were well tolerated by soft tissues. In a canine spinal fusion feasibility study by Cook et al. (18), gross failure of porous tricalcium phosphate implants occurred three to six weeks post implantation because of the poor mechanical properties of the device. However, histologic evaluation revealed a complete lack of foreign-body or inflammatory response to the material in spite of the device failure. Recently, Goodman et al. (46) implanted HA and titanium alloy particulate into rabbit tibiae in an attempt to model the cellular response to potential debris released from implants. These authors found that the materials were substantially more biocompatible than particles of polymethylmethacrylate or polyethylene implanted as controls, and the HA particles were still associated with the bony remodeling reported with larger forms of the material. All of these findings confirm the excellent biocompatibility of HA.

Although the efficacy and the benign nature of calcium phosphate materials are widely reported, a few negative reactions, such as an inflammatory response to an HA suspension in a few early animal (rat) studies also have been reported (29,77). In addition, clinical problems have been experienced with the migration of granules used in ridge augmentation because of difficulty in attaining mechanical stability at the implant site (81,82). In one study, high rates of dehiscence and infection with highly porous HA were reported but were attributed to the physical form of the material as well as to trauma (81).

These few negative reports are in sharp contrast to many animal studies that demonstrate the biocompatibility and functional success of calcium phosphate ceramics in dentistry and orthopedic applications. Cullum et al. (24) applied dense HA in maxillary alveolar cleft defects in 12 mongrel dogs and by eight weeks demonstrated no inflammation and repair of the cleft defect. In a 16-week study of nine dog mandibles, Block and Kent (7) compared the osteoinductive abilities of HA alone to HA mixed with autogenous bone from the posterior iliac crest. Both implant groups showed bony ingrowth and an absence of inflammatory cells, but the HA/bone mixture demonstrated a higher level of bone development. Frame et al. (38) found that the addition of particulate HA to resorbable plaster of paris did not interfere with the healing and consolidation of an augmented maxillary ridge. Denissen et al. (28) and Frame (37) separately concluded that HA is an ideal biomaterial for alveolar ridge augmentation because of its flexibility, acceptable mechanical strength, high degree of biocompatibility, and low incidence of related adverse reactions at bone sites adjacent to the material. Klein et al. (67) implanted porous calcium phosphate cylinders in rabbit tibiae and, at three, six, and nine months after implantation, found that all specimens were biocompatible and caused no inflammatory response regardless of the macro- or microporous structure or the calcium phosphate ratio of the implant. In studies evaluating the use of HA in reconstructive middle ear surgery, van Blitterswijk et al. (4) found that events during *Staphylococcus aureus* - initiated infection in rats did not differ in the presence or absence of dense, macroporous HA. These investigators concluded that HA is appropriate for application in reconstructive middle ear surgery based on their experimental and early clinical results. In a three and one-half month follow-up study by Bucholz et al. (11) of interporous HA utilized to fill metaphyseal defects associated with tibial plateau fractures in humans, no inflammatory reaction was demonstrated.

The underlying basis for the lack of local or systemic toxicity with calcium phosphates is their chemical nature, as they contain only calcium and phosphate ions. Studies performed to determine the fate of the released ions were cited by Jarcho (58) and include the implantation of a bioresorbable tricalcium phosphate material in puppies (palate) and dogs (orbital, iliac, mandible, SC, IM, femur, and spine), and nonresorbable HA in dogs (alveolus). Analysis of serum and urine calcium and phosphate levels and/or SMA 12 parameters produced normal results. In addition, no abnormalities or pathological calcifications were found when tissue pathology, including fine detail kidney radiography, was performed on major organs. It must be assumed that too few ions are released from implants to affect the normal calcium or phosphate balance.

In his text, *Bioceramics of Calcium Phosphate*, de Groot (47) stated that the tracing of serum and urine levels in different animal models for evidence of the release of calcium and phosphate ions from resorbable and nearly nondegradable calcium phosphate materials indicated no abnormal findings. There was no evidence of pathological reactions to this material from histologic studies of the major organs, including the kidney. De Groot found that the regulatory system of the body appears to be capable of integrating any ions that are dissolved from these ceramics.

In addition to animal studies, extensive clinical data in dental applications support the biocompatibility of HA. For example, a study by Holmes et al. (55) presents data from 17 consented biopsies up to 16 months post implantation. A 24 month study by Rothstein et al. (82), which enrolled 198 patients, two studies by Kent et al. of 32 patients (63) and of 56 patients (64), a four-year study by Block and Kent (6) of 74 patients, and a five-year investigation by Cranin and Satler (23) of 50 patients, all confirmed the efficacy of the implant material without any observed adverse biologic effects.

According to Thomas et al. (89) calcium phosphate materials have been utilized safely in humans "in the augmentation of alveolar ridges, as bone graft extenders, and in spinal fusion applications". In addition, Zide et al. (95) have demonstrated that after application of particulate, dense, nonporous HA in intimate contact with the dura for reconstruction of cranial defects no clinical evidence of adverse reactions was reported at the one to three and one-half year follow-up evaluation (93).

Therefore, calcium phosphate ceramics have exhibited excellent biologic response in both animal and human studies. The data seem to support de Groot's view that, "From the standpoint of hard tissue response to implant materials, the calcium phosphate ceramics are probably the most compatible materials presently known" (47).

## Biodegradation

The factors that govern the rate and degree of bioresorption of calcium phosphate bioceramics have yet to be completely defined. Hoogendoorn et al. (56) cited studies that reach different conclusions on the resorption and degradation of HA and attributed the dissimilar results to the effect on dissolution properties of different procedures and different specifications for the materials used. Although the starting materials and the details of fabrication of calcium phosphate ceramics do not appear to affect the material's biocompatibility, they do appear to affect the resorption and degradation of the material. The bioresorbability of calcium phosphate materials appears to be dependent on chemical composition, crystal composition, the structure as a "material," and on the environment at the implantation site (66, 68). Jarcho (58) has proposed the existence of two different biologic resorption pathways: one involving solution-mediated processes (implant solubility in physiologic solutions) and the second involving cell-mediated processes (phagocytosis).

In general, *in vitro* biodegradation studies of calcium phosphate ceramics have shown that tricalcium phosphate dissolves at a more rapid rate than HA in a variety of solvents (58, 69). Comparison of the relative dissolution rates of human dental enamel and a dense HA ceramic in buffered lactic acid found that the dental enamel appeared to dissolve ten times faster than the HA ceramic on a weight/weight basis. However, when dissolution results were normalized for surface area, both were found to dissolve at an identical rate (58). The relative dissolution rates of dense HA and tricalcium phosphate ceramics in buffered acid (pH 5.2; 0.4 M lactate) and buffered basic (pH 8.2; 0.05 M edetate) media also have been compared. The materials utilized were well characterized as 100% pure and 100% dense, with very similar ceramic microstructures and similar preparations. In the acid medium, the tricalcium phosphate dissolved 12.3 times faster than the HA and in the basic medium, 22.3 times faster (58). Thus, for HA/tricalcium phosphate mixtures with similar material structure but differing crystal/chemical compositions (the result of differing chemical preparation methods), the bioresorption rate should be directly proportional to the content of tricalcium phosphate in the ceramic (58).

Hoogendoorn et al. (56) studied the stability of dense HA *in vivo* by evaluating long-term implantation of HA implants in dogs. These authors found minimal degradation of the implants after three and one-half years of implantation. After eight years of follow-up, Gumaer et al. (50) found that dogs implanted with HA granules and discs not only tolerated the implant well, without inflammation, but little resorption occurred overall. Frame (37) found that block form HA undergoes some degradation *in vivo*, the rate of which was dependent on differences in ceramic formation (i.e., calcium/phosphate ratio and presence of impurities), the crystallographic structure of the ceramic, and the porosity of the material.

In addition to chemical factors that affect bioresorbability, material structure and porosity can also affect biodegradation and, in some instances, can override the influence of the chemical factors. Surface area is a major factor in determining dissolution rates of any solid material and rates can best be expressed in terms of weight dissolved per unit surface area exposed. The many porous calcium phosphate ceramics investigated have had wide variations in material characteristics, including differing degrees and sizes of macroporosity (pores usually greater than 100 µm introduced for tissue ingrowth), different microporosity (pores less than 5 µm from a particular fabrication process), and different types of pore interconnectivity and organization. It is difficult, if not impossible, to measure or estimate with accuracy the surface area of these materials, or indeed to reproduce a given material accurately. Therefore, it is difficult to predict quantitative dissolution rates for porous calcium phosphate materials, and comparisons of the biodegradation rates measured *in vitro* may be misleading. Clearly, the dissolution of porous calcium phosphates *in vivo* is less predictable than for the fully dense material.

Controlled studies of porous HA and porous tricalcium phosphate implant materials prepared by naphthalene pore formation showed no significant bioresorption of the HA material after periods greater than one year post implantation, whereas resorption of the tricalcium phosphate material occurred (58). Several studies by Klein et al. (67) to evaluate the influence of the calcium to phosphate ratio, the crystallographic structure, and the degree of porosity and physiological environment on degradation showed that in rabbit tibiae solid HA suffered little degradation whereas ß-whitlockite displayed much greater degradation. By comparison, implants placed subcutaneously showed no evidence of resorption for both microporous HA and ß-whitlockite, whereas macroporous HA bioresorbed (68). Klein et al. (67) concluded that the physiologic environment significantly affects the biodegradation of calcium phosphate ceramics and that, in a given site, the chemical and crystal composition, microstructure, and porosity all affect dissolution rates.

For mechanically stable HA implants undergoing minimal dissolution, Bauer et al. (1) have supported Jarcho's thesis of a cell-mediated resorption process by showing osteoclastic remodeling of natural and synthetic HA probably controlled by Wolff's law of bone remodeling. Thus, for HA/bone interfaces subjected to stress, osteoclastic remodeling of bone and synthetic HA, followed by osteoblastic renewal of bone, may occur, whereas in areas suffering stress shielding, the synthetic material may be removed without replacement by bone. Recent work by Jansen et al. (57) on ceramic coatings showed a degradation of HA coating thickness in dogs at three months post implantation, with apposition of bone to the implant in some areas. These authors contend that the degradation of the HA coating does not cause a loss of the integration and is not detrimental to the implant's success. This removal of HA and bone by osteoclasts with replacement of bone by osteoblasts at the implant surface, suggests that solid HA or coated HA implants are involved in the remodeling process caused both by host factors and by the presence of the implant itself.

Although a complete understanding of the factors that influence the bioresorption of calcium phosphate implant materials has yet to be achieved, it is apparent that both chemistry and material structure contribute to dissolution. It can be stated that high density implants of crystalline HA have a lesser tendency to bioresorb because of their chemistry and their small surface area. Dense tricalcium phosphate implants exhibit a measurable dissolution rate. Porous tricalcium phosphate implants resorb at a greater rate than porous HA implants of very similar structure. Macroporosity increases the degree of dissolution. The presence of microporosity (in addition to macroporosity) may promote the bioresorption of all calcium phosphate materials. Finally, dissolution is affected by environment (pH), and resorption may be controlled by cellular activity.

### *In vivo* Reactions with Bone

The investigation and development of calcium phosphate implant materials have defined the highly biocompatible nature of these materials as well as their favorable biologic profile. The advantage of these materials are probably related to their chemical composition, which, when they are implanted in bone, allow calcium and phosphate ions to be derived from the implant and/or the surrounding bone. The composition of any solids deposited on the surface of the calcium phosphate implants are believed to be determined by the surrounding physiologic medium, and ultimately, in bone, this medium would generate calcium phosphate solids in the form of biologic apatite. The final result is that calcium phosphate implant materials become coated with a microscopic layer of bone mineral shortly after implantation in bone (58).

The histologic consequences associated with implantation in bone of calcium phosphate materials can be characterized as normal bone healing processes on and around the implant (58). Typically, bone is deposited directly on the surface of the implant without an intervening fibrous tissue membrane. In addition, normal calcification occurs at an implant site. One study performed by Jarcho (58) examined the healing process of dense HA implants placed in surgically created defects in dog femurs. Calcium and phosphorous content and Ca/P ratios were examined at the implant sites and compared with bone sites removed from the implant. Immediately adjacent to the implants, increasing Ca/P ratios (from 1.50 at one month to 1.62 at six months) and increasing calcium and phosphorous concentrations were observed. At six months, the implant site mineralization was found to be comparable to that of the surrounding bone (58).

Calcium phosphate implants apparently have the unique and potentially valuable ability to bond directly to bone. Initial animal studies were directed at the use of porous calcium phosphate implants, so that bony ingrowth and consequently mechanical stabilization would be achieved by ingrowth into the pores. Early examination of these porous implant sites focused on bone ingrowth and therefore did not readily reveal the bone-bonding phenomenon. However, Driskell et al. (32), in performing a scanning electron microscopic study of fractured samples of porous tricalcium phosphate implant sites, first noted, "the fracture lines propagated through the bone/ceramic interfaces," and concluded, "the evidence suggests that a chemical bond exists between the calcified tissue and the ceramic". Thereafter, with studies using dense implant materials, it became evident that calcium phosphate implants became strongly bonded to the appositional bone without need for a mechanical interlock. Jarcho (58) stated that a number of investigators subsequently observed this ability of bone to bond directly to the surface of calcium phosphate implants in their use of an array of materials and animal models.

Although the precise bonding mechanism and the chemical composition of the "cement" that bonds HA implants and bone have not been determined, optical and electron microscopic observations by several investigators have provided some information about the nature of the bond. According to Cormack (22), the bone-bonding substance is very similar in character to natural bone cementing substance: initially amorphous, thereafter progressively transforming to a crystalline state, heavily mineralized, and rich in mucopolysaccharides. Jarcho (58) reported that the initial appearance of the bonding zone and the first gross indication of bonding occurred with the first evidence of an acellular bone matrix from differentiating osteoblasts. In decalcified sections prepared for electron microscopy, implants were reported to be covered with a narrow (three to five microns wide) amorphous electron-dense band without distinct structural details. The probable removal of minerals during decalcification was suggested by needle-like clefts present in the amorphous layer. In addition, loosely arranged collagen bundles were observed between the amorphous zone and the cells.

Jarcho (58) has reported on electron microscopic examinations of undecalcified "early bonding" HA implant/bone sections. In one study, Jarcho stated that plate-shaped bone mineral crystals, which had deposited directly and irregularly on the surface of an HA implant, calcified the apparent amorphous zone. In a second study, similar findings were reported, but the bone mineral crystals were observed to deposit in an orderly, perpendicular palisade configuration directly on the HA implant's surface (Fig 1). The difference in these reports was attributed to dissimilarities in the sample preparation techniques (58). With maturation of the implant site over several months, the bonding zone diminished until it was restricted to a thin band of approximately 500-2000 Å between the implant and the normal-appearing bone. Examinations of decalcified sections by electron microscopy showed the thin band to be composed of the identical amorphous "ground substance" detected at earlier healing periods. Undecalcified sections revealed the band to be mineralized, with the crystals of the bonding zone merging into those that were laid down in a normal longitudinal fashion on nearby collagen fibers.

Studies of the *in vivo* response to calcium phosphate materials at the cellular level are numerous. For example, Block and Kent (7) examined the healing of mandibular ridge augmentations in nine dogs, using both HA alone and HA mixed with autogenous bone. Although bony ingrowth occurred in each instance, the extent of ingrowth was much greater with HA mixed with bone. In contrast, Bell and Beirne (2) found that HA and tricalcium phosphate, both alone and mixed with collagen, did not induce bony healing in rat mandible defects. The periphery of the defect showed bone ingrowth, but the entire graft did not fill with bone. The authors suggested that the implant was not osteoinductive but that promotion of healing may have been compromised by the implant's location.

The high level of biocompatibility of calcium phosphates as compared with other materials has stimulated studies evaluating the osteogenicity of calcium phosphate implants. In one study, Millipore chambers were used to compare the osseous response to dense HA implant materials in the form of

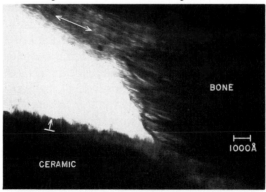

**FIG. 1.** Direct transmission electron micrograph of an undecalcified ultrathin section of a bone–HA implant interface, prepared by ion beam micromilling. Biological apatite is deposited directly on the surface of the implant in a perpendicular palisade fashion. The white space represents the area perforated by the ion beam. (Courtesy of John Kay.)

plugs or particles blended with hemopoietic marrow to the response in control chambers containing marrow only. Six weeks after implantation, a greater number of control chambers contained newly formed bone (90%) than did the HA/marrow-containing chambers (35%) (58). Frame (37) cited a number of studies demonstrating that HA biomaterials are not osteogenic, in that they do not induce bone formation in soft tissues or promote faster bone growth in bony implant locations. However, the same author stated that calcium phosphate materials, in some instances promote the growth of bone into areas that it would otherwise not occupy. A number of authors have described materials with this property by terms such as "osteoconductive" and "osteophilic." Jarcho (58) cited a series of controlled experiments in which surgically created defects were made in the orbital rims, mandibles, and iliac crests of dogs, and when left unfilled for periods up to one year displayed only minimal evidence of spontaneous repair. When porous bioresorbable tricalcium phosphate implants were used to fill similar defects, complete ingrowth of bone was observed at one year, with some of the resorbable implant remaining.

Many studies have been performed that investigated the "osteoconductive" properties of HA. Ricci et al. (79) compared the bone/ceramic interface of uncoated CP titanium vs. HA-coated titanium implants in a canine model and found that most HA-coated implants had a complete bridge of bone attached to the coating over a large contact area at twelve weeks after surgery. Holmes et al. (53, 54) described the permanence of porous HA as a bone graft substitute over the course of four years in canine mandibles and demonstrated the osseous incorporation and long term permanence of the HA matrix. Lieblich and Topazian (70) described a study that compared the repair strength of HA and HA with autogenous, corticocancellous bone in rabbit femora and humeri. At six and sixteen weeks, mechanical tests demonstrated increased strength of the humeri augmented with HA and the femoral bone augmented with the HA/ corticocancellous bone mixture as compared with the untreated control. In utilizing porous bioresorbable tricalcium phosphate materials, other investigators have observed that, by positioning the implant material so that it partially protruded from surgically created defects, bone could be induced to grow above original cortical bone levels. One example cited by Jarcho (58) showed that within a calcium phosphate ceramic, lateral bone growth of up to 7.5 mm was possible in the canine femoral shafts, whereas control defects similarly filled with a gelatin-based hemostatic compound displayed lateral bone growth of only 4 mm. Bucholz et al. (11) performed a study of interporous HA as a bone graft substitute in tibial plateau fractures and demonstrated that the material permitted bone ingrowth, was osteoconductive and, at the same time, underwent biogradation slowly in humans. A canine study by Russotti et al. (83) was conducted to assess the efficacy of HA/tricalcium phosphate particles in enhancing the biologic fixation of a porous-coated femoral component without interference fit. In this study, the HA/tricalcium phosphate materials demonstrated neither osteoconductive nor osteoinductive properties, perhaps owing to the absence of an initial stabilization and apposition to adjacent bone. However, Manley et al. (74) found that HA-coated implants are less affected than other press-fit implants by micromotion and lack of precise placement.

In summary, HA-coated implants are now known to be capable of bonding to bone, especially if initial stability is ensured. The material appears to be osteoconductive and becomes covered with bone as long as some bone contact is present at initial placement. In general, it is agreed that calcium phosphate materials do not stimulate osteogenesis but, unlike traditional biomaterials, are capable of conducting bone growth into implant surface shapes or bony defects.

## HYDROXYLAPATITE COATINGS AND SURFACE TREATMENTS

The mechanical properties of calcium phosphate implant materials have been found to be the primary limitation for their application in weight-bearing implants. These materials are brittle, have low impact resistance and low tensile strength. Table 1 details a comparison of the ranges of mechanical properties observed with calcium phosphate ceramics vs. those of currently used metallic materials and bone (58).

To overcome their limitations in physical properties, the application of calcium phosphates to metallic substrates takes advantage of both the strength of the metal and the biocompatibility of the ceramic. Whereas solid HA implants have been found to have low fatigue strength, HA coatings, applied by plasma spraying to titanium alloy substrates, appear to attain the fatigue properties of metal (44, 65).

**TABLE 1**. *The mechanical properties of bone and metallic and calcium phosphate implant materials**

| Material | Compressive tensile strength (MPa) | Strength (MPa) | Modulus ($10^3$ MPa) |
|---|---|---|---|
| Bone | | | |
|   Cortical bone | 138 | 69 | 13.8 |
|   Cancellous bone | 41–62 | 3.4 | - |
| Metals | | | |
|   316 L stainless | - | 552–1000 | 207–276 |
|   Co-Cr alloy | - | 669 | 207 |
|   Titanium | - | 345 | 110 |
| Calcium phosphates | | | |
|   Porous | 7-69 | 2.5 | - |
|   Dense | 207– 897 | 69 –193 | 34.5–103 |

* Modified from (58), with permission

### *In Vivo* Studies with Coated Implants

Early animal studies of calcium phosphate coatings in orthopedic applications demonstrated similar biocompatibility to solid ceramic materials. At post-implantation periods of up to 32 weeks, Cook et al. (21) found that adult mongrel dogs had good tolerance to uncoated, bead-blasted CP titanium implants and titanium alloy (Ti-6Al-4V) implants with an HA coating applied by plasma spraying. No evidence of inflammation, tissue reaction, or negative clinical indications to the implants was found. Jasty et al. (59) implanted tricalcium phosphate/HA-coated acetabular prostheses in dogs. Before sacrifice, at three or at six weeks, the dogs were ambulatory. After sacrifice, the dogs were found to have no infections or adverse tissue reactions. Geesink et al. (15) evaluated plasma-sprayed, 50 μm-thick, apatite-coated titanium cortical plugs in dogs and found radiographic and histologic evidence of new bone formation, bone remodeling, and bonding of the implant to bone at the six week follow-up and at subsequent evaluations. An inflammatory response observed at six weeks was absent after twelve weeks. Geesink considered this to be a normal reaction to surgical trauma. De Groot et al. (48) loosely inserted coated plugs in the lateral cortex of adult canine femora and found within six weeks that the defects in the periosteum and cortex around the implants were filled with bone. Light microscopy revealed new bone in close contact with the implant, the new bone displayed remodeling and the lacunae had osteoblasts, osteoclasts and osteoid. Cook et al.(47) also showed that HA-coated substrates encourage a faster, stronger bony attachment compared with the same uncoated metal substrate in canine transcortical implants. The same rapid proliferation of bone over the coated implants has been shown also in canine studies of HA-coated dental implants, loaded hip replacements, screws, and intramedullary rods (8, 52, 61, 62, 86).

Evaluation of the attachment strength between coated implants and bone has been shown by many authors. Cook et al. (21) evaluated the differences in mechanical strength at the bone–implant interface of bead-blasted CP titanium transcortical implant plugs and titanium alloy (Ti-6Al-4V) plugs with a plasma-sprayed HA coating, at three, five, six, 10 and 32 weeks after random implantation in adult mongrel dogs. They reported that the average interfacial shear strength of HA-coated implants, approximately 6–7 MPa, was significantly greater than that of uncoated titanium implants, which were around 1 MPa. The increased strength was related to the fact that the HA-coated titanium alloy supported bone mineralization directly at the surface, with no interposed fibrous tissue layer, in contrast to only isolated areas of direct bone to implant apposition in the uncoated bead-blasted CP titanium implants (21). De Groot et al. (48) studied the mechanical and biologic properties of coated cortical plugs inserted in the lateral cortex of adult canine femora. Histology showed an intact HA coating with good bone contact. Push-out tests showed that the uncoated plugs were loose in the bone. The apatite-coated surfaces apparently required a stress of 55 MPa and 62 MPa to remove the implants, at three and six months, respectively. These values are significantly greater than those reported by Cook et al. Boone et al. (10) pointed out that whereas de Groot et al. used formalin fixation of specimens at retrieval, Cook et al. tested their specimens "fresh." Therefore, formalin-induced shrinkage of bone produced artificially high shear values in the study of de Groot et al. However, both Cook et al.(21) and de Groot et al. (48) reported histologic findings of excellent implant biocompatibility and no evidence of a fibrous tissue seam between implant and bone.

Radiographic analysis by Geesink et al. (44) of hip implants coated with an HA/ calcium oxide mixture in dogs showed proliferation of bone on the implant surface from six weeks on. The implants were well-integrated to the surrounding bone, showed no radiolucent lines, and all spaces had disappeared by six weeks. Uncoated control implants showed no induction of new bone and a thick fibrous seam. Histologic evaluation verified that defects around the coated implants became filled with bone by the sixth week, that there was bone proliferation, close contact of the implant with cortical bone and that bonding of the coating to the implant was maintained through 12 months. In brief, although this coating was not as stable as that of HA alone, the calcium phosphate ceramic demonstrated new bone formation, bone remodeling and intimate interface with bone. In another study utilizing a canine endoprosthesis model, Thomas et al. (87) reported on HA-coated and uncoated, grooved and plasma-sprayed prostheses in adult dogs evaluated up to 52 weeks post implantation. They cited studies that found that HA coating on dense titanium surfaces demonstrated slightly increased and accelerated bone ingrowth and resulted in bone implant shear strengths up to seven times those of uncoated implants. The HA porous devices also appeared better organized and had higher mineralization.

Manley et al. (73,74) performed histologic and quantitative analyses of HA-coated and uncoated titanium (Ti-6Al-4V) alloy intramedullary implants subjected to functional shear loading in osteotomized canine femora. Twelve adult dogs were allowed unrestricted motion immediately post implantation and were sacrificed 10 weeks after the initial surgery. Radiologic evaluation revealed that the uncoated titanium implants had a large external callus around the osteotomy site, an acceptable level of stability and were surrounded by a thin fibrous seam (73) (Fig 2A.) The HA-coated implants had a slight callus formation around the osteotomy site, radiographic evidence of cortical atrophy adjacent to the defect and were surrounded by thick bony proliferation without evidence of a fibrous tissue seam (73) (Fig 2B). The authors found that the interfacial shear strength of the HA-coated implants increased fourfold relative to the uncoated titanium implant at only five weeks post implantation (74). The shear strength was enhanced for the HA-coated implants even when placement of the device was not precise, indicating that HA-coated implants were less affected by precise placement than other press-fit implants (74).

In another report, Manley et al. (72) compared intramedullary implants (grit-blasted titanium, porous titanium and smooth titanium with an 80 μm HA coating) press-fitted in 68 canine femora. Histologic evaluation showed that bone penetrated the porous titanium coatings and apposed the HA coatings at five weeks. The bone in direct apposition to the HA proliferated with time and extended to the surrounding osseous structures. The grit-blasted titanium implants without coating, in contrast, had a fibrous seam between the implant and the bone. The investigators concluded that bone apposition to HA-coated implants occurs even when functional loads cause micromotion between implant and bone (72). Søballe et al. (85) compared the effects of HA and titanium coatings on the skeletal fixation of unloaded titanium plugs implanted in noninterference and interference fit in six dogs. Each dog received both types of implants either press-fit or with a noninterference fit consisting of a 1mm gap around the implant. At four weeks post implantation, the titanium-coated implants inserted as a noninterference fit experienced a 65% reduction in fixation compared with the press-fit titanium implants. In contrast, HA-coated implants inserted with a gap demonstrated only a slight reduction in fixation. In addition, the noninterference fit, HA-coated implants experienced a 120% increase in bone/implant interface shear strength as compared with the titanium-coated cylinders. Histologic evaluation demonstrated that HA-coated implants had significantly more mineralizing bone in direct contact with the implant in noninterference fit ($p<0.001$) and press-fit ($p<0.01$) as compared with titanium-coated implants. Søballe et al. (85) concluded that although tight interference fit appeared to be an important factor for implant fixation, HA coatings can eliminate the negative influence of a noninterference fit between bone and implant.

The effectiveness of HA coatings in enhancing the attachment of porous-coated surfaces has been evaluated by a number of investigators. Thomas et al. (87) found that HA-coated and uncoated porous devices demonstrated similar bone ingrowth after six weeks. In a separate study, Thomas et al. (88) found that HA-coated and uncoated porous titanium alloy canine transcortical plugs had equivalent maximal long-term shear strengths, with no significant difference in shear strength after three, six and twelve weeks of implantation. Rivero et al. (80) observed, in a study of tricalcium phosphate-coated and uncoated porous titanium fiber metal implants in dogs, that at two, four and six weeks post implantation, the volume fraction of bone ingrowth was not statistically signifi-

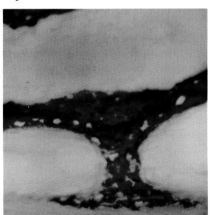 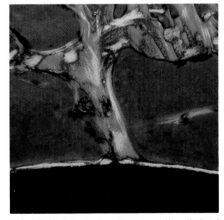

**FIG. 2A.** Histological section of an uncoated titanium alloy intramedullary rod after six weeks implantation in an osteotomized canine femur. A layer of intervening fibrous tissue is present between the implant and the surrounding bone.

**FIG. 2B.** Histological section viewed in polarized light of HA-coated titanium alloy intramedullary rod after six weeks, implantation in the same animal model. Bone is in direct apposition to the HA coating, without any intervening fibrous tissue between the implant and the bone.

cant between the control and coated implants. In addition, these authors found that there was no significant difference in bone/implant shear strength at any evaluation period except at four weeks. They stated that for both the coated specimens and the controls a positive correlation existed between the strength of implant fixation and the volume of bone ingrowth. In investigating porous cobalt chromium alloy plugs partially coated with HA and implanted into canine femora, Cook et al. (9) determined that the HA-coated samples demonstrated a statistically significant increase in the percentage of porous structure filled with mineralized bone at each evaluation period after four weeks (range $p=0.0012$ to $p=0.0001$), as well as a more rapid development of attachment strength. These authors concluded that although their findings are similar to those reported for smooth and grooved surfaces, HA-coated porous surfaces demonstrated enhanced biologic fixation over similar uncoated surfaces. Chae et al. (13) evaluated tricalcium phosphate-coated and uncoated porous cobalt chromium rods implanted in rabbit tibiae and found that although an extensive osseous response had occurred, the pull-out strengths of the coated specimens were not increased over the uncoated samples. The authors attributed their results to a number of factors, including the fit of the implants, implantation site, animal model, and ceramic characteristics. These studies demonstrate that HA does have the effect of increasing both the osseous response time and volume to porous coatings, however, the results also indicate that the ultimate attachment strength of both HA-coated and uncoated porous surfaces remains equivalent.

In summary, all studies of non-porous HA-coated implants demonstrated that the strength of the bone–implant interface exceeded that measured for uncoated implants. The thickness of the coating affected the strength, the thicker coatings being structurally weaker, with failure occurring within the ceramic coating rather than within the bone during mechanical tests. All studies also demonstrated a favorable biologic response to HA coatings with bone in intimate contact with the HA. By contrast, improvement gained by HA coating of porous metal implants was short term. In addition, it is unclear as yet whether the stress shielding of bone and coating by the porous metal will lead to cell-mediated removal of the HA as the basic studies reported earlier suggest.

## CLINICAL STUDIES

Clinical experience with HA coatings utilized in conjunction with orthopedic prosthetic implants continues to develop. Furlong and Osborn (40) began clinical trials in 1985 with a femoral stem incorporating a thick, 200 μm HA coating (Osprovit coating) and reported that more than 600 such femoral stems have been successfully implanted. These authors stated that "an interface lacking a separating fibrous membrane is the only guarantee for long term clinical success." They continued by stating that "the only biomaterial capable of creating a substantial continuity between itself and bone tissue is HA ceramic" (40).

Geesink (42) has reported his use of the Omnifit-HA total hip system with a thin 50 μm HA coating in 100 patients since 1986. At two-year follow-up, radiolucent lines around the coating were completely absent and endosteal densification of trabecular bone was observed in the distal region of the coating. He reported very few instances of thigh pain, as well as excellent clinical results as early as three months post implantation. In addition, there were no reports of delamination of the coating from the implanted prostheses. In 1990, Geesink (43) updated his findings utilizing the Omnifit-HA Hip System with clinical and radiographic results of 100 consecutive primary and revision cases with a mean follow-up of two years. At the 24 month follow-up, mean HHS were 97 points for primary hips and 99 points for revision hips, with a mean incidence of pain below 4%. Radiographic signs of bone ingrowth to the implant stem were visible in some patients at the six month follow-up and were present in 90% of cases at the one-year follow-up and in 100% of cases at the two-year follow-up. According to Geesink, enhanced biologic fixation is provided by the HA coating. This is demonstrated by a pattern of bony changes around the stems, consisting of endosteal bone apposition against the coating, proximal calcar atrophy, and reactive line formation around the distal uncoated portion of the implant. He stated that this pattern is similar to that described for well-ingrown, porous metal-coated devices (43).

Additional clinical experience with the Omnifit-HA Hip System has been reported. Drucker et al. (84) reported on 58 cases with up to one year of follow-up with this system, and stated that excellent clinical results were realized but that the limited follow-up precluded evaluation of bone remodeling changes. Manley and Koch (75) reported the use of the Omnifit-HA Hip System in two (United States and European) multicentric clinical trials with a total of 523 cases. Two-year follow-up data were reported for 236 HA-coated implant cases as well as for a control group of 49 patients implanted with Omnifit hip stems without an HA coating. The mean HHS for the coated stems was 96.1 points, as compared with 85.1 points for the non-HA stems. Radiographic evaluations at one year (213 hips) and two years (205 hips) were performed on the proximal HA-coated load transfer zones. At the one year follow-up, none of the Omnifit-HA stems exhibited reactive lines. At the two- year follow-up, 0.8% of the Omnifit-HA stems exhibited reactive lines in the targeted area as compared with 11.8% for the uncoated Omnifit stems. The authors stated that these data demonstrate that the implants were completely stable, with no sign of interface changes at the one-and two-year post-implantation evaluations. D'Antonio et al. (26,27) also reported their early clinical experience with the HA-coated Omnifit-HA Hip Stem at two-and three-year follow-up. In 92 cases at the two-year evaluation, D'Antonio et al. (26) reported a mean HHS of 95.2 points, an incidence of thigh pain of only 4.3% (four cases) and radiographic observations of a rapid bony response. In 142 cases with three year follow-up, the authors cited their continued excellent results and concluded that the clinical and radiographic findings support the proposition that these stems are well fixed proximally and exhibit excellent stress transfer (27). The few autopsy specimens available support this view also (1) (Fig 3).

Clinical studies have also been performed utilizing HA coatings on porous-coated hip prostheses (12,15,16, 36, 91,92). Vaughan et al. (91,92) reported on their early clinical results of 53 HA-coated Mallory–Head porous hip prostheses as compared with 50 uncoated Mallory–Head porous hip prostheses (91, 92). The HA-coated Mallory-Head porous prosthesis recipients were followed for a mean period of seventeen months (range 12 to 24 months), while the uncoated Mallory–Head porous systems were monitored for a mean of 48 months. The HA-coated Mallory–Head porous prosthesis group was reported with a mean HHS of 93.41 points, which is comparable to the uncoated Mallory–Head porous prosthesis group with a reported mean Harris Hip Score of 94 points. No subsidence, acetabular migration, or component failures were reported for either group. Radiographic evaluations of the HA-coated Mallory–Head porous prosthesis group demonstrated an absence of radiolucent lines and minimal signs of adaptive bone remodeling, while the uncoated group revealed a slightly increased incidence of radiolucent lines as compared with the HA-coated components. Cook et al. (15,16) observed similar results in their study comparing 85 HA-coated Long-term Stable Fixation (LSF) Hip Prostheses and 80 uncoated LSF components evaluated up to one year post implantation. These authors stated that although both pain relief and overall HHS rating improved for the two study groups after surgery, the HA-coated group demonstrated greater improvement at all evaluation periods. In addition, radiographically the HA-coated group displayed a lower incidence of radiolucencies than did the uncoated group. Emerson et al. (36) stated that their study results with HA-coated porous prostheses demonstrated that the HA-coated stems had an increase in proximal femoral density and more rapid clinical healing at six months than did uncoated stems. Therefore, these authors all concluded that early clinical results appear to support the early beneficial effects of HA porous-coated surfaces.

Several authors have reported on the experience with HA-coated APR Hip Systems. Dorr (30) reviewed the clinical and radiographic data presented by several authors comparing both HA-coated textured APR stems and HA-

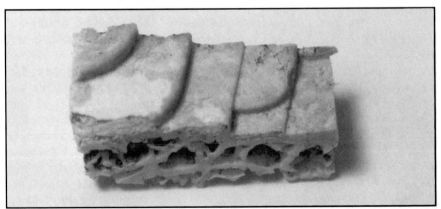

**FIG. 3.** Decalcified section of bone retrieved at autopsy from a patient who died of a myocardial infarction nine months post implantation of a press-fit HA-coated Omnifit femoral stem. The section demonstrates remodeling of bone that mirrors the HA-coated normalization steps of the implant.

coated porous APR II stems versus uncoated stems in revision and primary total hip arthroplasty. Studies that evaluated the HA-coated revision stems spanned the evolution of three stem designs. The final revision stem design consisted of an HA-coated porous long stem which was evaluated with up to two years of follow-up. For the 35 cases evaluated, the mean HHS was 87 points. Friedman et al. (39) reported on 111 HA-coated non-porous APR I stems that were compared with 21 uncoated APR I stems and were followed for a minimum of two years. The HA-coated stems had statistically superior HHS (mean: 90; $p<0.05$) as compared with the uncoated stems at the three, six, and twelve month evaluations, as well as demonstrating only a 7% radiolucency rate medially vs. a 25% radiolucency rate in the same region for the uncoated stems (39). In a study that compared press-fit HA-coated APR Primary Hip System components vs. uncoated APR prostheses, Dorr and Smith (31) reported a mean HHS at two years of 93 points for the 98 HA-coated APR cases as compared with a mean HHS of 87 points for the 17 cases in the un-coated APR group. Again, few radiolucencies were observed for the HA-coated group. Within this study, one HA-coated hip prosthesis recipient died three months post implantation. Evaluation of the retrieved prosthesis by light microscopy demonstrated osteoid on approximately 20% of the coated surface of the femoral component and on 40% of the coated acetabular surface. Backscattered electron images revealed bone spicules connecting the bone graft and surrounding cancellous bone to the HA coating (31). Therefore, the authors concluded that these results illustrate that HA-coated joint prostheses enhance early skeletal attachment and confirm its osteoconductive properties and biologic fixation.

Further studies have been published that describe histologic observations related to HA-coated hip implants retrieved at autopsy. Bauer et al. (1) evaluated five Omnifit-HA Hip Stems and their surrounding bone tissue retrieved after implantation periods ranging from 4.5 to 25 months. The cause of death in each case was unrelated to the implants. The histologic findings of these authors suggest the presence of cortical and cancellous remodeling in accordance with Wolff's Law and focal loss of HA in areas of bone resorption. Although clear histological differences related to time *in situ* were not detected, the presence of hyperplastic bridges of bone in areas of force transmission was observed. Bone apposition to the implant surfaces was observed at a level ranging from 32% to 78% of the available surface per histologic section, with the majority of the bone formation near the endosteal surfaces of the implants. Bauer et al. (1) concluded that the lack of a fibrous tissue membrane surrounding the implants suggests that each prosthesis was mechanically stable at the time of retrieval.

Hardy et al. (51) examined specimens of HA-coated femoral prostheses retrieved from four patients who had died within nine months of the total hip arthroplasty procedure. Histologic examination distinguished a difference in bone response in the proximal femur and the femoral shaft: the proximal cancellous bone retained its normal architecture and contained large amounts of stromal tissue, whereas the bone tissue adjacent to the HA coating contained immature trabecular bone. Microscopic examination demonstrated that there was no interposition of fibrous tissue between the new bone layer and the HA-coated surface. In the uncoated areas of the stem, a layer of fibrous tissue oriented parallel to the implant surface covered the titanium alloy. This fibrous tissue tapered off and disappeared at the transition point between the uncoated and HA-coated titanium surfaces and was replaced by new bone. Although the observation period was short, no HA resorption or variations in HA thickness were observed. Using roentgenogram, backscattered electron (BSE) imaging, and light microscopy, Bloebaum et al. (9) analyzed an HA-coated hip implant retrieved from a patient who died three weeks after implantation. Results of the BSE analysis revealed bone apposition on approximately 10% of the HA-coated femoral component surface and on 20% of the coated acetabular component surface. The observations of these authors suggest that bidirectional bone remodeling had occurred and that it appeared to improve skeletal attachment as compared with unidirectional bone remodeling. Furlong et al. (41) reported on their observations related to the histologic study of three post-mortem HA-coated hip stems retrieved after 10 days, 17 days and 7 weeks, respectively. Analysis showed complete restoration of the bone marrow with islands of woven bone visible and adjoining the HA coating. The seven-week specimen was reported to show bonding osteogenesis and bridging trabeculae that had matured into lamellar bone. The authors concluded that HA seems to affect the differentiation and proliferation of osteogenic cells directly, reducing by half the time required for osteogenesis to occur and thereby obtaining an apparent permanent mechanical fixation within a few days or weeks. Finally, Søballe et al. (84) reported on an HA-coated hip stem retrieved from a 98-year-old, osteoporotic woman after 12 weeks of implantation due to recurrent dislocation. Histologic sections and microscopic examination showed a thin layer of new bone in direct contact with the HA coating. Moreover, quantitative analysis demonstrated that 45% of the proximal, 54% of the intermediate, and 45% of the distal surfaces of the fully coated prosthesis were covered by bone. Therefore, although long term follow-up has yet to be achieved, the early clinical, radiographic and histologic results with HA-coated orthopedic hip implants are extremely favorable.

## SUMMARY

Extensive literature on calcium phosphate biomaterials studied *in vitro*, *in vivo* and clinically now exists. A broad understanding of the material's chemical, physical, physiochemical, and biologic characteristics has been gained. Although solid HA exhibits unacceptable mechanical properties as a load-bearing implant, thin HA coatings on metallic substrates achieve the strength properties of the underlying material while taking advantage of the biocompatibility of HA. As a biomaterial, HA [$Ca_5(PO_4)_3(OH)$] has consistently proven to be nontoxic, nonallergenic, biocompatible, and elicits no inflammatory response, regardless of whether it is implanted in bead or block form or as a coating on a substrate. No adverse system effects have been reported. Studies have shown that the application of HA to an implant eliminates the development of the fibrous seam that is normally generated with uncoated implants. The coating appears to be bonded to bone and to become part of the natural remodeling process around the implant. It is probable that the prevention of fibrous tissue formation around an implant is essential for long term prosthetic stability. Therefore, a material such as HA that inhibits production of the fibrous seam is highly desirable for use in orthopedic implant applications. To date, clinical results with thin coatings of HA have been extremely successful and continued success is anticipated.

## REFERENCES

1. Bauer TW, Geesink RGT, Zimmerman R, McMahon JT. Hydroxyapatite-coated femoral stems. Histological analysis of components retrieved at autopsy. *Journal of Bone and Joint Surgery*. December 1991; 73A (10): 1439-52.
2. Bell R, Beirne OR. Effect of HA, tricalcium phosphate, and collagen on the healing of defects in the rat mandible. *Journal of Oral and Maxillofacial Surgery*. 1988; 46: 589-94.
3. Black J. Ceramics and composites. In: *Orthopaedic Biomaterials in Research and Practice*: New York, NY: Churchill Livingstone Inc.; 1988: 191-211.
4. van Blitterswijk CA, Bakker D, Grote JJ, Daems WT. The biological performance of calcium phosphate ceramics in an infected implantation site: II. Biological evaluation of hydroxyapatite during short-term infection. *Journal of Biomedical Materials Research*. 1986; 20: 1003-1015.
5. van Blitterswijk CA, Grote JJ, Kuypers W, Blok-van Hoek CJG, Daems WT. Bioreactions at the tissue/hydroxyapatite interface. *Biomaterials*. July 1985; 6: 243-51.
6. Block MS, Kent JN. Long-term radiographic evaluation of HA- augmented mandibular alveolar ridges. *Journal of Oral and Maxillofacial Surgery*. 1984; 42: 793-96.
7. Block MS, Kent JN. Healing of mandibular ridge augmentations using HA with and without autogenous bone in dogs. *Journal of Oral and Maxillofacial Surgery*. 1985; 43:3-7.
8. Block MS, Kent JN, Kay JF. Evaluation of HA-coated titanium dental implants in dogs. *Journal of Oral and Maxillofacial Surgery*. 1987; 45: 601-07.
9. Bloebaum RD, Merrell M, Gustke K, Simmons M. Retrieval analysis of a hydroxyapatite-coated hip prosthesis. *Clinical Orthopaedics and Related Research*. June 1991; 267: 97-102.
10. Boone PS, Zimmerman MC, Gutteling E, Lee CK, Parsons JR, Langrana N. Bone attachment to hydroxyapatite coated polymers. *Journal of Biomedical Material Research: Applied Biomaterials*. 1989; 23(A2): 183-99.
11. Bucholz RW, Carlton A, Holmes R. Interporous hydroxyapatite as a bone graft substitute in tibial plateau fractures. *Clinical Orthopaedics and Related Research*. March 1989; 240: 53-62.
12. Cates HE, Keating EM, Gittins M, Faris PM, Bissacotti JF, Ritter MA. Early clinical results of hydroxyapatite-coated total hip arthroplasty. *Seminars in Arthroplasty*. October 1991; 2(4): 317-22.
13. Chae JC, Collier JP, Mayor MB, Suprenant VA, Dauphinaus LA. Enhanced ingrowth of porous-coated CoCr implants plasma-sprayed with tricalcium phosphate. *Journal of Biomedical Materials Research*. 1992; 26: 93-102.
14. Ciccotti MG, Rothman RH, Veress SA, Hozack WJ, Moriarty L, Beight J. Clinical and roentgenographic evaluation of hydroxyapatite- coated and uncoated porous total hip arthroplasty: a preliminary report. *Seminars in Arthroplasty*. October 1991; 2(4): 280-88.
15. Cook SD, Enis J, Armstrong D, Lisecki E. Early clinical results with the hydroxyapatite-coated porous long-term stable fixation total hip system. *Seminars in Arthroplasty*. October 1991; 2(4): 302-08.
16. Cook SD, Enis J, Armstrong D, Lisecki E. Early clinical results with the hydroxyapatite-coated porous LSF total hip system. *Dental Clinics of North America*. January 1992; 36(1): 247-55.
17. Cook SD, Kay JF, Thomas KA, Jarcho M. Interface mechanics and histology of titanium and HA-coated titanium for dental implant applications. *International Journal of Oral and Maxillofacial Implants*. 1987; 12(1): 15-22.

18. Cook SD, Reynolds MC, Whitecloud TS, Routman AS, Harding AF, Kay JF, Jarcho M. Evaluation of HA graft materials in canine cervical spine fusions. *Spine*. 1986; 11(4): 305-09.

19. Cook SD, Thomas KA, Dalton JE, Volkman TK, Whitecloud TS, Kay JF. HA coating of porous implants improves bone ingrowth and interface attachment strength. *Journal of Biomedical Materials Research*. 1992; 26: 989-1001.

20. Cook SD, Thomas KA, Kay JF, Jarcho M. Hydroxyapatite-coated porous titanium for use as an orthopedic biologic attachment system. *Clinical Orthopaedics and Related Research*. May 1988; 230: 303-12.

21. Cook SD, Thomas KA, Kay JF, Jarcho M. Hydroxyapatite-coated titanium for orthopedic implant applications. *Clinical Orthopaedics and Related Research*. July 1988; 232: 225-43.

22. Cormack, D.H. ed.: *Ham's Histology ed. 9*. Philadelphia, PA: J.B. Lippincott Co.; 1987: 283-87.

23. Cranin AN, Satler, NM. Human mandibular alveolar ridge augmentation with HA: final report of a five year investigation. *10th Annual Meeting of the Society for Biomaterials*. April 27-May 4, 1984; Washington, DC: 324.

24. Cullum PE, Frost DE, Newland TB, Keane TM, Ehler WJ. Evaluation of HA particles in repair of alveolar clefts in dogs. *Journal of Oral and Maxillofacial Surgery*. 1988; 46: 290-6.

25. Daculsi G, LeGeros RZ, Nery E, Lynch K, Kerebel B. Transformation of biphasic calcium phosphate ceramics *in-vivo*: ultrastructural and physicochemical characterization. *Journal of Biomedical Materials Research*: 1989; 23: 883-94.

26. D'Antonio JA, Capello WN, Crothers OD, Jaffe WL, Manley MT. Early clinical experience with HA-coated femoral implants. *Journal of Bone and Joint Surgery*. August 1992; 74A (7): 995-1008.

27. D'Antonio JA, Capello WN, Jaffe WL. HA-coated hip implants: multi-center three-year clinical and radiographic results. *Clinical Orthopaedics and Related Research*. December 1992; 285: 102-15.

28. Denissen HW, van Dijk HJA, de Groot K, Klopper PJ, Vermeiden JPW, Gehring AP. Biological and mechanical evaluation of dense calcium hydroxyapatite made by continuous hot pressing. In: Hastings GW, Williams DF, eds. *Mechanical Properties of Biomaterials*. New York, NY: John Wiley & Sons Ltd.; 1980: 489-505.

29. Dieppe PA, Huskisson EC, Crocker P, Willoughby DA. Apatite deposition disease. A new Arthropathy. *Lancet*: February 7, 1976; 7954: 266-269.

30. Dorr LD. Clinical total hip replacement with hydroxyapatite from 1984 to 1991. *Seminars in arthroplasty* October 1991; 2(4): 289-4.

31. Dorr LD, Smith C. Clinical results for the calcitite-coated press-fit APR hip system. *Dental Clinics of North America*. January 1992; 36(1): 239-46.

32. Driskell TD, Hassler CR, McCoy LR. The significance of resorbable bioceramics in the repair of bone defects. *Proceedings of the 26th Annual Conference England Medical Biomaterials*. 1973; 15: 199.

33. Drobeck HP, Rothstein SS, Gumaer KI, Sherer AD, Slighter RG. Histologic observations of soft tissue responses to implanted, multifaceted particles and discs of HA. *Journal of Oral and Maxillofacial Surgery*. 1984; 42: 143-49.

34. Drucker DA, Capello WN, D'Antonio JA, Hile LE. Total hip arthroplasty using a hydroxyapatite-coated acetabular and femoral component. *Orthopaedic Review*. February 1991; 20(2): 179-92.

35. Eggli PS, Müller W, Schenk RK. Porous hydroxyapatite and tricalcium phosphate cylinders with two different pore size ranges implanted in the cancellous bone of rabbits. A comparative histomorphometric and histologic study of bony ingrowth and implant substitution. *Clinical Orthopaedics and Related Research*. July 1988; 232: 127-38.

36. Emerson RH, Head WC, Peters PC. Comparison of the early healing course of porous titanium with hydroxyapatite-coated porous titanium hip implants: clinical considerations for the use of hydroxyapatite coating in total hip replacement. *Seminars in Arthroplasty*. October 1991; 2(4): 295-301.

37. Frame JW. Hydroxyapatite as a biomaterial for alveolar ridge augmentation. *International Journal of Oral and Maxillofacial Surgery*. 1987; 16: 642-55.

38. Frame JW, Rout PGJ, Browne RM. Ridge augmentation using solid and porous hydroxylapatite particles with and without autogenous bone or plaster. *Journal of Oral and Maxillofacial Surgery*. 1987; 45: 771-7.

39. Friedman RJ, Dorr LD, Gustke KA, Braunohler WM, Savory CG, Guyer WD, DeAndrade RJ. Effects of HA on total hip arthorplasty. *37th Annual Meeting, Orthopaedic Research Society*. March 4-7, 1991; Anaheim, CA: 538.

40. *The Furlong® Hydroxyapatite Ceramic Coated Total Hip Replacement.* London, England: Joint Replacement Instrumentation Ltd., 1987; 16 pp.
41. Furlong RJ, Osborn, JF. Fixation of hip prostheses by hydroxyapatite ceramic coatings. *Journal of Bone and Joint Surgery.* S eptember 1991; 73B(5): 741-45.
42. Geesink RGT. Experimental and clinical experience with hydroxyapatite-coated hip implants. *Orthopaedics.* September 1989; 12(9): 1239-42.
43. Geesink RGT. Hydroxyapatite-coated total hip prostheses. Two-year clinical and roentgenographic results of 100 cases. *Clinical Orthopaedics and Related Research.* December 1990; 261: 39-58.
44. Geesink RGT, de Groot K, Klein CPAT. Bonding of bone to apatite-coated implants. *Journal of Bone and Joint Surgery.* January 1988; 70B(1): 17-22.
45. Geesink RGT, de Groot K, Klein CPAT. Chemical implant fixation using hydroxyl-apatite coatings. The development of a human total hip prosthesis for chemical fixation to bone using hydroxyl-apatite coatings on titanium substrates. *Clinical Orthopaedics and Related Research.* December 1987; 225: 147-70.
46. Goodman SB, Davidson J, Fornasier VL. The histological reaction to titanium alloy and hydroxyapatite particles implanted in the rabbit tibia. *Fourth World Biomaterials Congress.* April 24-28, 1992; Berlin, Germany: 317.
47. de Groot K. *Bioceramics of Calcium Phosphate.* Boca Raton, FL: CRC Press, Inc.; 1983.
48. de Groot K, Geesink R, Klein CPAT, Serekian P. Plasma sprayed coatings of HA. *Journal of Biomedical Materials Research.* 1987; 21: 1375-81.
49. Gumaer KI, Salsbury RL, Sauerschell RJ, Slighter RG, Drobeck HP. Evaluation of hydroxyl-apatite root implants in baboons. *Journal of Oral and Maxillofacial Surgery.* 1985; 43: 73-9.
50. Gumaer KI, Sherer AD, Slighter RG, Rothstein SS, Drobeck HP. Tissue response in dogs to dense HA implantation in the femur. *Journal of Oral and Maxillofacial Surgery.* 1986; 44: 618-27.
51. Hardy DCR, Frayssinet P, Guilhem A, LaFontaine MA, DeLince PE. Bonding of hydroxyapatite-coated femoral prostheses. Histopathology of specimens from four cases. *Journal of Bone and Joint Surgery.* September 1991; 73B(5): 732-740.
52. Hayashi K, Uenoyama K, Matsuguchi N, Sugioka Y. Quantitative analysis of *in-vivo* tissue responses to titanium-oxide and hydroxyapatite-coated titanium alloy. *Journal of Biomedical Materials Research.* 1991; 25: 515-23.
53. Holmes RE, Hagler HK. Porous HA as a bone graft substitute in mandibular contour augmentation: a histometric study. *Journal of Oral and Maxillofacial Surgery.* 1987; 45: 421-29.
54. Holmes R, Hagler H. Porous hydroxyapatite as a bone graft substitute in maxillary augmentation. A histometric study. *Journal of Cranio-Maxillo-Facial Surgery.* 1988; 16: 199-205.
55. Holmes RE, Wardrop RW, Wolford LM. HA as a bone graft substitute in orthognathic surgery: histologic and histometric findings. *Journal of Oral and Maxillofacial Surgery.* 1988; 46: 661-71.
56. Hoogendoorn HA, Renooij W, Akkermans LMA, Visser W, Wittebol P. Long term study of large ceramic implants (porous hydroxyapatite) in dog femora. *Clinical Orthopaedics and Related Research.* July/August 1984; 187: 281-8.
57. Jansen JA, van de Waerden JPCM, Wolke JGC, de Groot K. Histologic evaluation of the osseous adaptation to titanium and hydroxyapatite-coated titanium implants. *Journal of Biomedical Materials Research.* 1991; 25: 973-89.
58. Jarcho M. Calcium Phosphate Ceramics as Hard Tissue Prosthetics. *Clinical Orthopaedics and Related Research.* June 1981; 157: 259-78.
59. Jasty M, Rubash HE, Paiement G, Bragdon C, Parr J, Harrigan TP, Harris WH. Stimulation of bone ingrowth into porous surfaced total joint prosthesis by applying a thin coating of tricalcium phosphate-hydroxyapatite. *13th Annual Meeting of the Society of Biomaterials.* June 2-6, 1987; New York, NY: 251.
60. Kay JF, Golec TS, Riley RL. Hydroxyapatite-coated subperiosteal dental implants: design rationale and clinical experience. *Journal of Prosthetic Dentistry.* September 1987; 58(3): 339-43.
61. Kay JF, Manley MT, Stern LS, et al.: The effect of HA coatings on fixation of loaded metallic devices - a preliminary study. *Proceedings of the European Society of Biomaterials.* September 14-17, 1986; Bologna, Italy: 30.
62. Kent JN, Block MS, Kay J, Jarcho M., Finger IM. HA coated and non-coated dental implants in dogs. *12th Annual Meeting of the Society of Biomaterials.* May 29-June 1, 1986; Minneapolis, MN: 16.

63. Kent JN, Quinn JH, Zide MF, Finger IM, Jarcho M, Rothstein SS. Correction of alveolar ridge deficiencies with nonresorbable HA. *Journal of the American Dental Association*. December 1982; 105: 993-1001.

64. Kent JN, Quinn JH, Zide MF, Guerra LR, Boyne PJ. Alveolar ridge augmentation using nonresorbable HA with or without autogenous cancellous bone. *Journal of Oral and Maxillofacial Surgery*. 1983; 41: 629-42.

65. Kester MA, Manley MT, Taylor SK, Cohen RC. Influence of thickness on the mechanical properties and bond strength of HA coatings applied to orthopaedic implants. *37th Annual Meeting, Orthopaedic Research Society*. March 4-7, 1991; Anaheim, CA: 95.

66. Klein CPAT, Driessen AA, de Groot K. Relationship between the degradation behavior of calcium phosphate ceramics and their physical-chemical characteristics and ultrastructural geometry. *Biomaterials*. May 1984; 5: 157-60.

67. Klein CPAT, Driessen AA, de Groot K, van den Hooff A. Biodegradation behavior of various calcium phosphate materials in bone tissue. *Journal of Biomedical Materials Research*. 1983; 17: 769-84.

68. Klein CPAT, van der Lubbe HBM, Driessen AA, de Groot K, van den Hooff A. Biodegradation behavior of various calcium-phosphate materials in subcutaneous tissue. In: Vincenzini P, ed. *Ceramics in Surgery*. Amsterdam, The Netherlands: Elsevier; 1983.

69. Lee DR, Lemons JE, LeGeros RZ. Dissolution characteristics of commercially available HA particulate. *15th Annual Meeting of the Society for Biomaterials*. April 28-May 2, 1989; Lake Buena Vista, FL: 161.

70. Lieblich SE, Topazian RG. Changes in bone strength after augmentation with HA or HA/bone. *Journal of Oral and Maxillofacial Surgery*. 1987; 45: 1055-7.

71. Malawista SE, Duff GW, Atkins E, Cheung HS, McCarty DJ. Crystal-induced endogenous pyrogen production. A further look at gouty inflammation. *Arthritis and Rheumatism*. September 1985; 28(9): 1039-46.

72. Manley MT, Gaisser DM, Uratsuji M, Stulberg BN, Bauer TW, Stern LS. Fixation of porous titanium and smooth HA interfaces in a loaded model. *34th Annual Meeting, Orthopaedic Research Society*. February 1-4, 1988; Atlanta, GA: 332.

73. Manley MT, Kay JF, Uratsuji M, Stern LS, Stulberg BN. HA coatings applied to implants subjected to functional loads. *13th Annual Meeting of the Society of Biomaterials*. June 2-6, 1987; New York, NY: 210.

74. Manley MT, Kay JF, Yoshiya S, Stern LS, Stulberg BN. Accelerated fixation of weight bearing implants by HA coatings. *33rd Annual Meeting, Orthopaedic Research Society*: January 19-22, 1987; San Francisco, CA: 214.

75. Manley MT, Koch R. Clinical results with the hydroxyapatite-coated Omnifit hip stem. *Dental Clinics of North America*. January 1992; 36(1): 257-62.

76. Metsger DS, Driskell TD, Paulsrud JR. Tricalcium phosphate ceramic - a resorbable bone implant: review and current status. *Journal of the American Dental Association*. December 1982; 105: 1035-8.

77. Nagase M, Baker DG, Schumacher HR. Prolonged inflammatory reactions induced by artificial ceramics in the rat air pouch model. *The Journal of Rheumatology*. 1988; 15(9): 1334-8.

78. Parsons JR, Liebrecht P, Ricci JL, Salsbury R, Alexander H, Weiss AB. Enhanced stabilization of orthopaedic implants with spherical HA particulate. *12th Annual Meeting of the Society of Biomaterials*. May 29-June 1, 1986; Minneapolis, MN: 134.

79. Ricci JL, Spivak JM, Alexander H, Blumenthal NC, Parsons R. Hydroxyapatite ceramics and the nature of the bone-ceramic interface. *Bulletin of the Hospital for Joint Diseases Orthopaedic Institute*. 1989; 49(2): 178-91.

80. Rivero DP, Fox J, Skipor AK, Urban RM, Galante JO. Calcium phosphate-coated porous titanium implants for enhanced skeletal fixation. *Journal of Biomedical Materials Research*. 1988; 22: 191-201.

81. Rooney T, Berman S, Indresano AT. Evaluation of porous block HA for augmentation of alveolar ridges. *Journal of Oral and Maxillofacial Surgery*. 1988; 46: 15-18.

82. Rothstein SS, Paris D, Sage B. Use of durapatite for the rehabilitation of resorbed alveolar ridges. *Journal of the American Dental Association*. October 1984; 109: 571-74.

83. Russotti GM, Okada Y, Fitzgerald RH, Chao EYS, Gorski JP. Efficacy of using a bone graft substitute to enhance biological fixation of a porous metal femoral component. In: *The Hip: proceedings of the 15th open scientific meeting of The Hip Society*. 1987; 120-54.

84. Søballe K, Gotfredsen K, Brockstedt-Rasmussen H, Nielsen PT, Rechnagel K. Histologic analysis of a retrieved hydroxyapatite-coated femoral prosthesis. *Clinical Orthopaedics and Related Research*. November 1991; 272: 255-8.

85. Søballe K, Hansen ES, Brockstedt-Rasmussen H, Pedersen CM, Bünger C. Hydroxyapatite coating enhances fixation of porous coated implants. A comparison in dogs between press fit and nointerference fit. *Acta Orthopaedica Scandinavica.* 1990; 61(4): 299-302.

86. Thomas KA, Cook, SD, Anderson RC, Haddad RJ, Kay JF, Jarcho M. Biological response to HA coated porous titanium hips. *12th Annual Meeting of the Society of Biomaterials.* May 29-June 1, 1986; Minneapolis, MN: 15.

87. Thomas KA, Cook SD, Haddad RJ, Kay JF, Jarcho M. Biologic response to HA-coated titanium hips. A preliminary study in dogs. *Journal of Arthroplasty.* March 1989; 4(1): 43-53.

88. Thomas KA, Cook SD, Kay JF, Jarcho M, Anderson RC, Harding AF, Reynolds MC. Attachment strength and histology of HA coated implants. In: Saha S, ed. *Biomedical Engineering V. Recent Developments. Proceedings of the Fifth Southern Biomedical Engineer ing Conference.* New York, NY: Pergamon Press; 1986: 205-11.

89. Thomas KA, Kay JF, Cook, SD, Jarcho M. The effect of surface macrotexture and hydroxy lapatite coating on the mechanical strengths and histologic profiles of titanium implant materials. *Journal of Biomedical Materials Research.* 1987; 21: 1395-414.

90. Tracy BM, Doremus RH. Direct electron microscopy studies of the bone- HA interface. *Journal of Biomedical Materials Research.* 1984; 18: 719-26.

91. Vaughan BK, Lombardi AV, Mallory TH. Clinical and radiographic experience with a hydroxyapatite-coated titanium plasma-sprayed porous implant. *Seminars in Arthroplasty.* October 1991; 2(4): 309-16.

92. Vaughan BK, Lombardi AV, Mallory TH. Clinical and radiographic experience with a hydroxyapatite-coated titanium plasma-sprayed porous implant. *Dental Clinics of North America.* January 1992; 36(1): 263-72.

93. Zide MF, Kent JN, Machado L. HA cranioplasty directly over dura. *Journal of Oral and Maxillofacial Surgery.* 1987; 45: 481-86.

*Hydroxylapatite Coatings in Orthopaedic Surgery,*
edited by R. G. T. Geesink and M. T. Manley.
Raven Press, Ltd., New York, © 1993.

# A New Concept of Prosthetic Fixation

## Ronald Furlong, F.R.C.S.

The time has come for surgeons to give up pretending to believe that long-lasting prosthetic fixation can be achieved simply by implanting a stem, often of bizarre design, into the femoral shaft.

For years, where the use of cement has been abandoned, surgeons have been subjected to report after apologetic report indicating that by use of a stem of this design or that one, the complaint of postoperative midthigh pain has been reduced to 5% or thereabouts. This is indeed successful compared with the 25% to 30% prevalence of thigh pain three years after implantation with some "successful" all-metal, noncemented designs. But is it really a success?

In their hearts, surgeons know that ultimately "gate post" fixation must fail because of the physiology of functional adaptation. Had the proposal of "gate post" fixation been made to either Wilhelm Roux or Julius Wolff, he would have known the consequence instantly. Friedrich Pauwels did know the answer as does the house-surgeon who removes a Steinmann pin with his thumb and forefinger three months after insertion. The time has arrived for surgeons to clarify their thoughts and squarely face the problem, which is how to secure permanent fixation of a prosthetic device in the femur.

In this context, the word "permanent" is understood to mean the remaining life span of the patient. The term "fixation" is taken to mean a state of coalescence or continuity between prosthesis and bone. These criteria are established to demonstrate what will be demanded. It may be that such high and demanding standards of fixation are not required, but that is another matter and is irrelevant here.

In a clinical sense it is assumed that only by the high standard stated above can full, free, and painless function be enjoyed for the lifetime of the patient after total hip replacement.

Let us examine the situation in relation to "press fit" used to obtain fixation. "Press fit" is a friction-induced type of micromechanical interlocking, produced by means of elastic and plastic deformation of the trabeculae that are contacted, i.e., involved; this temporarily prevents implant/bone motion. Elastic deformation implies that trabeculae are subjected to sustainable stress. It is because of their high elasticity that this stress has not exceeded the limit of their ultimate bending strength. The trabeculae have remained intact. If the load-bearing capacity of the trabecular bone is exceeded either by peak stresses or by long subjugation to load, plastic deformation supervenes.

Trabeculae that have been overstressed, fractured, or damaged by reaming or other surgical manipulation during preparation of the implant cavity are, in principle, a disadvantage because plastic deformation is unphysiological and is therefore followed by necrosis of the involved bone. The devitalized tissue is inevitably resorbed with the result that the friction-form locking first achieved, becomes ineffective and the prosthesis loosens. Relative movement increases considerably at the interface between prosthesis and bone. Such interface movement provokes the formation of a fibrous membrane which has an unfavorable effect on load transfer. It also has been found that femoral reaming, even with the best surgical tools, may produce only a 30% contact between metal and bone. As metal is not osteotropic, the resultant 70% of space between femur and implant inevitably becomes filled with connective or fibrous tissue. Once the interface has been formed as a fibrous intervening layer, the way for osseous growth is barred and only osteogenesis at a distance or, at best, "contact osteogenesis," can be achieved.

With this sequence in mind, surgeons are compelled to look for alternative means of prosthetic fixation. Such an alternative is at hand and involves the use of an hydroxylapatite (HA) ceramic-coated, biomechanically designed prosthesis.

An HA ceramic-coated prosthesis is now advocated because it becomes physiologically integrated with bone. The word "osseointegration" has recently become debased in meaning. Originally coined by dentists, it was used to denote the particular efficacy of an implant peculiar to dentistry. Later investigators used the term to describe bone growth toward titanium to a distance of less than 1 μm, which it will do in conditions of absolute stillness. Because the intervening space is so narrow, it contains no cells and is no longer visible by light microscopy. When the term "osseointegration" re-emerged, confusion arose because the state described is no more than "contact osteogenesis." Here the word will be used in its first meaning, i.e., to denote tissue continuity or coalescence.

HA ceramic (HA-C) was first used in a clinically serious manner by Johannes Friedrich Osborn, a maxillofacial surgeon practicing in Hamburg. The fractured mandible is often comminuted and compounded, so that complications jeopardizing union are almost inevitable. Osborn found that if the fracture site was immobilized by external fixation the fracture would readily unite when HA-C granules were used to replace loose fragments and to restore continuity to the bone. He was impressed by the readiness with which the HA-C was covered and penetrated by bone. This bioactivity of osteotropism is responsible for the new bone formation, during the course of which an interface develops on the pattern of bonding osteogenesis (Fig. 1).

By this time the ceramic and mineralized bone can no longer be distinguished because the HA-C becomes part of the bone tissue itself. In the case of both Osprovit granules and Osprovit coating, this identical phenomenon can be observed in human bone evaluated histologically. Through growth and modeling, after some months, the interface reaches a final state that is characterized osteologically by coalescence and biomechanically by a substantial bond. This is the essence of the success of the HA-C coated prosthesis, because where there is osteotropism there is life.

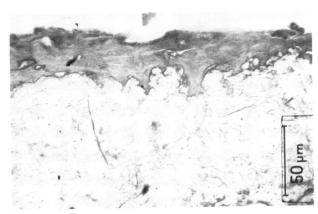

**FIG. 1** Hydroxylapatite ceramic is both covered and penetrated by bone, the result of osteo-tropism.

The statement by McKee, "An important problem is fixation of the prosthesis. This involves the attachment of dead to living tissue," is no longer relevant, because the dead has been animated by osteotropism. Henceforth, there are two living partners involved in the integration of the HA-coated prosthesis, the stem and the host bone. The situation is created of a fresh fracture about to unite and success is assured.

Surgeons have long realized that sound *per primam* bony union is best secured in conditions of contact, stillness, and stressing. So it is with the integration of HA with bone. Osborn was well aware of this, as shown by the way he treated the fractured mandible supplemented with HA. However, he was skeptical as to whether these physical conditions could be transferred to the femur. He set himself the task of finding a hip prosthesis with built-in stability by virtue of a biomechanical design. This he would coat with HA, using the plasma-flame process and, with luck, after implantation there was sufficient stability to ensure the three-month mechanical fixation necessary to provide contact, stillness, and stressing, permitting union to take place.

In 1983, taking inspiration from the glass stopper of a decanter, I designed a coned prosthesis. I believed that because such a stopper does not descend, rotate nor lean due to its conical shape, neither would a hip prosthesis if a cone were built into its design. I felt it would mechanically fix into the mouth of the medullary canal at operation. Osborn recognized the potential of my femoral stem and soon this prosthesis, coated with HA, was available for clinical evaluation (Fig. 2).

Osborn had mastered the intricacies of the plasma-spray method of coating a metal and, after animal experimentation, he decided to use a 200 μm thick coating of HA. According to his studies, Osborn estimated that because of osteotropic consumption the thickness of the Osprovit coating is reduced by approximately 40 to 60 μm by the time coalescence is established. Therefore, a coating thickness of 200 μm was chosen. This concept of a thick coating was vindicated when it was reported that after some 12–20 months 50–60 μm of

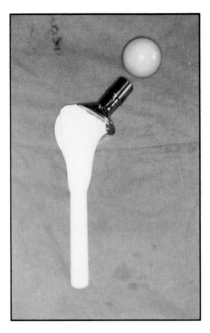

**FIG 2.** The whole of the intraosseous prosthesis is coated.  The jammed cone secures mechanical fixation.

coating had been used as a result of modeling processes.  A metal-to-bone contact took place when the HA layer was only 50 μm thick.

Therefore, the coating, named by Osborn "Osprovit," is 200 μm thick and has a bond strength of 40 MPa and a porosity of 15% to 20%.  No suggestion of instability of the coating *in situ* has arisen after 11,000 implantations over a seven-year period.

Given that a metal-bone interface will not provide permanent fixation, because only compressive and not tensile forces are transferred across this type of interface, the whole of the intraosseus femoral stem is coated.  The coalescence of the HA to bone provides fixation but the design of the prosthesis ensures the permanence of that fixation, because of the primary mechanical fixation obtained from the moment of implantation.

## FIXATION OF THE BODY OF THE PROSTHESIS

Implantation of the prosthesis is performed as follows. An x-ray template is used to determine the dimensions of the prosthesis.  At operation, a space in the metaphysis of the femur is cautiously and sparingly prepared to receive the prosthesis.  The prosthesis becomes impacted into the mouth of the medullary tube.  Impaction must be firm.  On a clinical note, the surgeon will observe that at the moment of impaction the note of the hammer "hardens."  From this moment the prosthesis is immobile and the mechanical fixation is absolute.

From his experience with jaw fractures, Osborn insisted that three months of immobility between fragments was necessary to secure the effect of osteotropism that would simulate primary bone union. From the moment of implantation, the body of the prosthesis is surrounded by and compressed by mature trabeculae, some in a state of elastic deformation and some damaged by the procedure of implantation. Osteotropism soon covers the HA surface.

Osteotropism becomes effective and the coated surface of the prosthetic body is covered with bone and penetrated to a depth of 10–20 µm. When the reparative phase of the damaged trabeculae is completed, they become attached to the bony "shell" on the HA surface. Other trabeculae not in contact with the prosthesis reach out to make contact and this process is also initiated from the surface of the prosthesis.

Within two to three months order is re-established and the trabeculae, as a result of functional adaptation, reorder themselves into the best vectorial alignment to transmit the stresses of body load. In this connection it is noticable that, at the point of attachment of a trabecula to either bone or HA, no sign of frictional or shear stressing is apparent. It would appear that the body-weight stressing that, at first sight, appears to be longitudinal in direction is in fact lateral or normal. Therefore, the vectorial aspect of the established trabeculae is one of lateral compression.

Clinical and radiologic evidence extending over seven years led to the belief that the stressing to which the elastic supportive trabeculae are subjected is physiologic because no pathologic alteration in the distribution of the trabeculae has been observed over this time. It can be justly claimed, therefore, that implantation of HA-coated prostheses is permanent as far as histologic evidence is concerned.

## FIXATION OF THE STEM OF THE PROSTHESIS

Concerning the stem of the prosthesis, the principle of fixation is similar to that used in the body of the prosthesis, but its application is different.

In essence, sufficient room should be created around the cylindrical stem to allow the development of vectorially arranged elastic trabeculae that will cradle the prosthesis while permitting micromotion. The medullary tube is reamed out to a diameter 2 mm larger than the diameter of the stem to be used. This ensures a gap of 1 mm surrounding the stem. However, if a gap of 2 mm surrounding the stem is created, this is no disadvantage. The medullary cavity is reamed gently and the debris is not removed. In theory, because of impaction of the cone the prosthesis should be completely immobile and should occupy the center of the lumen, having no contact with bone. The phenomenon of trabecular growth soon begins, rapidly supporting the stem while the cone is still effective. When the stability given by the impacted cone diminishes, the vectorial trabeculae give the stem total support. In this situation the trabeculae develop in direction and magnitude according to the quality of the local stressing and have been seen in histologic specimens nine weeks after implantation (Fig.3).

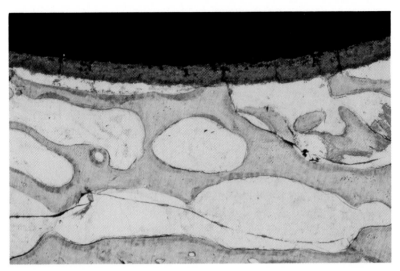

**FIG 3.** The forces attaching trabeculae to HA are compressive and at right angles, not tangential.

The trabeculae are not clearly visible on x-ray until almost a year after implantation. At that time they can be seen in profusion in locations of significant stress. Often they are seen in the metaphyseal cancellous bone surrounding the body of the prosthesis. They may be present on both sides of the metal, either just proximal or distal to the cone. The stem itself often does not seem to be attached by trabeculae to the host bone, but the tip of the prosthesis is always surrounded by supportive trabecular bone. Sometimes the stem is in contact with the cortical bone of the shaft, which may be considerably thickened for a distance of several inches proximal or distal to the point of contact.

At this level the trabeculae are always transverse in direction, indicating that the prosthesis still retains a tilting moment into either valgus or varus. When trabeculation at the tip is present on both sides, this indicates that both tensile and compressive stresses are in action.

In view of this finding, it seems bizarre that some surgeons do not use fully-coated prostheses. The half-coated prosthesis lacks the ability to accept or transmit tensile stresses. Therefore, to deprive an area of HA at which tensile stresses are at work seems strange, since HA is the only medium that can transmit tensile stresses.

The cradling of the prosthesis implies the capability of accepting micromovement without separate movement of particles (Fig. 4). Relative movement between the bone and the prosthesis is inevitable. This is more closely related to the cold hard facts of geometry than to the relative elasticity of the participants. Because this micromotion *is* inevitable it must be accommodated, and this is achieved by the elasticity of the prosthesis-bearing trabeculae. Provided the deformation of the trabeculae under load remains within the

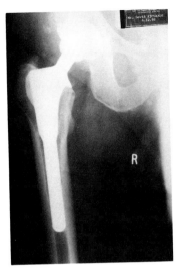

**FIG. 4.** Trabeculae, both medial and lateral, by their elasticity cradle the body of the prosthesis.

elastic limit, physiology is satisfied. The fact that the stressing is within elastic limits is underscored by the fact that a follow-up period of six years has failed to demonstrate clinically, by radiology or by autopsy, that anything other than physiologic stressing exists in the upper end of the femur.

Apart from the relationship of the bone to the prosthesis, it is advantageous to preserve the hollow status of the femur. The hollowness of the bone exhibits a different type of elasticity from that of solid bone, as when the upper end of the femur is filled with a prosthesis and cement, stiffening it as though it were solid. Such a state is pathologic, rather than physiologic. Pathology is an ongoing state whereas physiology is stable.

For the reasons described above it is claimed that the concepts pertaining to this type of fixation are unique and are not to be compared or confused with any other mode of fixation. It is clear, however, that the fixation mode of the future must lie in the realm of physiology rather than in the present mode of pathology.

*Hydroxylapatite Coatings in Orthopaedic Surgery,*
edited by R. G. T. Geesink and M. T. Manley.
Raven Press, Ltd., New York, © 1993.

# Variations in Hydroxylapatite Crystallinity: Effects on Interface Reactions

Clemens A. van Blitterswijk, Ph.D., Yvonne P. Bovell, B.S.,
Jim S. Flach, M.S., Henk Leenders, B.S.,
Ineke van den Brink, B.S., and Joost de Bruijn, B.S.

Hydroxylapatite (HA) coatings on metal substrates have found widespread clinical application (1-3). These composites provide sufficient mechanical strength, provided by the metal, and favorable interactions with bone, caused by the ceramic. Although clinical evaluations have proven the efficacy of an HA- coated device versus press-fit implantation of the metal prosthesis alone, several factors concerning the functioning of the coating still remain unclear.

One unclear factor, which is receiving increased attention lately, is whether a coating should provide long term performance or if its function is only temporary. Those in favour of long-term performance seem to feel that since the clinical improvement of coated versus noncoated devices is clearly caused by the HA coating, the dissolution of that coating could potentially reduce the initial benefit. On the other hand, one might also reason that the HA coating provides a rapid integration of the prosthesis in bone and after the establishment of such a proper integration, the actual presence of a coating would no longer be required. The latter assumption is supported by the fact that some studies show comparable push-out values for noncoated versus HA-coated titanium prostheses after *long term* implantation (4), whereas a much better bonding was initially obtained by HA-coated implants.

Irrespective of the desire for coating longevity, one aspect which remains essential is the ability of the coating to bond to bone in the shortest possible time. Bone-bonding has been defined as follows: the establishment by physicochemical processes of a continuity at the interface between implant and bone matrix (5). In the case of calcium phosphate ceramics, this continuity is generally thought to be composed of a carbonate-containing apatite layer, with an organic component that has been deposited on the ceramic surface (6). In decalcified sections, this interfacial zone has an electron dense morphology (6,7-13) which explains why it is frequently referred to as an electron-dense layer, although bonding zone, lamina limitans-like layer and cement-line are also used.

Up to now, it has not been clear how this calcium phosphate precipitate is exactly formed, but the series of events proposed by Legeros et al. (6) seem to provide a sound hypothesis: 1. Partial dissolution of the ceramic macrocrystals. 2. Increase of the concentration of calcium and phosphate in the micro environment. 3. Formation of carbonate apatite microcrystals. 4. Association of these microcrystals with an organic matrix.

If this assumption is correct, it provides an interesting conflict. If one favours a coating with longevity, it needs to have a low dissolution rate. This, however, is likely to slow down the processes involved with the electron-dense carbonate apatite deposit, and might thus delay the occurrence of bone-bonding. It has been demonstrated by several authors that the calcium phosphate precipitate is indeed a precursor of bone-bonding.

Summarizing the above, one can state that there seems to be an inherent conflict between manufacturing a slowly resorbing HA coating and obtaining a rapid bond with bone. In order to investigate this phenomenon further, a series of experiments in which the dissolution properties of HA coatings were varied by altering the crystallinity was started. The coatings were evaluated in *in vitro* assays and by implantation.

## Materials

In these experiments, we used four series with different variations in crystallinity. The first series (series A) comprised three HA coatings on a titanium-vanadium alloy substrate. Coating crystallinities, as determined by X-ray diffraction were 5%, 53% and 78% (Fig. 1 a-c). The first two coatings were both manufactured by plasma-spraying using different parameters, whereas the last coating was an amorphous plasma-sprayed coating that was subsequently subjected to a heat treatment (600°C), thus increasing the crystallinity.

The second series (series B) was produced in a similar way as series A, however crystallinities of 15%, 43% and 69% were obtained.

The third series of coatings with varying crystallinity (series C), differed from the previous two in that it concerned bilayered coatings, on a titanium alloy substrate, that had all been subjected to heat-treatment. The first layer was

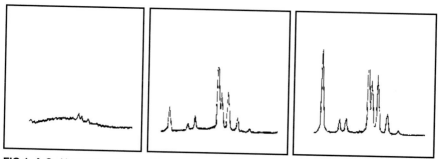

**FIG 1. A-C.** X-ray diffraction spectrograms of the 5%(a), 53%(b) and 78%(c) crystalline hydroxylapatite coatings.

plasma-sprayed as an amorphous coating and was subjected to heat-treatment at 600°C. X-ray diffraction showed this coating to be 100% crystalline. On top of this coating, another layer was plasma-sprayed which was initially amorphous and was then submitted to heat treatments at increasing temperatures (400°C-600°C) resulting in top-coatings with crystallinities of 10%, 24%, 38%, 66%, 86% and 100%.

The fourth variation in crystallinity (series D) did not concern coatings but discs of stoichiometric HA calcined at 600 and 900°C (average grain size ± 0.1 μm and microporosity 40-50%) or sintered at 1250°C (average grain size 3.1 μm, microporosity ± 3%).

## Coating Morphology

During the *in vitro* and *in vivo* experiments, the morphology of the coatings in series A and B was investigated by both scanning and transmission electron microscopy. Scanning electron microscopy showed that all surfaces were initially relatively smooth but closer examination revealed that the coatings with intermediate crystallinity possessed a slightly higher surface roughness. Transmission electron microscopy demonstrated a more prominent difference. The highly amorphous coatings were predominantly composed of tiny electron dense crystals. Similar crystals were also seen in the coatings with higher crystallinity but, in these cases, they formed a matrix in-between larger electron dense domains. These domains were relatively small but high in frequency for the heat treated material, whereas they were much larger but lower in frequency for the materials with intermediate crystallinity (Fig. 2a,b).

From these data it may be concluded that the morphology of the coating reflects the manufacturing procedure. The amorphous coatings are largely based on feedstock powder that was completely molten during plasma spraying, and was frozen into an amorphous structure because of the rapid cooling upon striking the substrate surface. Apparently the tiny crystals are no longer detected by x-ray diffraction. In contrast, the coatings with intermediate

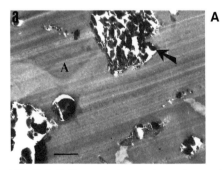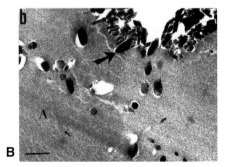

**FIG. 2. A,B** Transmission electron micrographs showing the composition of the 53% (a) and 78% (b) coating. The 53% coating shows relatively large crystalline domains (arrow) in an amorphous matrix (A) as opposed to smaller domains seen for the heat-treated 78% coating. bar(μm)= 0.38

crystallinity that were not subjected to heat treatment and were plasma-sprayed with less extreme parameters, still possessed relatively large crystalline domains, reflecting the partially non-molten feedstock powder. The smaller crystalline domains in the heat-treated coatings were not present after plasma-spraying but formed during the heat-treatment procedure.

## Degradation Studies

The degradation of the coatings was investigated in several experimental models. The first concerned exposing the coatings of series B to $a$-MEM medium supplemented with 15% fetal bovine serum, antibiotics, 10 mM ß-glycerophosphate and 50 µg/ml ascorbic acid. This medium is routinely used for osteoclast cultures. The analysis by atomic absorption spectrometry of retrieved medium indicated that the 15% and 43% crystalline HA coatings showed a similar calcium release which was significantly higher than that observed for the heat-treated 69% crystalline coating (Fig. 3).

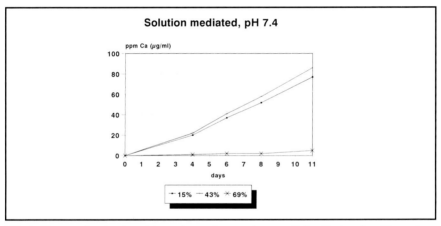

**FIG. 3.** Diagram showing the calcium release of a range in crystallinity of hydroxylapatite coatings that were exposed to cell-culture medium.

In a similar experiment, the coatings of series C, which were all subjected to some form of heat treatment, were exposed to a similar culture medium as mentioned above for series B but with the addition of 10-8 M dexamethasone. The results that were obtained by atomic absorption analysis of the medium for calcium are plotted in Fig. 4 and strongly suggest a direct relation between the extent of crystallinity and degradation rate. The higher the crystallinity, the lower the degradation.

In another model, the coatings of series A were implanted subcutaneously into rats and investigated after 2, 4, 13 and 52 weeks by light microscopy, scanning and transmission electron microscopy and image analysis.

Light microscopy revealed that even after one year, irrespective of the type of coating, HA was still present on the titanium substrate. Image analysis,

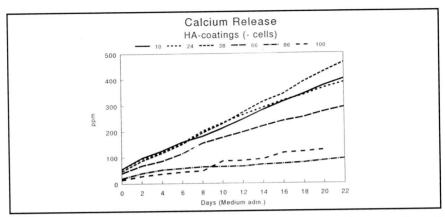

**FIG. 4.** Similar diagram as shown in Fig. 3 with a slightly different crystallinity range and a small variation in the medium (see text).

however, demonstrated that differences in degradation rate did exist although predominantly in the first postoperative intervals (Fig. 5). The 5% crystalline HA coating showed the most degradation (36 μm after six weeks) followed by the 53% crystalline coating (17 μm at six weeks); the 78% crystalline heat-treated coating hardly showed any degradation at all. After implantation intervals longer than six weeks no noteworthy degradation was observed for any of the coatings.

Scanning electron microscopy of the surface of the coatings, after hypo-chlorite treatment to remove the interfacial tissues, showed distinct differences (Fig. 6). After 1 year, the 5% crystalline coating was still relatively smooth although some crack formation and a fine granular deposit could be observed (Fig. 6a). The surface of the 53% crystalline coating was rough and revealed irregularly shaped rather large protrusions (Fig. 6b). The 78% crystalline heat-treated material only showed focal areas of degradation, where many protrud-

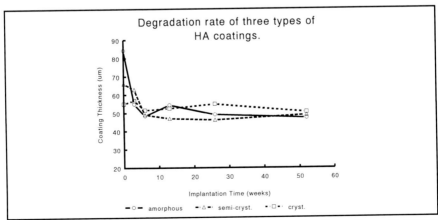

**FIG. 5.** Diagram showing the coating thickness of three hydroxylapatite coatings with different crystallinities after subcutaneous implantation.

ing needle shaped crystals were seen (Fig. 6c). These findings corresponded well with the transmission electron microscopical data, which were indicative of a smooth coating with apparent areas of calcium phosphate precipitation (demonstrated by x-ray microanalysis) in the case of the 5% crystalline material (Fig. 7a). In contrast, the 53% crystalline coating showed protrusion and even detachment of large electron dense crystalline domains from the coating surface, similar to those described under the heading "coating morphology". The heat-treated material did not show any distinct changes of its surface (Fig. 7b).

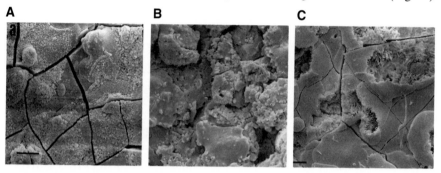

**FIG.6. A-C**  Scanning electron micrographs of the surface of three hydroxylapatite coatings with increasing crystallinity rates. Note the differences between the 5% (a), 53% (b) and 78% (c) coatings. bar($\mu$m)= 6.5

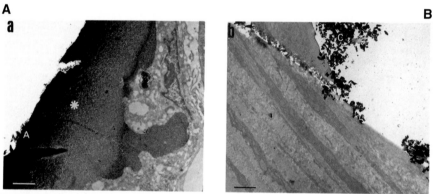

**FIG.7. (A.)**  Transmission electron micrograph of the tissue/hydroxylapatite interface for an amorphous coating (A), an apparent calcium phosphate deposition (*) can be observed at the coating surface. bar($\mu$m)= 2.1  **(B.)** Transmission electron micrograph of the interface between 78% crystalline hydroxyapatite (C) and fibrous tissue. No noteworthy changes have occurred at the interface. bar($\mu$m)= 2.1

## Degradation Conclusions

The results described above generally confirm the hypothesis that increased crystallinity of coatings will lead to a decrease in degradation rate. If degradation occurred it would mainly involve the amorphous matrix that was present in all coatings. Dissolution of the amorphous matrix caused the detachment of non-dissolved, more-crystalline domains, thus accelerating the overall degradation rate. The deviating behavior of the 43% crystalline coating in Fig. 12, where it shows more resorption than expected, may be explained by the fact that the top of this coating contains much amorphous material and the evaluation interval was short. It was not clear why degradation apparently stopped after six weeks of subcutaneous implantation for all tested coatings. This latter finding might be interpreted in a way that, at longer implantation intervals, biological calcium phosphate precipitation equals or exceeds the physicochemical calcium release from the amorphous phase of the coating.

## Cellular Aspects of Degradation

Although the previous section demonstrated that dissolution of plasma-sprayed HA coatings can occur and is at least partially dependent on the crystallinity of the coating, it was not clear whether this dissolution was a purely physicochemical process or also cell-mediated.

Up to date, it is known that macrophages and multinucleated cells play a role in the degradation of calcium phosphate ceramics (8,10,14-18). To our knowledge it has not been demonstrated that this role exceeds the mere phagocytosis of already detached or relatively loose fragments. In addition to the role of phagocytes in calcium phosphate degradation, it has been suggested by several authors that resorptive osteoclast activity could be a contributing factor in HA coating degradation (17,19-21). Unfortunately, in most reports this assumption is largely based on only morphological observations and not on enzymatic characteristics, the combination of which seems essential to determine the exact nature of these cells. In other reports such an enzymatic analysis was performed but the coating was not a stoichiometric HA or the analysed material was no coating at all.

In order to obtain more information on the cellular component in HA coating degradation, we performed the following studies.

In the first study, we cultured rat bone marrow cells on series B under culture conditions favorable for osteoclast differentation (22). In this experiment, a similar calcium release was detected by atomic absorption for the 15% and 43% crystalline materials whereas the lowest calcium release was found for the 69% crystalline material (Fig. 8). These data did not significantly deviate from studies in which the coatings were exposed to medium without cells, suggesting that these cells did not play an important role in coating degradation. This was further confirmed by investigation of the coating surface which revealed no clear signs of cell-mediated degradation. Determining the number of tartrate resistant acid phosphatase (TRAP) positive cells (indicative for osteoclasts) on the surface of the coatings revealed that most of these cells were seen on the 43% crystalline material (Fig. 9). This indicated that osteoclast-like cell formation was not predominantly controlled by the amount of calcium being released from the coating nor did the number of TRAP positive cells affect coating degradation.

Since under normal conditions osteoclasts do not function solitarily but in

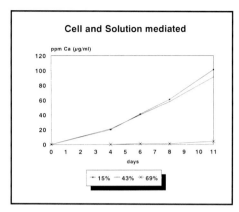

**FIG. 8.** Diagram showing the release of calcium from various coatings after incubation with osteoclast-like cells.

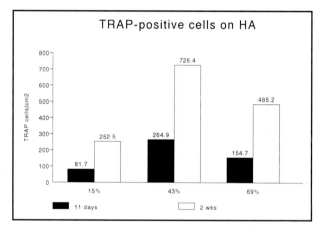

**FIG. 9.** Diagram of the amount of TRAP positive cells in a culture of bone marrow cells on hydroxylapatite coatings with different crystallinities.

a complex biological system, we tried to mimic the natural situation more closely by bringing an osteoblast component into the cultures.

For these experiments a two-stage culture was used on series D, calcined and sintered HA discs (23). The first stage comprised the culture of rat bone marrow cells under culture conditions favoring osteoblast differentiation (24).This was supposed to result in the deposition of a mineralized matrix on each of the three substrates. However, a distinct mineralized matrix was only found on the densely sintered HA. The nature of this deposition will be discussed in more detail in later sections of this chapter. After removal of the cells grown during the first stage, by trypsin treatment, a new population of rat bone marrow cells was cultured but under conditions that allowed differentiation into TRAP positive cells. Earlier studies by Davies et al.(22) have shown that these osteoclast-like cells were able to resorb the mineralized matrix that had been deposited during the first-stage culture. As a control study the first stage was omitted for series D and only the culture conditions favoring TRAP positive cell formation were used.

In the control experiment without the first stage culture, no indications of cell-mediated resorption were seen by scanning electron microscopy, in spite of the presence of TRAP positive cells. This situation changed for the two-stage culture, where discrete cell-mediated resorption could be observed on the calcined materials. Both the materials calcined at 600°C and 900°C showed characteristic scalloped resorption lacunae with scanning electron microscopy (Fig. 10), which were not observed on the sintered HA in the two-stage culture (Fig. 11) or on any of the materials from series D, in the one-stage osteoclast-like cell culture. These data indicate that osteoclasts are indeed able to resorb specific types of artificial calcium phosphate although this resorptive activity is not solely dependent on the ceramic substrate but on the interactions with factors secreted by other cells as well. Although distinct cell-mediated resorption of HA was demonstrated in this two stage culture model, the results still support the finding that dense highly crystalline HA materials are not subject to major degradation in the studies described in this paper.

## Conclusions on Cell-mediated Resorption

Several publications have reported data suggestive for cell-mediated resorption of different calcium phosphate substrates (8,14,15-21). The data derived from these studies are hard to compare due to the use of different materials and varying methods of analysis. In our opinion, none of these studies, although sometimes suggestive, provide sufficient evidence that HA coatings are subject to cell-mediated resorption in addition to mere physicochemical processes. The studies described in this report seem to confirm the absence of cell-mediated resorption on HA coatings but an interesting aspect emerged from the two-stage culture on series D. Apparently, the surface of calcium phosphate substrates can be modified by osteoblast-containing cultures in such

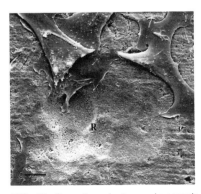

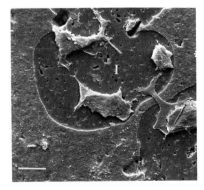

**FIG. 10.** Scanning electron micrograph showing a resorption lacunae (R) on a pressed calcined (600°C) hydroxylapatite plate after a two-stage culture. bar(μm)= 9.4

**FIG. 11.** The surface of a sintered hydroxylapatite plate after the two-stage culture. Although resorption of the mineral deposition (*) has occurred, no change of the implant surface (I) was observed. bar(μm)= 14

a way that TRAP-positive cells are stimulated to resorb the substrate. This interaction between different cell types involved in bone-remodeling deserves further attention in future studies on the resorption of HA coatings.

## Interface Reactions

As already stated above, bone bonding is caused by a continuity at the interface between biomaterial and bone matrix. The formation of an electron dense layer at the bone/biomaterial interface (containing both carbonate apatite and an organic component) (6,8,12) seems to play an important role in this process. The dissolution characteristics of an HA coating are likely to affect the precipitation of the carbonate-apatite at its surface and also, most probably, the morphological appearance of the electron-dense layer. Therefore, an experiment was started to investigate how variations in crystallinity, i.e. disso-lution rate, of HA coatings would affect the appearance of the interface in general and the electron-dense layer in particular.

The coatings from series B were subjected to a culture of rat bone marrow cells under circumstances favorable for differentiation into osteoblasts. In accordance with several other studies (12,13,22), the incubation of these cells on the HA substrate caused the formation of a globular afibrillar matrix followed by the incorporation of collagen fibers and their subsequent mineralization. The investigation of the interfacial zone between these mineralized areas and the coating indeed showed that the type of interface formed depended on the rate of crystallinity.

In the case of the 15% and 43% crystalline coatings, an amorphous zone of approximately 1 μm wide was frequently seen interposed between the depos-ited extracellular matrix and the bulk of the coating. This zone was less dense than the underlying ceramic and contained material of an apparently organic nature, in addition to calcium phosphate. On top of this amorphous zone, mono- or multilayered electron dense layers were located at the interface with the mineralized matrix (Fig. 12). Conversely, the 69% heat-treated coating lacked such an amorphous zone and was generally characterized by a single electron dense layer at the interface with a thickness of 20 - 60 nm at the interface (Fig. 13). For both the 15% and 43% crystalline coatings and the heat treated coating, the use of ruthenium red staining demonstrated the presence of glycosaminoglycans in this electron dense interfacial zone. In routine stain-ing, this zone also showed tiny needle shaped calcium and phosphorus contain-ing crystals. Another observation of interest was that the 43% and 69% crystalline HA coatings only showed a parallel orientation of collagen fibers along the interface, whereas the most amorphous 15% crystalline material also showed a perpendicular deposition of fibers.

## Conclusions on Interface Reactions Related to Crystallinity

From the above findings, it became clear that variations in crystallinity indeed resulted in differences at the interface. The bulk of the most crystalline

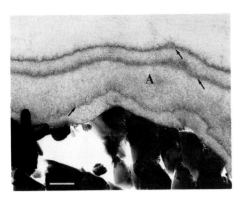

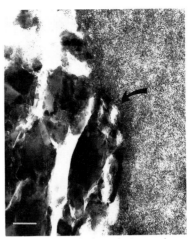

**FIG. 12.** Transmission electron micrograph of the surface of a 43% crystalline material after incubation in a mineralizing bone marrow culture. Note the amorphous zone (A) and the multilayered electron dense layer (arrows). bar($\mu$m)= 1

**FIG. 13.** Transmission electron microscopy of the surface of a 69% crystalline hydroxylapatite coating under similar conditions as in Fig. 12. Just a monolayered electron dense layer (arrow) can be seen. bar($\mu$m)= 14

coating was in immediate contact with the electron-dense deposit at the interface with the mineralized matrix. In contrast, the more amorphous materials showed the occurrence of an amorphous zone in-between the electron-dense layer and the more dense bulk of the coating. Such an amorphous zone has been described before for HA (8,12) and up to date its actual meaning is not clear. Taking into consideration the following data, it might well be that the amorphous zone represents a calcium phosphate dissolution/precipitation zone, in other words, a dynamic interface: 1. In this experiment, the amorphous zone was found for materials with the highest dissolution rate and was absent with the most crystalline coating. 2. Its density was less than the bulk coating and it contained an organic component, in addition to a calcium phosphate matrix. 3. It was located underneath the electron-dense layer that is usually present at the HA/bone interface.

In this respect, it was interesting to observe that only the most amorphous material showed perpendicularly-aligned collagen fibers along its interface. This is a characteristic ascribed to bioglasses or glass ceramics (25,26), the most bioactive materials known to date, but more recently for loaded HA implants, as well (27).

## General Discussion

The dissolution rate of calcium phosphate ceramics has always been the subject of discussion. Even on HA and tricalcium phosphate-sintered blocks, which have been investigated for over two decades now, no consensus on the rate of degradation exists (8,14,28-31). Therefore, it is not surprising that the resorption of HA coatings, which have much more recently become the subject of interest, is still largely unclear. Some publications report a relatively fast degradation (32) whereas others still show remnants of the coating after years of implantation (2,33). The current investigation has shown that although other factors may also be of importance for degradation, variations in HA crystallinity significantly affect the rate of degradation. With comparable coating structures, the higher the rate of crystallinity, the lower the degradation rate will be. Furthermore, it was demonstrated that dissolution of the amorphous matrix of a coating will lead to mechanical detachment of the more crystalline fragments, thus causing a more rapid degradation than would be expected by calcium phosphate dissolution alone. Interconnection of the crystalline fragments in a coating may reduce this problem. Dissolution of the coating was associated with the occurrence of an amorphous zone in-between the electron dense zone and the bulk of the coating, which potentially represents a dynamic interface in which calcium phosphate dissolution and precipitation take place. This zone has also been demonstrated for calcium phosphates with different crystal structures from HA (34.) Finally, this study demonstrated that interactions between different cell types which are located at the bone/calcined HA interface, osteoblasts and osteoclasts, can potentially affect the degradation rate and degradation mechanism. So far, we have not been able to demonstrate this phenomenon for HA coatings as well.

To date it is still not clear whether the degradation of the HA coating represents an eventual clinical problem or whether it is an essential aspect in bone-bonding.

Several authors have stated that the deposition of a carbonate apatite layer on the surface of bioactive materials is an essential component in the bone-bonding process (6,35.) This has not only been said for calcium phosphate ceramics but also for Bioglass (25), glass ceramics (36,37) and for Polyactive, a bone-bonding PEO/PBT copolymer (38,39,40). In the case of both HA and Polyactive, the important role of such a calcium phosphate precipitation has been demonstrated by the fact that bonding osteogenesis (41) could only be found after a calcium phosphate precipitation on the materials surface had occurred (38,40,42). Even the discussion of whether or not titanium would potentially be able to bond to bone seems to be largely based on a calcium absorption on its surface after long-term implantation (43,44,45). All these data would suggest that bone-bonding can only occur after the deposition of a biological apatite layer at the bone/biomaterial interface. This presumption, in combination with the hypothesis ventilated by Legeros et al. (6), which considers the dissolution of calcium from the biomaterial surface an essential step in the formation of a carbonate apatite layer at the surface, makes it very likely that some critical amount of coating degradation is essential to obtain rapid bone-bonding.

Although this relation between calcium release and speed of bone-bonding has been established for Bioglass (46) and AW-glass ceramic (36), it has never been definitively proven for calcium phosphate ceramics. The data that are currently available, however, provide some circumstantial evidence. With increasing tricalcium phosphate content, biphasic (HA/TCP) ceramics showed more alkaline phosphatase production (indicative for increased bone metabolism) (40). There seems to be a relation between the amount of HA available in composites and the degree of bone-bonding (48,49). In a rat bone-marrow culture, fluoroapatite, which degrades very slowly, showed a slower deposition of the apatite containing electron-dense layer on its surface as compared to a regular HA coating (34). Furthermore, the current study demonstrated that variations in crystallinity of HA coatings not only affected the degradation rate but also the mineralized matrix/coating interface (50). A Bioglass-like collagen interdigitation was obtained at the interface of the most amorphous, i.e. fast degrading, HA coating. Unfortunately, no data exist as yet that unequivocally confirm this hypothesis (that greater dissolution provides faster bonding) for *in vivo* implantation of HA coatings in bone. Fluoroapatite, with its low dissolution rate, did not show less bone-bonding as compared to HA coatings (32) and it has never been shown that more amorphous coatings do indeed show a beneficial effect at the interface with bone. Furthermore, densely sintered HA blocks generally show a good integration with bone and the occurrence of an electron-dense calcium phosphate deposit on their surface (8,15). It should be emphasized that most of these studies did not specifically investigate short-term interface reactions and this is where the most beneficial effect of calcium phosphate dissolution is to be expected.

In summary it can be stated that several data are available which suggest that a certain amount of coating dissolution is desirable for an optimal functioning of the coating. *In vivo* confirmation of this assumption has not as yet been obtained, nor has it been well investigated. With the current status of knowledge, we should be careful of any modification of the clinically successfully applied coatings since we do not possess sufficient knowledge on the underlying bone-bonding mechanism. Highly crystalline coatings, for instance, might be interesting in reducing degradation but we do not know what the effect will be on short-term bone-bonding performance which is the ultimate property of HA-coated versus noncoated devices.

## REFERENCES

1. Geesink RGT. Hydroxyapatite-coated total hip prostheses. Two-year clinical and roentgenographic results of 100 cases. *Clinical Orthopaedics* 1990; 261: 39-58.
2. Hardy DCR, Frayssinet P, Guilhem A, Lafontaine MA, Delince PE. Bonding of hydroxyapatite coated femoral prostheses. Histopathology of specimens from 4 cases. *Journal of Bone and Joint Surgery* 1991;73B: 732-40.
3. Denissen HW, Kalk W, de Nieuport HM, Maltha JC, van den Hooff A. Mandibular bone response to plasmasprayed coatings of hydroxylapatite. *International Journal of Prosthodontics,* 1990 3: 53-8.
4. Jansen JA, van der Waerden JPCM, Wolke JGC, de Groot K. Histologic evaluation of the osseous adaption to titanium and hydroxyapatite-coated titanium implants. *Journal of Biomedical Materials Research* 1991;25: 973-89.
5. Williams DF, Black J. Definitions in biomaterials, *Consensus Conference in Chester;* 1991.
6. LeGeros RZ, Orly I, Gregoire M, Daculsi G. Substrate surface dissolution and interfacial biological mineralization. *The Bone-Biomaterial Interface,* Davies, J.E. Ed., University of Toronto Press; 1991: 76-88.
7. Jarcho M. Calcium phosphate ceramics as hard tissue prosthetics. *Clinical Orthopaedics and Related Research,* 1981; 157:259-78.

8.  van Blitterswijk CA, Grote JJ, Kuijpers W, Blok-van Hoek,CJG Daems WTh. Bioreactions at the tissue/hydroxyapatite interface. *Biomaterials;* 1985; 6:243-51.
9.  Ganeles J, Listgarten MA, Evian CA. Ultrastructure of durapatite-periodontal tissue interface in human intrabony defects. *Journal of Periodontology,* 1986, 57(3):133.
10. van Blitterswijk CA, Hesseling SC, Grote JJ, Koerten HK, de Groot K. The biocompatibility of hydroxyapatite ceramic: A study of retrieved human middle ear implants. *Journal of Biomedical Materials Research;*1990; 24:433-53.
11. Sautier J-M, Nefussi R-R, Forrest N. Ultrastructural study of bone formation on synthetic hydroxyapatite in osteoblast cultures. *Cells and Materials,* 1991; 1(3):209-17.
12. de Bruijn JD, Klein CPAT, de Groot K, van Blitterswijk CA. The ultrastructure of the bone-hydroxyapatite interface *in vitro. Journal of Biomedical Materials Research* 1992; 26(10):1365-82.
13. Davies JE, Nagai N, Takeshita N, Smith DC. Deposition of cement-like matrix on implant materials. *The Bone-Biomaterial Interface,* Davies, J.E. Ed., University of Toronto Press; 1991: 285-94.
14. van Blitterswijk CA, Grote JJ, Kuijpers W, Daems WTh, de Groot K. Macropore tissue ingrowth: a quantitative and qualitative study on hydroxyapatite ceramic. *Biomaterials;* 1986; 7:137.
15. van Blitterswijk CA, Grote JJ. Biological performance of ceramics during inflammation and infection. *Critical Reviews in Biocompatibility;* 1989; 5(1):13-43.
16. Koerten HK, van Blitterswijk CA, Hesseling SC, de Bruijn JD, Grote JJ, Daems WTh. Formation of extracellular deposits by macrophages exposed to poorly degradable biomaterials. *Interfaces in Medicine and Mechanics II,* Williams, K.R., Toni, A., Middleton, J., Pallotti, G. Eds., Elsevier Applied Science, London; 1991: 160-68.
17. Muller-Mai CM, Voigt C, Gross UM. Incorporation and degradation of hydroxyapatite implants of different surface roughness and surface structure in bone. *Scanning Microscopy;*1990; 4(3):613-24.
18. van Blitterswijk CA, Koerten HK, Hesseling SC, Terpstra RA, de Groot K, Grote JJ. Calcium phosphates during inflammation. *Bioceramics,* Heimke, G. Ed., German Ceramic Society, Cologne; 1990; 2: 41-8.
19. Gross UM, Muller-Mai CM, Voigt C. Comparative morphology of the bone interface with glass ceramics, hydroxyapatite, and natural coral. *The Bone-Biomaterial Interface,* Davies, J.E. Ed., University of Toronto Press; 1991: 308-20.
20. Bauer TW, Geesink RGT, Zimmerman R, McMahon JT. Hydroxyapatite coated femoral stems, Histological analysis of components retrieved at autopsy. *Journal of Bone and Joint Surgery* 1991; 73A(10):1439-52.
21. Ogura M, Sakae T, Davies JE. Resorption of calcium hydroxyapatite substrata by osteoclast-like cells in vitro. *Bioceramics 4,* Bonfield et al. Eds., Butterworth-Heinemann, London; 1991; 4:121-6.
22. Davies JE, Chernecky R, Lowenberg B, Shiga A. Deposition and resorption of calcified matrix *in vitro* by rat marrow cells, *Cells and Materials,* 1991; 1 (1):3-15
23. de Bruijn JD, Bovell YP, Davies JE, van Blitterswijk CA. Osteoclastic resorption of calcium phosphates is potentiated in post-osteogenic culture conditons. *Journal of Biomedical Materials Research* (submitted).
24. Maniatopoulos C, Sodek J, Melcher AH. Bone formation in vitro by stromal cells obtained from bone marrow of young adult rats. *Cell Tissue Research,* 1988; 254:317-30.
25. Hench LL, Splinter RJ, Allen WC, Greenlee TK. Bonding mechanisms at the interface of ceramic prosthetic materials. *Journal of Biomedical Materials Research* 1971: 117-41.
26. Davies JE, Matsuda T. Extracellular matrix production by osteoblasts on bioactive substrata in vitro. *Scanning Microscopy;* 1988; 2 (3):1445-52.
27. Søballe K, Hansen ES, Rasmussen HB, Bünger C. Hydroxyapatite coating converts fibrous anchorage to bony fixation during continuous implant loading. *38th Annual Meeting Orthopaedic Research Society,* 292, 1992.
28. Klein CPAT, Driessen AA, de Groot K. Biodegradation behavior of various calcium phosphate materials in bone tissue. *Journal of Biomedical Materials Research* , 1983; 17:769-84.
29. Jarcho M, Kay JF, Gumaer KI, Doremus RH, Drobeck HP. Tissue, cellular and subcellular events at a ceramic hydroxyapatite bone interface. *Journal of Bioengineering* 1977;1: 79.
30. Nery EB, Lynch KL, Hirthe WM, Mueller KH. Bioceramic implants in surgically produced infrabony defects. *Journal of Periodontology* 1975; 46:328-47.
31. van Blitterswijk CA, Grote JJ, Koerten HK, Kuijpers W. The biological performance of calcium phosphate ceramics in an infected implantation site: III Biological performance of ß-whitlockite in the non-infected and infected middle ear of the rat. *Journal of Biomedical Materials Research* 1986; 20:1197.

32. Dhert, WJA, Klein CPAT, Jansen JA, van der Velde EA, Vriesde RC, Rozing PM, de Groot K. A histological and histomorphometrical investigation of fluoroapatite, magnesium whitlockite and hydroxylapatite plasma-sprayed coatings in goats. *Journal of Biomedical Materials Research* 27 (1): 127-38.

33. Geesink RGT, de Groot K, Klein CPAT. Bonding of bone to apatite-coated implants. *Journal of Bone and Joint Surgery;* 1988; 70B(1):17-22.

34. de Bruijn JD, Davies E, Klein CPAT, de Groot K, van Blitterswijk CA. Biological responses to calcium phosphate ceramics. *Bone-bonding,* Ducheyne, P, Kokubo, T, van Blitterswijk, CA Eds., Reed Healthcare Publishers, Leiderdorp;1992:57-72.

35. Andersson OH, Karlsson KH. Silica gel thickness and calcium phosphate formation at the surface of bioactive glass. *Bone-Bonding Biomaterials,* Ducheyne P, Kokubo T, van Blitterswijk CA. Eds., Reed Healthcare Communications, Leiderdorp; 1992: 79-84.

36. Kokubo T, Ito S , Huang ZT, Hayashi T, Sakka S, Kitsugi T, Yamamuro T. Ca,P rich layer formed on high strength bioactive glass ceramics A.W. *Journal of Biomedical Materials Research* 1990; 24:331-43.

37. Neo M, Kotani S, Fujita Y, Nakamura T, Yamamuro T, Bando Y, Yokoyama M, Ohtsuki C, Kokubo T. Differences in bone-bonding mechanisms between surface active ceramics & resorbable ceramics: Scanning and transmission electron microscopic study. *Bioceramics 4,* Bonfield et al. Eds., Butterworth-Heinemann, London; 1991; 4:165-70.

38. van Blitterswijk CA, Bakker D, Hesseling SC, Koerten HK. Reactions of cells at implant surfaces. *Biomaterials;* 1991; 12:187-93.

39. van Blitterswijk CA, Hesseling SC, van den Brink J, Leenders H, Bakker D. Polymer reactions resulting in bone-bonding: A review of the biocompatibility of Polyactive. *The Bone-Biomaterial Interface,* Davies, JE, Ed., University of Toronto Press; 1991: 295-307.

40. Okumura M, van Blitterswijk CA, Koerten HK, Bakker D. Bonding osteogenesis in porous polymers (Polyactive) and hydroxyapatite. *Transactions 4th World Conference on Biomaterials;* 1992: 52.

41. Osborn JF, Newesely H. Dynamic Aspects of the implant-bone-interface. *Dental Implants,* Springer verlag, Heimke, G. Ed.; 1980: 111-23.

42. Okumura M. Personal communication; 1992.

43. Hanawa T. Titanium and its oxide film: A substrate for formation of apatite. *The Bone-Biomaterial Interface*; 1991: 49-61.

44. Ducheyne P, Healy K. Titanium immersion induced surface chemistry changes and the relationship to passive dissolution and bioactivity. *The Bone-Biomaterial Interface,* Davies, JE Ed., University of Toronto Press; 1991: 62-7.

45. Li P, Ohtsuki C, Kokubo T, Nakanishi K, Soga N, Nakamura T, Yamamuro T. A role o f hydrated silica, titania and alumina in forming biologically active apatite on implant. *Transactions 4th World Conference on Biomaterials,* 1992: 4.

46. Hench LL. Surface reaction kinetics and adsorption of biological moieties: A mechanistic approach to tissue attachment. *The Bone-Biomaterial Interface*; 1991: 33-48.

47. Caplan AI. Cell mediated bone regeneration. *The Bone-Biomaterial Interface,* Davies, Ed., University of Toronto Press; 1991: 199-204.

48. de Bruijn JD, van Sliedregt A, Duivenvoorden AM, van Blitterswijk CA. *In vitro* bone formation associated with apatite coated polyactide. *Cells and Materials,* 1992: 2 (4): 329-37.

49. Verheyen CCPM, de Wijn JR, van Blitterswijk CA, Rozing PM, de Groot K. Hydroxylapatite/poly(L-lactide) composites. An animal study on push out strengths and interface histology. *Journal of Biomedical Materials Research* in press.

50. de Bruijn JD, Davies JE, Flach JS, de Groot K, van Blitterswijk CA. Ultrastructure of the mineralized tissue/calcium phosphate interface *in vitro*. In: *Tissue-inducing biomaterials.* Cima L and Ron E. Eds. Materials Research Society Symposium Proceedings, 1992; 252:63-70.

*Hydroxylapatite Coatings in Orthopaedic Surgery,*
edited by R. G. T. Geesink and M. T. Manley.
Raven Press, Ltd., New York, © 1993.

# Developments in Bioactive Coatings

Klaas de Groot, Ph. D., John A. Jansen, D.D.S., Ph.D.,
Joop G.C. Wolke, B.E.,
Christel P.A.T. Klein, Ph.D., D.V.S. and
Clemens A. van Blitterswijk, Ph.D.

Many materials have been used for the construction of medical and dental implants. Of these materials, the metal titanium, either commercially pure or alloyed with other metals (Al, V), and the ceramic hydroxylapatite (HA) have been proven to be the most suitable. Especially in combination, coatings of HA on titanium implants have been very successful. This is due to the biocompatibility of HA coatings, which allow a fast direct bond with living bone, combined with the mechanical strength of titanium or its alloys (1).

In several studies, HA coatings were shown to hasten the initial biological response to the implanted devices and form a good biological base for bone ongrowth. HA coatings will resorb over time, but after periods of one year, titanium itself is able to form a bond with bone almost like apatite itself (2). Hence, it is currently assumed that HA coatings (a) have the principal function to reduce the time needed for bone bonding from (at least) one year for titanium to a few weeks and (b) allow bone bonding to take place with less precise surgical techniques than required for noncoated implants.

The question arises whether bioactive coatings, like those obtained by plasma spraying HA on titanium substrates, can be improved further. In this chapter we will try to take a look at possible future developments. We will do so by identifying and answering the following questions:

- Which other bioactive materials could be used as a coating?
- Which other techniques, besides plasma spraying, can be used to apply a coating?
- Which surface treatments, other than just depositing a thin layer of some bioactive material onto a substrate, can be used?

## BIOACTIVE COATINGS OTHER THAN HYDROXYLAPATITE

### Calcium Phosphate Coatings Other Than Hydroxylapatite

One of the goals of the research on bioactive coatings is to further improve their characteristics. Factors of coating stability, biodegradation, coating/tissue interface and coating/implant interface are points of interest; furthermore, the plasma-spray features of the material are important with respect to a large-scale, standardized applicability.

Davis (3) stated in a study in rats that dense fluorapatite (FA) is biocompatible and not visibly degradable when implanted in soft tissue. With respect to bone-bonding capacities, Heling (4) implanted sintered plugs of fluorapatite in tibiae of guinea pigs and found bonding of the bone with the implants without signs of inflammation. Lugscheider (5) compared the plasma-spray characteristics of HA with FA and found that HA is not stable at the high plasma temperatures and that dissociation can be seen in the X-ray diffraction pattern. FA however, was thermo-stable and did not show dissociation, and thus with respect to plasma-spray characteristic was superior to HA. Furthermore, the effects of adding magnesium to beta-whitlockite (MW) was investigated by Klein (6), and rebound biodegradation was reduced.

Based upon the above-mentioned phenomena, our group studied *in vivo* the applicability of FA and magnesium whitlockite coatings and compared them with HA coatings and blasted uncoated titanium implants (BL) (7).

Using a stereo microscope with a magnification of 2 x, the part of each implant that was visible in the medullary channel was judged. The following system, assigning numbers, was used for scoring the amount of coating visible:

0 =     No coating visible
1 =     Less than 10% coating visible
2 =     Between 10% and 90% coating visible
3 =     Over 90% coating visible

This scoring system gives only a gross idea of the degradation of coating at the medullar part of the implants, but large differences in degradation behavior can be assessed. From this analysis, FA does not visibly disappear after 12 weeks, while both HA and MW have disappeared partially (Figure 1).

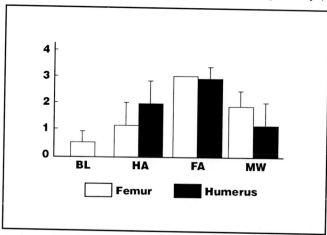

**FIG. 1.**   Mean scores of coating appearance ± standard deviation at medullar site for femora and humeri separately. Numbers corresponded with coating visibility (0=no coating; 1=< 10%; 2=between 10% and 90% coating visible).

Nevertheless, for both femur and humerus, HA and FA have the same push-out strength, both higher than BL and NW (Fig. 2).

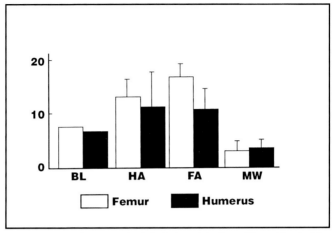

**FIG. 2.** Mean push-out strengths ± standard deviation of the four different implant types at 12 weeks. Data for femur and humerus are separated; b=8.

The position of an implant in either femur or humerus does not affect the push-out strength. Another conclusion is that, with respect to the FA implants, there is a difference in mean push-out strength between femur and humerus. Therefore, we had to compute further effects for femur and humerus separately. These findings have important relevancies for ceramic implant research, because several investigators implanted materials at different positions and in different bones. Although the position of an implant in a bone does not affect push-out strength, the bone type in which an implant is placed is of importance. First, this makes comparisons of push-out data between various investigators difficult, and second, the choice of which bone to implant a new material in can influence the data. Because of this, we would especially emphasize the care that has to be taken when extrapolating results to human applications.

Comparing the four different implant types with each other, we found that the FA- and HA-coated implants give higher strength values than the MW-coated and blanc implants (BL). Combining these findings with the coating appearance at the medullar site of the implants, FA coating gives the highest push-out strengths and lowest degradation.

### Bioactive Glasses as a Coating

Bioglass has been shown to bond to living bone because of its controlled surface reactions, leading to a calcium phosphate layer on its surface in an aqueous environment. This layer has been shown to have an HA structure (8).

Early experiments (9) to apply bioglass coatings have failed due to catastrophic failure of the coating (in *in vivo* animal experiments). Since then, no successful animal tests have been reported with bioglass coatings.

Although the similarity between the surface of a bioglass (after the controlled surface reactions have taken place) and the surface of bulk apatite would suggest the same bioactivity, *in vitro* cell cultures have shown that there exists a difference with respect to individual osteoblast morphology and osteoblast expression: osteoblasts cultured upon bioglass showed a better osteoblast-like morphology and a generally better expression of osteoblast phenotype in comparison with bulk HA (10).

Obviously, the difference between the two types of HA-i.e., produced by controlled bioglass surface reactions and by sintering starting powders, respectively-plays an important role. On the other hand, it has been recently suggested (11) that silica-containing calcium phosphate glasses may be toxic when implanted as dust particles (5-10 μm) in mice, probably due to the highly toxic effect of dissolved silicium ions, $Si^{4+}$. The conclusion has to be made that bioglasses are still promising as coating material because of their superior *in vitro* cell culture behavior, but that the possibility of toxicity of silica components needs much more investigation.

## Bioactive Polymer Coatings

Recently, it has been shown that a certain class of polymers, chemically known as poly (ethylene oxide)/poly (tetramethylene terephtalate) segmented copolymer, further referred to as "Polyactive" (the trade name), has bonebonding properties. To evaluate this further, Okumura et al., evaluated thin films of 0, 3 x 5 x 15 mm³, of two types of Polyactive: the ratio of ethylene oxide and tetramethylene terephthalate being 70/30 and 55/45, respectively.

Implants were soaked in marrow cell suspensions. Implants alone (control) and combined with bone marrow cells were implanted subcutaneously in the back of syngeneic Fischer rats. The implants were harvested 1, 2, 3, 4, 6, and 8 weeks after the surgery. Undecalcified sections of the implants were studied by fluorochrome labeling. The histological sections were observed under light microscopy or fluoromicroscopy and stained with either Villanueva bone stain, sudan black, alizarin red, or toluidine blue. The bone/biomaterial interface was examined by SEM-EDMA and TEM. Polyactive itself showed extensive areas of calcification stained with alizarin red even one week after implantation. The calcification area was larger in 70/30 Polyactive at the first period (Fig. 3).

All Polyactive materials showed calcification however, only marrow cell–loaded Polyactive revealed new bone formation beginning at three weeks postimplantation. Although the early bone formation usually started away from the polymer surface, osteoblasts were deposited on the surface of calcified Polyactive later and subsequently the bone formation proceeded to the centripetal direction toward the center of pores (bonding osteogenesis).

Compared with 55/45 Polyactive, 70/30 Polyactive showed the earliest appearance of calcification and bonding osteogenesis (Figs. 3, 4). SEM-EDMA analysis of the bone/Polyactive interface showed high levels of calcium and phosphorus both in the calcified polymer and bone at the interface, suggesting

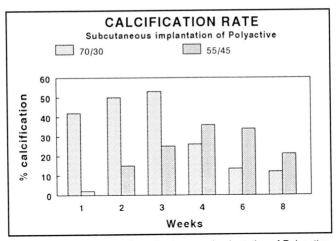

**FIG. 3.** Calcification rate of a subcutaneous implantation of Polyactive.

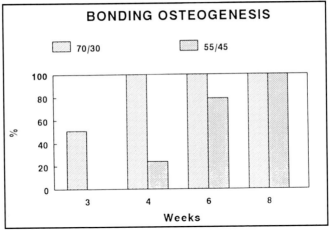

**FIG. 4.** Bonding osteogenesis of an implantation of Polyactive as it appeared in histological sections.

a chemical bonding. Undecalcified sections for TEM showed direct bone bonding to the calcified Polyactive. In addition, an electron-dense structure observed at the HA/bone interface was detected at the bone/polymer interface.

Control HA without marrow did not show any bone formation. SEM study of the HA surface showed newly formed calcium phosphate precipitation on the material surface two weeks after implantation. Composite grafts of HA and marrow revealed primary bone formation on this newly formed Ca–P layer. Active osteoblasts faced to the ceramic surface then produced osteoid, which became mineralized bone. A fluorochrome labeling study showed the consistent centripetal bone growth in all HA–marrow composites.

It is thus clear that the cell-mediated heterotopic osteogenesis following the bonding osteogenesis theory is found not only in porous HA and tricalcium phosphate ceramics, but also in Polyactive. This polymer, combined with marrow cells, showed osteoblasts deposition on the calcified polyactive and subsequent centripetal bone growth in a way similar to bioactive hydroxl-apatite ceramics. In addition, 70/30 Polyactive, which calcified first, showed earlier consistent bonding osteogenesis. These results suggest the bioactive property of Polyactive. (That is, Polyactive can sustain the bone marrow cells differentiation into osteogenic cells on its calcified surface and the differenti-ated cells (osteoblasts) causes bonding osteogenesis, apparently related to the calcification of Polyactive itself.)

Because of the unique bone-bonding properties of this polymer, an experi-ment was performed to coat dental implants with it. A stress analysis showed that flexible polymer coatings may have an advantage as compared with HA: the use of such coatings may lower more than four times the normal compres-sive stress on the cortical bone around the neck of the dental implant.

In conclusion, coatings of bioactive bone-bonding polymers are very likely to receive increased attention in the future.

## COATING TECHNIQUES OTHER THAN
## AIR PLASMA SPRAYING

### Flame SprayTechniques Other Than Air Plasma Spraying

Besides air plasma spraying (APS), two other spray technologies have been evaluated in our research group: vacuum plasma spraying (VPS) and high-velocity oxygen fuel (HVOF) (13).

In the present study, we will discuss the mechanical and physical aspects using the three different systems. The HA coatings were examined by X-ray diffraction, infrared spectroscopy, surface morphology, and solubility in differ-ent buffers.

HA powder was obtained from Merck. The powder was granulated (1–2 mm) and sintered under inert atmosphere. Thereafter the granules were crushed, milled, and sieved. For plasma-spraying a particle size distribution of 1–125 μm was used.

Plasma-spraying conditions were as follows:

For plasma spraying, Metco-MN, Metco-VPS, and Metco-DJ systems were used. The spray conditions were:

|  | APS | VPS | HVOF |
|---|---|---|---|
| Arc current (AmP) | 400 | 500 | - |
| Arc voltage (V) | 60 | 50 | - |
| Arc gas | nitrogen | | |
| Gasses HVOF | oxygen/propylene/air | | |
| Spray rate (gr/min) | 12-16  14-20 | 14-20 | |
| Spray distance (cm) | 8 | 24 | 15 |
| Ambient pressure (mbar) | 1000 | 100 | 1000 |
| Coating thickness (μm) | 2 | 8 | 5 |

Prior to the plasma spraying, all samples were sandblasted, followed by ultrasonic cleaning and drying at 100°C.

Surface roughness measurements showed that surface roughness did depend on the equipment for spraying the coatings. The HA–APS coating had the roughest surface. Furthermore, tensile strength measurements showed a somewhat higher tensile strength for the HA–VPS coating and failure modes in the interface glue/coating. Hence, we believe that adhesion is mostly governed by the physical and thermal state of the (partially) molten particles when they reach the metallic substrate, during the spraying process.

X-ray diffraction shows that the most crystalline structure is obtained from a HVOF system (Figs. 5–8). We believe this to be due to the higher particle velocities and low energy of the flame: this gives less decomposition of the HA powder and, as a result, a more crystalline structure. The SEM photographs show that the HA–HVOF has the highest porosity. This is in agreement with the results of the X-ray diffractions. When the particles retain too short in the flame, they do not melt enough to obtain a dense coating. Evaluation of cross sections of the different coatings showed that the density decreased in the sequence HA–APS > HA–VPS > HA–HVOF.

IR scans show again that the particles in the HVOF flame hardly melt, indicated by presence of the OH band at 640 cm$^{-1}$. To obtain a dense coating it is necessary that the particles melt at least partially.

Finally, the *in vitro* solubility tests in Gomori's buffer show clearly that *in vitro* HA-HVOF is less soluble than HA-APS and HA-VPS, but in citrate there is no difference between HA–VPS and HA–HVOF (Fig. 9). It must be emphasized that *in vitro* solubilities are not predictive for behavior *in vivo*, as shown by Klein's animal studies (14) on HA.

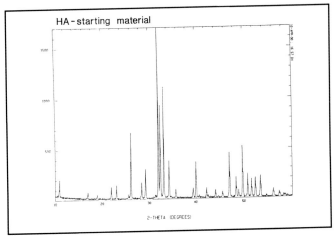

**FIG. 5.** XRD pattern of sintered HA starting powder.

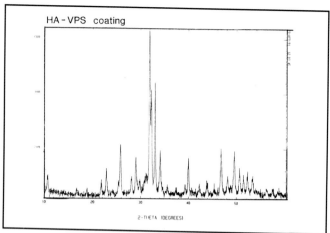

**FIG. 6.** XRD pattern of HA–APS coating.

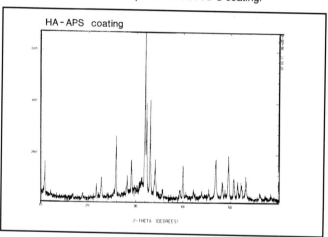

**FIG. 7.** XRD pattern of HA–VPS coating.

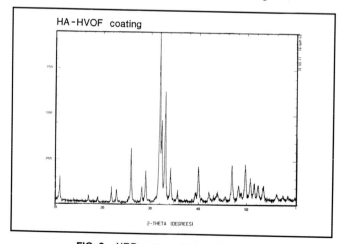

**FIG. 8.** XRD pattern of HA–HVOF coating.

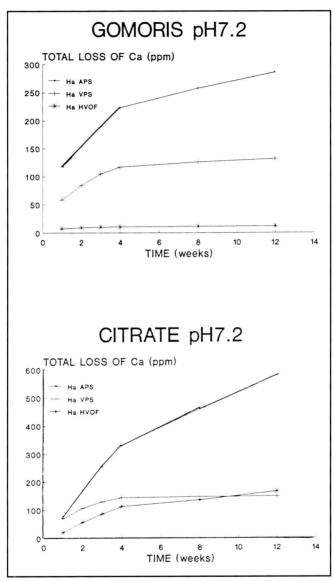

**FIG. 9.** Results of solubility tests in different buffers.

## Coating Techniques Other Than by Means of Flame Spraying

Besides flame spraying to apply coatings, various other techniques are used such as dip coating followed by sintering, electrophoretic deposition, immersion coating and hot isostatic pressing, but in our opinion the only one that has a very promising future is sputter coating.

Sputtering is the process whereby, in a vacuum chamber, atoms or molecules of a material are ejected from a target by the bombardment of high-energy ions. The dislodged particles deposit on a substrate, also placed into the vacuum chamber. There are several sputter techniques, e.g., diode sputtering, radiofrequent (RF) or direct current (DC) sputtering, ion-beam sputtering and reactive sputtering. All these techniques are variants of the same above-mentioned physical phenomena. However, a drawback inherent to all these techniques is that the deposition rate is very low; hence, the process itself very slow. By using a magnetically enhanced variant of RF sputtering, these problems can be solved. This method is called magnetron sputtering.

In a preliminary study, Jansen et al. (15) investigated the possible application of magnetron sputtering for the production of ceramic films on metal and plastic substrates. Radiofrequent (RF) magnetron sputter-coating was performed using a commercially available sputter unit (Edwards ESM 100). Copper discs, plasma-spray-coated with HA, were used as target material. The apatite powder (Ca/P ratio 1.67) used for the coating of the targets was obtained commercially from Merck and had a particle size between 1 and 125 μm. The chemical composition and purity of the target-coating was confirmed by X-ray crystal diffraction (XRD).

Only minimal line broadening can be seen, which indicates a well-crystallized material. Plasma spraying does not alter the crystallographic structure, only a little line-broadening is visible.

Before sputtering the substrates were cleared by etching with argon ions. The sputtering process was performed using standard conditions. The deposition rate of ceramic on the substrates was 90 mm during 10 minutes of sputtering. Coating thicknesses of 0.02 – 6.5 μm were produced.

The deposited films were characterized as follows: (a) the appearance and the integrity of the coating was examined with a scanning electron microscope, (b) a scanning electron microscope equipped with an energy-dispersive X-ray detector was used to obtain information about the elemental composition of the surface of the coated specimens, (c) X-ray diffraction (XRD) was used to evaluate the crystallographic structure, (d) Ca and P concentrations were determined by atomic adsorption spectrometry, and (e) bonding to substrate of the coating was tested by tensile bond tests.

SEM examination of the sputtered coating on the various materials showed an excellent coverage of the substrate surfaces. Coatings had a uniform thickness and a columnar structure without any porosity in the interface.

Energy-dispersive X-ray analysis demonstrated that the sputtered coatings contained mainly calcium (Ca) and phosphorus (P). Further, titanium (Ti) and aluminium (Al) were detected. The detected titanium and aluminium originate from the titanium/alloy substrate surface. Semiquantitative analysis of the X-ray pattern for the relative amount of calcium and phosphorus revealed that the Ca/P ratio of the sputtered coating was 1.93. X-ray patterns indicated that the sputtered coating was a well crystallized calcium phosphate ceramic. Although it was not possible to match the Ca/P structure with one of the diffraction data of the Joint Committee on powder Diffraction Standards (Joint Committee), further investigations revealed that the X-ray diffractogram was very similar to the X-ray diffractogram of intact tooth enamel.

The tensile strength measurements demonstrated that it was impossible to measure the real bond strength of the sputtered coating to the underlying substrates. The bond failure occurred in all investigated specimens at > 53 MPa in the glued interface. The measurements of the amount of calcium and phosphorus by atomic adsorption and colorimetry demonstrated that the Ca/P ratio was 2.5.

SEM examination of rat palatal epithelial (RPE) cell cultures demonstrated that there were no differences in cellular behavior between untreated and sputter-coated substrates. For all incubation periods, the cells spread and grew equally well on all the test surfaces.

SEM study of animal implants showed, at the cortical level, a close adaptation of bone to the implant surface. These results demonstrated that it is possible to form a dense, adherent ceramic coating onto metal and plastic substrates. The X-ray diffraction pattern for the obtained coating appeared to be similar to the X-ray diffraction pattern of the apatite crystals in intact tooth enamel.

The biocompatibility experiments demonstrated again the well-known fact that calcium phosphates with other Ca/P ratios of between 1.50 and 1.67 (HA) can also be biocompatible.

The *in vivo* experiments, in which the sputter-coated implants were investigated by EDMA after insertion into rabbit tibia, showed that the Ca/P ratio of the coating decreases after three months of implantation. This phenomenon can be caused by a gradual change in composition of the surface of the sputtered film (e.g., by dissolution, precipitation, or ion exchange reactions as discussed elsewhere in this chapter for bioactive surfaces (19)).

In summary, based on the results of this preliminary study, it can be concluded that magnetron sputtering is a promising method for forming a biocompatible ceramic coating onto a metal or plastic substrate. The advantages of magnetron sputter-coating above other sputtering processes include the high deposition rate, the excellent adhesiveness and the ability to coat implants with difficult surface geometries. Still, several questions have to be resolved before magnetron sputtering can be applied to routinely produce crystalline pure Ca/P ceramic coatings on implant surfaces. These questions (e.g., the endurance and the Ca/P ratio of the coating) require further *in vitro* and *in vivo* studies.

## THE FUTURE

In the preceding paragraphs, we have discussed various coatings and coating techniques. We have reached the conclusion that HA plasma-sprayed coatings are certainly not the end: FA and bioactive polymers have been identified as new biomaterials for the near future. Furthermore, high-velocity oxygen fuel spraying, but not vacuum plasma spraying, is basically superior to air plasma spraying in terms of price, coating density, and degree of crystallinity. Another promising technique for obtaining ceramic coatings is magnetron sputtering.

However, all of these developments, which are likely to appear on a routine basis in the near future (between now and, say, five years), are still based on the principle that some bioactive layer must be deposited onto an implant by means of some external technology.

Several developments, however, may point to a quite different direction:

- Bioglass is historically the first example of a biomaterial that, only after immersion in body (or other aqueous) fluids, obtains an HA layer, due to diffusion of calcium (and possibly phosphate ions) out of the bulk onto the surface of the glass;

- The polymer "Polyactive" follows another path: calcium and phosphate ions diffuse from the outside body fluid into the polymer gel and start precipitating directly at and below its surface;

- A similar calcification process has been found with other polymer gels: Klein et al. (16) described that Ca alginate gels after implantation show a thin subsurface mineralized layer, and Swart et al . (17) found that poly-hydroxyethyl methacrylate phosphate gels (a polymer gel with negatively charged phosphate groups) show similar behavior;

- Recently, Li et al. (18) (from Kokubo's research group at Kyoto University) found that silicium hydroxide gels (and possibly other metal hydroxide gels), after immersion in simulated body fluids (SBF), obtain under "certain conditions" a calcium phosphate surface layer due to precipitation of calcium and phosphate ions in SBF. These "certain conditions" are thought to be (a) presence of negative charges, (b) availability of a "suitable" pore structure.

- Any calcium phosphate surface not formed in the body itself will change its composition after implantation due to its intrinsic thermodynamic instability; it has been shown (19) that completion of such a subtle change of man-made calcium phosphate surfaces into physiologically stable HA is necessary for the bone-bonding process to start; this may be the reason that the time for bone-bonding to occur may differ from one bioactive surface to the other (for example, it has been suggested that some bioglasses require less time than some apatites to allow bone-bonding).

- Titanium itself has been shown to have bone-bonding capacities after extended implant times: Klein et al. (2) found that after one year of implantation, titanium plugs had push-out strength values similar to those of HA-coated plugs after several weeks. This phenomenon suggests a gradual change of the Ti surface after implantation, similar to the *in vitro* produced silicium gels by Li et al. (18).

Considering these arguments, it seems possible to suggest the following method for obtaining bone-bonding surfaces: create a surface with the required negative density and pore structure such that either after immersing in SBF or after a short implantation period (= immersing in real body fluid), a physiologically stable HA layer is formed at and within this surface. This apatite surface should be produced on metals, polymers, and ceramics, examples being titanium with a titanium hydroxide-structured porous surface, "Polyactive" and bioglass or man-made apatite, respectively, and thus allow bone bonding.

In summary: for the future we foresee two lines of research:

- Short term (0-5 yr):    further improving, in terms of fast bony
                          ingrowth, the selection of bioactive
                          materials and coating technologies;

- Long term (0-10 yr):    studies of optimal electrical charge
                          distributions and porosities for surfaces,
                          such that they turn into physiological
                          HA surfaces after immersion in
                          simulated body fluid (or after implantation).

## REFERENCES

1.  De Groot K., Medical applications of calcium phosphate bioceramics (Review article), *Journal of the Ceramics. Society of Japan*, 1991, 99: 943-53.
2.  Wolke JGC, Klein CPAT, de Groot K., Bioceramics for maxillo facial applications, In: *Bioceramics for the human body*, A Ravaglioli and A Krajewski (Ed.), Elsevier Science Publishers, 1991, 166-80.
3.  Davis SD, Gibbons DF, Martin RL, Levitt SR, et al. Biocompatibility of ceramic implants in soft tissue, *Journal of Biomedical Materials Research*, 1972, 6:425-33.
4.  Heling L, Heindel R, Merin B., Calciumfluorapatite: A new material for bone implants. *Journal of Oral Implants*, 1981, 9: 548-52.
5.  Lugschneider E, Weber TH, Knepper M., *Production of biocompatible coatings of hydroxyapatite and fluorapatite*, Presented at National Thermal Spray Conference, Cincinnati, 1988.
6.  Klein CPAT, de Groot K, Driessen AA, van der Lubbe HBM., A comparative study of different beta-whitlockite ceramics in rabbit cortical bone with regard to their biodegradation behavior, *Biomaterials*, 1986, 7: 144-6.
7.  Dhert WJA, Klein CPAT, Wolke JGC, et al. Fluorapatite, magnesiumwhitlockite and hydroxylapatite coated titanium plugs: mechanical bonding and the effect of different implantation sites, In: *Ceramics in Substitutive and Reconstructive Surgery*, P Vincenzini (Ed.), Elsevier Science Publishers, 1991, 385-94 .
8.  Ogino M, Chuchi F, Hench LL. Compositional dependence of the formation of calcium phosphate films on bioglass, *Journal of Biomedical Materials Research*, 1980, 14: 55-64 .
9.  Griss P, Werner E, Heimke G, Raute-Kreinsen U. Vergleic hende experimentelle Untersuchungen an $AL_2O_3$- Keramik und mit mod. Bioglas (LL Hench) beschichteter $AL_2O_3$-Keramik, *Archives of Orthopaedic and Traumatic Surgery.*, 1978, 92: 199-208.
10. Vrouwenvelder WCA, Groot CG, de Groot K. Behaviour of fetal rat osteoblasts cultured *in vitro* on bioactive glass and non reactive glasses, *Biomaterials*, 1992, 13: 381-92.
11. Nagase M, Abe Y, Chigira M, Udagawa E. Toxicity of silica-containing calcium phosphatase glasses, demonstrated in mice, *Biomaterials*, 1992, 13: 172-5.
12. Van Blitterswijk CA, et al. Interfacial reactions leading to bone bonding with PEO/PBT copolymers (Polyactive), In: *Bone-Bonding Biomaterials,* Ducheyne, Kokubo, van Blitterswijk, Eds., Reed Healthcare, Leiderdorp, The Netherlands, 13-30 (1992).

13. Wolke JGC, de Groot K, Kraak TG, et al. The characterization of HA coatings sprayed with VPS, APS and DJ Systems, In: *Thermal Spray Coatings: Properties, Processes and Applica tions,* ASM International, 1991, 481-90.
14. Klein CPAT, de Blieck-Hogervorst JMA, Wolke JGC, de Groot K. Studies of the solubility of different calciumphosphate ceramic particles in vitro, *Biomaterials*, 1990, 11: 509-12.
15. Jansen JA, unpublished results, manuscript in preparation.
16. Klein CPAT, van der Lubbe HBM, de Groot K. A plastic composite of alginate with calcium phosphate granulate as implant material: an in vivo study, *Biomaterials,* 1987, 8: 308-10.
17. Swart JGN, Driessen AA, de Visser AC. Calcification and bone induction studies in heterogenous phosphorylated hydrogels, In: JD Andrade, *Hydrogels for medical and related applications*, American Chemical Society (Publishers),1976, 151-7.
18. Li P, Ohtsuki C, Kokubo T, et al. Apatite formation induced by silica gel in a simulated body fluid, Submitted, *Journal of the American Ceramics Society,* 1992.
19. Hyakuna K, Yamauro T, Kotoura Y, et al. Surface reactions of calcium phosphate ceramics to various solutions, *Journal of Biomedical Materials Research*, 1990, 24: 471-88.

*Hydroxylapatite Coatings in Orthopaedic Surgery*,
edited by R. G. T. Geesink and M. T. Manley.
Raven Press, Ltd., New York, © 1993.

# Biomechanical Aspects of Hydroxylapatite Coatings on Femoral Hip Prostheses

## Rik Huiskes, Ph.D. and Harrie Weinans, Ph.D.

The presumed advantage of a hydroxylapatite (HA) coating on noncemented prostheses is its fast postoperative osseous integration. This produces strong and lasting bonds between implants and bone, suitable for transferring hip joint loads to the bone without interface failure or relative motions. The biomechanical questions related to this behavior, and its presumed advantages, are whether the early integration process is reproducible, whether relative interface motions due to early prosthetic loading may prevent it, and whether the eventual bonds are indeed strong enough to prevent long-term interface failure. Although the osseo-inductive capacities of HA coatings have been documented in animal experimental and human retrieval studies (1,2), it has also been shown convincingly that integration will not occur when relative motions are beyond certain threshold levels (3). The extent of these early motions depends on surgical, patient and prosthetic parameters, such as implant fit, hip joint loads, and mechanical implant characteristics, i.e., stiffness and interface friction properties. It is important to quantify the mechanical interrelationships and effects of these parameters on the osseous integration.

The same can be said about the probability of late mechanical interface loosening. The likelihood of interface failures depends on the balance between interface stress and interface strength. Whereas interface strength is a function of the biologic bonding characteristics, the HA resorption characteristics and the bonding strength between coating and implant, interface stress depends on surgical, patient, and prosthetic parameters, similar to those that determine the early relative interface motions mentioned above. These effects, too, require quantification. Although it is now often suggested that HA coatings resorb over time, whether this will cause late loosening depends equally on surgical and design factors, because it is not only the interface strength but also the stress that matters.

In addition to interface biomechanics, the long-term behavior of the reconstruction is governed by adaptive bone remodeling. The stresses and strains that occur within a bone depend on its external loads, its shape, and its internal structural organization. This implies that when a part of the bone is replaced by an implant of different mechanical properties, the stresses and strains within the remaining bone change, even if the external loads remain the same. In accordance with Wolff's law, a process of strain-adaptive bone remodeling then takes place, changing the shape and internal structural organization of the bone to adapt to the new mechanical requirements. Although this adaptive remodeling is obviously an important biologic asset, it does not necessarily have positive effects when implants are involved. The reason for this apparent contradiction is simply that the implant does not adapt with its host bone.

A notorious adverse effect of adaptive bone remodeling is resorption around femoral hip stems. After a stem is placed in the intramedullary canal of a femur, two important changes occur in the load-transfer mechanism (4). First of all the hip joint load is no longer transferred downwards through the metaphyseal trabecular structures and the cortex but now involves the implant–bone interface. Second, the load that was earlier carried by the bone alone is now shared with the stem. This phenomenon, called "load sharing," causes "stress shielding"of the bone; i.e., the bone is shielded by the stem from the stress to which it is normally subjected. As a result, the bone stresses become subnormal and the bone resorbs to adapt to this new situation. Hence, contrary to common usage, "stress shielding" is not synonymous with bone resorption but rather is its cause.

An example of the stress-shielding mechanism, as it can be determined in finite-element models, is shown in Fig. 1. The bone stresses are shown here as they occur in reconstructions with a noncemented femoral stem, relative to what they would have been  preoperatively case for the same external loads. The stress shielding is evident and clearly reduces from proximal to distal. Below the tip of the stem the stresses are again normal. Stress shielding is more severe for noncemented stems than compared for cemented ones (5). This is mainly due to the difference in flexibility of the two reconstructions. Because noncemented stems are bulkier, and therefore stiffer than cemented ones, they remove a larger share of load from the bone and thus create more stress shielding. It is to be expected that, as a consequence,  more adaptive bone resorption will also be seen around noncemented stems, and this is indeed

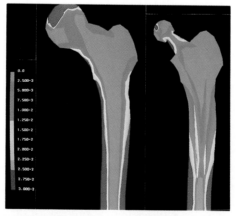

**FIG. 1.**     Stress shielding around a noncemented stem; shown are strain-energy-density patterns (related to stress patterns) in the bone before and after the replacement, for the same loading case.

generally observed in the clinical setting.

Stress shielding and bone resorption around noncemented stems have worried clinicians for a long time, particularly because it is not known where and when this slow process ends. Its adverse effects may be that the prosthesis breaks out of the bone when its holding power is reduced below a certain minimum and the patient makes an unfortunate step, or that not enough bone stock is available in case a revision is needed. However, very few problems of this kind have been reported in the literature.

The degree of stress shielding depends not only on stem flexibility but also on other mechanical factors. As a result, the amount of bone resorption is also multifactorial. Table 1 gives an overview of prosthetic design, surgical and patient parameters that can potentially affect the extent of long-term bone resorption around noncemented stems. The purpose of this chapter is to investigate these relationships, using strain-adaptive bone-remodeling analysis. Because of their important implications for osseous integration and risk of interface failure, the effects of these parameters on interface mechanics are also discussed.

**TABLE 1.**  *A few selected prosthetic, surgical, and patient factors that influence adaptive bone resorption and interface mechanics around femoral stems*

| Design Factors | Surgical Factors | Patient Factors |
| --- | --- | --- |
| Stem shape | Interface fit | Bone quality |
| Stem stiffness | | Bone reactivity |
| Coating placement | | Weight |
| Features | | Activity |

## WOLFF'S LAW

The concept of strain (or stress) adaptive bone remodeling was first emphasized in the literature of the last century, a development that culminated in what we now know as "Wolff's law." Although the implications of this "law" are basic assets of orthopaedic surgery and most orthopaedic surgeons have acquired an intuitive appreciation of its significance, the law itself and its scientific background are hardly known at all.

Wolff's law (6) is not a law in the sense of a quantitative, falsifiable statement in line with the tradition of the physical sciences, but rather consists of a series of observations. The most important of these are the "trajectorial hypothesis" and the concept of adaptive remodeling (or "Transformation" in the original German). The first one was based in particular on the work of the anatomist Meyer and the engineer Culmann, who discovered a remarkable similarity between the trabecular structure of the proximal femur and the patterns of stress trajectories calculated in a mathematical model of this structure, using the new theory of graphic statics developed by Culmann. As argued by Roesler (7,8), it is evident from his text that Wolff did not really understand the mechanical implications of that similarity, and hence did not interpret it correctly. The second observation, adaptive remodeling, had been discussed extensively in the earlier writings of Roux (9). Dibbits (10) convincingly argued, based on an extensive review of the literature from those days, that Wolff had never accepted Roux's adaptive remodeling theories earlier and maintained that bone is a static entity once it is formed by interstitial growth. He refused to acknowledge or appreciate advances in histology and biology, such as indications that bone is subject to continuous resorption and formation (10). Nevertheless, he adopted Roux's ideas in his 1892 book and became known later as the conceiver of the law. This "law"–Wolff called it a mathematical law, which it definitely is not–he summarized in five parts. The first two concern the trajectorial theory (incorrectly interpreted, as Roesler wrote). The next three state roughly that the internal architecture of a bone remodels after pathological alterations of its external shape have occurred (he shows a number of examples from his surgical practice and postmortem anatomic studies in his book), that bones have "functional shapes" in both normal and pathologic conditions, and that the "remodeling force" can be used for therapeutic ends. It may have been due to the fuzziness around its emergence or the unclarity of its form that it has taken such a long time before the "law" and the challenge contained in its last statement were addressed scientifically. In 1881, Roux suggested that the adaptive remodeling process was governed by a "quantitative self-regulating mechanism"(9), nothing else, Roesler wrote, "but what nowadays would be described as a biological control process" (8). Although the existence of such a process had never been denied, the presumption of a load, stress or strain mediator for such a process was generally accepted, and the mathematical tools to analyze such a process were available, it was "...not until the late seventies of this century that Cowin and co-workers (11, 12) proposed a first quantitative form of 'Wolff's Law'..." (8). Much progress has been made since then, particularly owing to the combination of finite element analysis with mathematical remodeling rules (13-15).

## Strain-Adaptive Bone-Remodeling Analysis

Strain-adaptive bone-remodeling analysis takes Roux's concept of a quantitative self-regulating mechanism or biologic control process, as a basis, according to which bone cells locally appraise loads and mediate bone formation and resorption. A schematic representation of this model is shown in Fig. 2A. The sensor cells, we assume, are the osteocytes (16), and the actors the osteoclasts and osteoblasts, although these assumptions are not critical for the remodeling theory. The sensors measure a strain-related mechanical signal and compare that with a normal reference value. If the signal is too high, the sensor mediates the actors to form bone; when it is too low, bone is resorbed. This process continues until the mechanical signal is again normalized. The values of the signal in each location of the bone depend on the external loads and the mechanical properties of the bone, i.e., on its shape or geometry and on its internal structural organization or architecture. While the remodeling process is enacted, and shape and architecture are changing, the signal values change as well, providing the feedback control loop for the sensors which govern the process.

The computer model used to simulate this process is illustrated schematically in Fig. 2B. Stresses and strains are determined in a finite element model of the bone, representing its shape and architecture (i.e., density patterns) and simulating its external loads. The model is then used iteratively whereby, during each iteration, the mechanical signals (S) are determined from the stresses, strains, volumes, and masses in each element and compared to reference values $(S_{ref})$. Using a mathematical remodeling rule, the local amounts of bone mass per element to be formed or removed are calculated and adjusted in the finite element model by changing the element volumes or densities.

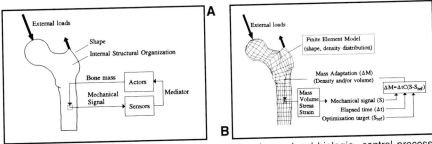

**FIG. 2.** Adaptive bone remodeling can be considered as a local biologic control process, governed by a mechanical signal, and appraised by sensors (osteocytes), that mediate actors (osteoclasts and osteoblasts) to regulate bone mass (**A**). Such a process can be described by a computer-simulation model in which a mathematical remodeling rule is coupled to a finite-element model (**B**).

Of course, the values of many of the parameters needed in such a computer-simulation model are unknown or uncertain. Of some quantities and relationships, e.g., the remodeling signal and the mathematical remodeling rule, we do not even know the character. This problem is approached in a way typical for modeling in physical sciences, by trial and error. First, sensible assumptions are made for quantities, values and relationships. These are then tried in the computer-simulation model relative to remodeling configurations of which the solution is known. The theoretical and real solutions are compared, and if they do not match the model parameters are adjusted accordingly until we are satisfied that its predictions are valid. In this way we have triggered and verified our model and its parameters relative to the density distribution of the normal femur (17,18), as illustrated in Fig. 3, and to three series of canine experiments with different types of hip prostheses (19-21), illustrated in Fig. 4. We are now confident that the model and its predictions make sense.

We use the elastic energy stored per unit of mass in the bone by the external loads as the remodeling signal, calculated as the product of the stress and strain tensors determined in the finite-element procedure, divided by the actual density. As illustrated in Fig. 3, this quantity gives an excellent representation of local bone loading, to the extent that normal bone density patterns can be predicted in bone growth and maintenance analyses (17, 18). The mathematical remodeling rule, in which the signal values are compared to their normal references, is a nonlinear one, in the sense that a threshold level, or dead zone, for bone reactions to abnormal loads is adopted (15). This implies that, locally,

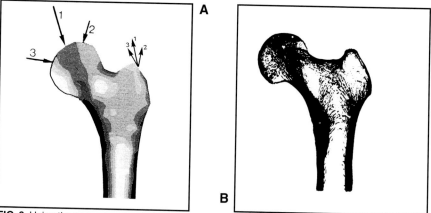

**FIG. 3.** Using the computer-simulation model illustrated in Fig. 2A, the normal density distribution of the femur, according to Wolff's law, can be predicted (18). Density distribution of a computer simulation (**A**) compared with the density distribution in a midfrontal section (**B**).

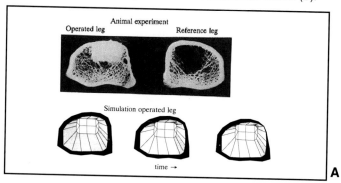

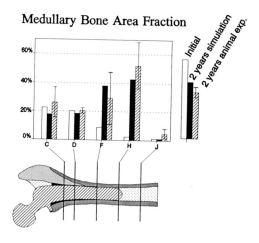

**FIG. 4.** By simulating animal experiments with canine hip replacement, the postoperative morphologic changes in cortical area and intramedullary density due to adaptive remodeling could be predicted, both in qualitative detail (**A**), and as quantitatively relative to averages and variations in an animal series (**B**) (19,20).

bone must be under or overloaded by at least a certain percentage before it reacts. This percentage depends on bone reactivity, and was established at average values of 35 for the dogs (19) and 75 for humans (22). This dead zone represents the "mean effective strain" (MES) concept of Frost (23).

For the reference signal values we use the distribution of elastic energy per unit of mass as it occurs in a normal bone subjected to typical loads. The procedure for simulating bone remodeling around hip stems is then illustrated in Fig. 5: finite-element models are made of the intact femur and the same femur with a prosthesis, which are subjected to the same external – hip and muscle – loading cycles. The model with the implant is subjected to the remodeling simulation procedure, whereby the element signal values after each time step are compared to those in the intact model, and the element-density values are adjusted accordingly for the next time step. This process continues until the signal values in the replacement model are again equal to those in the intact one, minus the threshold level. Some elements will not reach that stage because they have either resorbed completely in the process or reached the maximal density value of cortical bone. An example of such an end-stage density configuration is shown in Fig. 6 (24). The resorption patterns, particularly at the proximal side around this fully bonded titanium prosthesis, are evident, and are very similar to what can be seen on long-term postoperative radiographs.

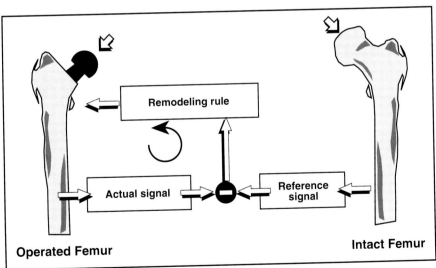

**FIG. 5.** In the analyses presented here, two finite-element models are applied. One, of the intact femur, provides for the reference values of the mechanical signal. In the other, with the prosthesis, bone density is gradually adapted to equalize the actual signal values to the reference ones. When this is accomplished, a new equilibrium has been established.

## The Effects of Prosthetic, Surgical, and Patient Factors

The bone-remodeling computer-simulation model is a versatile tool, particularly to investigate how remodeling and resorption patterns relate to all kinds of parameters, such as those listed in Table 1. The model is then used in a relative fashion, comparing one parameter value to another while other parameters remain unchanged. In this way the pure effects of a single factor can be evaluated, and the imprecisions inherent to models become of lesser importance. Some examples are shown in the remainder of this chapter, whereby effects of parameters on bone resorption and on interface mechanics are discussed. Bone resorption patterns are presented in the Gruen zones 1 through 7 (25), illustrated in Fig 7.

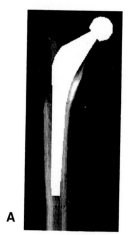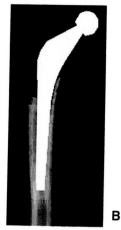

**A**                                                                **B**

FIG. 6. Result of a remodeling analysis as in Fig 5. Both pictures show density distributions in a three-dimensional finite-element model, projected in the frontal plane, simulating a radiograph; *(A* )the situation before remodeling has started (immediately postoperative), (**B**) after a new equilibrium has been established. Bone resorption, predominantly proximally, is evident.

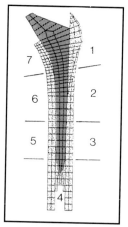

FIG 7. The Gruen zones (25) in which the bone-remodeling patterns are quantified in the parametric analysis (Tables 2-4).

## Stem Stiffness

The stiffness, or flexibility, of a stem depends on its shape and dimensions, and on the elastic modulus of its material. Bobyn and co-workers (26) performed experiments with dogs, implanting two kinds of hip stems with different stiffnesses, one made out of solid titanium and the other hollow. After two years the amount of bone resorption was evaluated postmortem and was shown to be much less around the flexible stem, thus confirming the assumed relationship between stiffness, stress shielding, and bone resorption.

In our computer-simulation analysis we look at the effects of material stiffness only; therefore stem shape and dimension remain constant. In each case the same external loading cycle is assumed and the stem is taken as fully bonded (osseointegrated) to the bone along its entire length. The only difference is the material, which is either a cobalt–chromium alloy (elastic modulus 210 GPa), titanium (elastic modulus 110 GPa), or a hypothetical "isoelastic" material with a similar elastic modulus as cortical bone (20 GPa). The results of the simulation analyses for these three cases are presented in Table 2 (27). Evidently, the effects are quite extensive. The drastic reduction in resorption from cobalt–chromium to titanium material (a reduction in stiffness by a factor of about two) from 76% to 54% resorption at the proximal, medial side, illustrates that titanium is a much better material for the bulky, noncemented prosthetic stems. The resorption reduces almost to nil in the case of an isoelastic material.

The results listed in Table 2 relate to analyses with two-dimensional FE models (27), but have also been confirmed in three-dimensional ones (22). In that case, for instance, it was found that the resorption reduces from about 67% to about 34% in the bone around the proximal third of the stem, when a change is made from titanium to an isoelastic material. Although 2-D and 3-D results are not well comparable in an absolute sense, relatively speaking the same trends were found.

**TABLE 2.** *Bone loss due to adaptive remodeling for three different stem materials (27)*

| Stem material (Elastic Modulus, GPa) | | Proximal | | Middle | |
|---|---|---|---|---|---|
| | | Medial | Lateral | Medial | Lateral |
| CoCrMo | (210) | -76% | -45% | -29% | -32% |
| Titanium | (110) | -54% | -38% | - 4% | -14% |
| "IsoElastic" | ( 20 ) | -7% | -1% | 0% | +2% |

Hence, it is evident that a flexible stem is advantageous for reduction of bone resorption. However, in what way does it affect interface mechanics, the process of osseous integration, and the probability for late interface failure and loosening? Because so little is known quantitatively about the integration and resorption processes of the HA coatings and their relationships with interface strength, these questions are not easily answered at present. However, it is obvious that the beneficial effects of flexible stems on proximal bone resorption are the result of higher load transfer at the proximal side. This implies higher interface stresses proximally, and more chances for initial interface motions. Figure 8 shows a relative comparison between the amounts of stress shielding and maximal proximal interface stresses for stem moduli between 20 and 110 GPa (22). When stiffness reduces, stress shielding reduces as well, but interface stresses soar. Conversely, the 110 GPa (titanium) stem produces more stress shielding but only half the interface stresses of the 20 GPa (isoelastic) stem. Although this has not been documented here, it is fairly obvious that the effects on relative interface motions are very similar, in the sense that they are higher for the flexible stems. Therefore, although flexible stems have definite advantages for bone resorption, without additional means of initial stability and enhancement of interface strength it is questionable whether they would really be clinically successful.

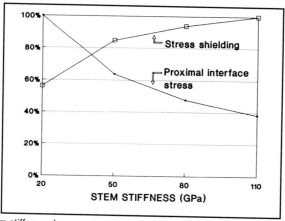

**FIG. 8.** When stem stiffness decreases, stress shielding also decreases, but proximal interface stresses increase; hence, although flexible stems produce less resorption, they increase the likelihood of interface failure and motions (22).

## Coating Placement and Integration

There are different philosophies about the placement of coatings. Coating the surface over the full length of the stem, enhancing the probability of integration, is one; limiting the coating to the proximal part only, enhancing proximal load transfer and reducing stress shielding, is another. There are two questions to be answered before a sensible choice between these alternatives can be made. The first concerns the relationship between coating location and the reproducibility of integration, of which, obviously, very little is known as yet. The second question, addressed here, concerns the relationship between ingrowth location, stress-shielding and interface mechanics. Evidently, in reality, the bonding patterns over the stem surface can be quite diverse, ranging from true biochemical integration to essentially unconnected.

In the analyses we disregard the subtleties and assume either a solid bond or a contact without friction between bone and implant. The first condition occurs, in the model, at the locations where the surface is coated; and the second prevails where the surface is not coated. The configurations thus analyzed and compared are full stem-length coating, one-third proximal coating, small-band proximal coating, and uncoated (press-fitted), as illustrated in Fig. 9. Again, all other parameters remain the same, i.e., identical loading cycles and a titanium stem. The results of the simulations are shown in Table 3 (24). Relative to the fully bonded stem (which is the same case as the titanium stem in Table2), one-third proximal coating reduces the amount of bone resorption at the proximal sides from 54% to 50% and from 38% to 22%. This is significant, but not so dramatic as sometimes hoped for. We see more reduction of bone loss around the midregion of the stem, which is caused by stress-transfer concentrations occurring at the edge of the coated region, as shown in Fig. 10. If coating is assumed only as a small band under the resection plane, we see a dramatic reduction of bone loss, e.g., to 18% and 13% at the proximal sides.

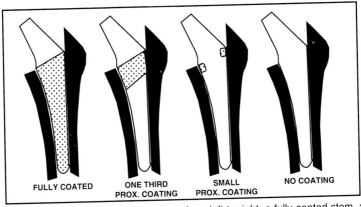

FULLY COATED    ONE THIRD PROX. COATING    SMALL PROX. COATING    NO COATING

**FIG. 9.** Four different coating configurations, from left to right: a fully coated stem, a one-third proximally coated stem, a small proximal coating, and no coating at all (24).

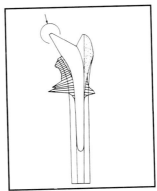

**FIG. 10.** Shear stresses at the stem–bone interface for a proximally coated stem; stress concentrations occur precisely at the edge of the coating, enhancing bone formation (Reproduced with permission from Huiskes R, Weinans H, Dalstra M. Adaptive bone remodeling and biomechanical design considerations for noncemented total hip arthroplasty. *Orthopedics* 1989;12:1255-67).

When we assume no bonding at all (Table 3), we do not obtain further reductions relative to the third case of the small proximal coating. When we compare the unbonded case with the one of the proximal one-third coating, we see that bone loss reduces from 50% to 35% in the proximal–medial region, and from a 5% loss to a 3% gain in the midlateral region, but no reductions are seen in the other regions. This confirms that the load-transfer mechanism of unbonded, press-fitted stems is very different from that of bonded ones, even if the bonding occurs in a small area only (5). What makes them so different is the fact that the unbonded stem subsides elastically when loaded, thereby stressing the interface, while the bonded stem is held in its position.

**TABLE 3.** *Bone loss due to adaptive remodeling for four different coating configurations, illustrated in Fig. 9 (24)*

| Bonding characteristics | Proximal | | Middle | |
|---|---|---|---|---|
| | Medial | Lateral | Medial | Lateral |
| Fully coated | -54% | -38% | -4% | -14% |
| One-third prox. coated | -50% | -22% | 0% | -5% |
| Small-band prox. coated | -18% | -13% | -5% | -4% |
| Uncoated | -35% | -26% | -13% | + 3% |

In summary, coating placement and bonding conditions have distinct effects on stress-shielding and bone resorption. Relative to a fully bonded configuration, bone resorption can be limited either by concentrating the coating on the proximal side or by having an uncoated smooth surface instead. In the first case, load transfer is concentrated at the proximal side and, as in the case of the flexible prosthesis discussed earlier, this implies not only less stress-shielding but also higher proximal interface stress concentrations, hence a higher probability of interface failure. It is obvious that in the case of the small proximal coating band (see Table 3), these stresses may become excessive (24). Again, a compromise must be found between acceptable resorption and acceptable loosening risks, by applying a coating that is located proximally but is still extensive enough to carry the interface loads.

The second way of limiting resorption relative to the case of full bonding, by press-fitting an unbonded prosthesis, also has its vagaries for interface mechanics. Because of its lack of bonding, the implant moves (subsides) relative to the bone each time the hip joint is loaded (5). Although this relative displacement stresses the surrounding bone, thereby reducing the amount of stress-shielding, it also produces continuous interface motions which may eventually cause interface–bone resorption and implant loosening.

## Implant Fit

Implant fit is considered a surgical parameter, although of course its precision and reproducibility can also be influenced by the design of stem and instrumentation. To evaluate the effect of this factor we compare three different configurations (Fig. 11): one with a precise (line-to-line) interference fit of the stem over its full length, one in which there is a 1 mm gap at the distal interface–hence, the case in which the distal bone has been overreamed by 2 mm, or the distal stem has been undersized by 2 mm – and one in which there is a proximal gap of 1 mm, hence proximal overreaming or undersizing by 2 mm. Again, all other parameters remain the same, i.e., the same loading cycle, titanium stem material, and no interface bonding. Thus, the first case is the same as the last one in the previous analysis.

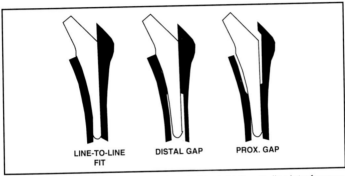

LINE-TO-LINE FIT     DISTAL GAP     PROX. GAP

**FIG. 11.** Three different configurations of fit, from left to right: line-to-line interference fit, distal gap (overreamed or undersized), and proximal gap (24).

The results of the remodeling analysis are shown in Table 4 (24). Relative to the precise interference fit, the distal gap causes load to be transferred more proximally, reducing bone loss to about the same amounts as the small-band proximal coating case in the previous analysis (see Table 3). Conversely, proximal overreaming or undersizing produces dramatic amounts of bone loss, up to 91% in the proximal–medial region. This is the worst case of resorption in our entire series, and is a nice illustration of the importance of surgical technique relative to implant design.

**TABLE 4.** *Bone loss due to adaptive remodeling for three different cases of fit, illustrated in Fig. 11 (24).*

| Fit characteristics | Proximal | | Middle | |
|---|---|---|---|---|
| | Medial | Lateral | Medial | Lateral |
| Line-to-line fit | -35% | -26% | -13% | +3% |
| Distal overreamed | -18% | -13% | +1% | +6% |
| Proximal overreamed | -91% | -48% | -34% | -7% |

## Patient Factors

Many patient factors can interfere with the bone-remodeling process, systemic and local, behavioral, physiological, or pathologic. We have summarized all factors in relation to their effects on three parameters (Table 1), hip joint loading, bone physical quality, i.e., density and stiffness, and bone reactivity, by which is meant the threshold strain deviation, or mean effective strain deviation, to which the bone reacts, represented in our models by the width of the dead zone.

Of these three parameters, we have not analyzed the effects of hip joint loading, probably because it seems so trivial. Obviously, increased hip joint loads increase the bone stresses proportionally. Because the bone-remodeling process is nonlinear–or so it is assumed in our models–the reduction of bone resorption is not necessarily nonlinearly proportional with the increase of load. In any case, there will be a reduction. However, there are also increases in relative interface motions immediately postoperatively, and perhaps a less effective integration process, with higher stresses and chances for interface failure, late postoperatively.

The effects of the other two patient parameters were evaluated relative to a three-dimensional finite-element model, based on a bone of which the normal density distribution was determined from CT scans (22). A fully-bonded titanium stem was inserted in the model, and the long-term remodeling patterns were determined with the simulation analysis. The results for this (reference) case are illustrated in Fig. 12, in which the resorption patterns are evident. To simulate a denser, hence also stiffer, bone, the normal preoperative density values measured were multiplied by a factor of two, albeit keeping the maximal density at the initial value of 1.73 g/cm$^2$, representing cortical bone. The result is a stiffer bone, for which the simulation analysis was repeated, keeping all other parameters the same. In the third analysis the original bone-density values were again used, but this time the threshold level for bone reaction was reduced from 75% to 35% of the normal signal values, thus simulating a bone with about twice the degree of reactivity.

The results are shown in Table 5, this time for four regions in the bone around the prosthesis, at the level of the Gruen zones 1 plus 7, 2 plus 6, 3 plus 5, and 4, respectively. Notable is the drastic reduction in resorption patterns for the stiffer bone, e.g., from 67% to 11% in the most proximal region, and the drastic increase for the bone with the higher reactivity, e.g., from 67% to 82% in this same proximal region.

Because these parametric variations are both rather hypothetical in extent we do not really know the real variability in bone stiffness or in bone reactivity, therefore it is not really possible to interpret them in terms of actual patient conditions. However, these examples nicely illustrate three important general points. The first is that in clinical series the extent of bone resorption will vary, even if prosthetic and surgical factors are equal in all cases, because of differences in patient factors. This may sound trivial, but it does suggest that to optimize results of joint replacements these patient factors should, ideally, be somehow evaluated preoperatively. The second point is that the younger patients, with presumably higher bone reactivities, could experience more postoperative bone loss, even if they are more active than older ones. The third point is probably the most important. The reduction in amounts of bone resorbed in the case of the stiffer bone indicates that bone stiffness is at least as influential a parameter as stem stiffness. This makes sense, of course, because

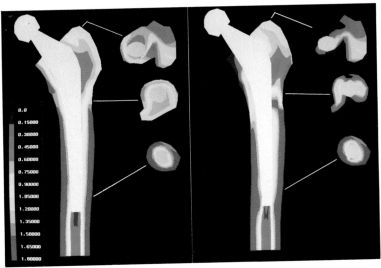

**FIG. 12.** Immediate postoperative density distribution, as based on CT scan, on the left, and density distribution after long-term remodeling simulation on the right, corresponding with the "normal" bone in Table 5 (22).

**TABLE 5.** *Bone loss due to adaptive remodeling in three different kinds of bones, a "normal" one (see Figure 12), one with a higher bone density and one with a higher reactivity (22)*

| Bone characteristics | Proximal | Upper middle | Lower middle | Distal |
|---|---|---|---|---|
| "Normal" | -67% | -35% | -4% | +5% |
| Dense (stiff) bone | -11% | -3% | -1% | +1% |
| High reactivity | -82% | -64% | -27% | 0% |

the load-sharing mechanism of stem and bone is governed by the ratio of stem and bone stiffnesses rather than by each separately (28). Recently, Engh and co-workers (29) published a report of bone-density measurements around hip stems in retrieved postmortem specimens, using dual-energy x-ray absorptiometry analysis, which produces accurate estimates, contrary to conventional radiographic measurement techniques. They compared results to those obtained from the contralateral femur, which was assumed to represent a density distribution similar to that of the treated femur preoperatively. They found 7% to 52% bone loss around the stem relative to the contralateral bone, with the largest part–a range of 30% to 80% and a mean of 45%–in the proximal region. They also found a good inverse correlation between the amount of bone loss in the treated bone and the density of the contralateral one (Fig. 13), thus confirming the relationship found in the model. Since it is possible in principle to estimate the density of bones preoperatively, this presents a means of customizing implant stiffness to the patient.

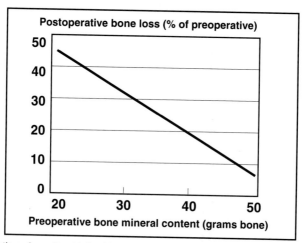

**FIG. 13.** Illustration of results obtained by Engh and co-workers (29) from precise radiodensity measurements in five postmortem specimens. An inverse correlation was found between postoperative bone loss around noncemented femoral stems and preoperative bone density, estimated by measurements of the contralateral bone. These findings confirm the predictions of the computer-simulation model (Table 5) in a qualitative sense.

## Discussion

The simulation model we developed is nothing more than a simple mathematical description of the concept of bone as a "quantitative self-regulating mechanism," suggested by Roux in 1881 (9), combined with finite-element analysis to make it applicable to the morphologic complexities of bone structures. Although the finite-element models are still crude relative to these structures and the remodeling model features a number of assumptions, the results it produces are surprisingly realistic. As said, the morphologic adaptations around canine prostheses in a number of experimental series could be predicted in detail (19-21), but predictions for human cases also are confirmed in the clinic. Earlier, these predictions had been called unrealistic, based on information from postoperative radiographs. However, these conventional radiographs are very imprecise. Recent radiographic studies, using precise objective measurement methods, have shown that the extent of bone resorption around hip stems predicted, on the order of 30% to 80%, is also found in reality (29-31). Effects of implant stiffness on bone resorption, predicted by the model, are similar to those found in animal experiments (26, 32).

The simulation model is particularly useful to analyze and explain the quantitative relationships between the morphologic changes and the various prosthetic, surgical and patient factors that affect them. Generally speaking, the results of the analyses performed for that purpose and discussed in this chapter are not surprising. Anything feasible that increases the external loads on the joint or lets them be transferred to the bone as far proximal as possible, such as flexible stems, small proximal coatings, and distal interface gaps, increases proximal bone stresses, reduces stress shielding, and diminishes bone resorption, but at a price. All these measures also tend to increase early interface motions, hence less effective osseus integration, and interface stresses (hence a higher probability of late interface failure and loosening). It seems that we are caught between a rock and a hard place, and compromises are required. Since stem loosening is a real problem and bone resorption only a potential one (remember that clinical problems as a result of it have not been reported as yet), it would probably be wise to stay on the conservative end where it concerns interface stress enhancing techniques or designs. Of course, conflicting design requirements are great candidates for computer optimization, and these methods will certainly be used in the near future, in combination with the simulation models discussed here.

Not all parameters were considered here, an important one of which is the shape of the stem, which was more or less similar in all analyses. Neither were design features, such as a prosthetic collar, analyzed. These factors can certainly have extensive effects on both bone resorption and interface mechanics.

Effects that were surprising, at least to us, are the dramatic influences of proximal fit and bone initial density (or stiffness) on the amount of bone resorption. It seems that these are parameters that can successfully, and safely, be considered to minimize bone loss. The degree to which uncoated, press-fitted stems limit resorption relative to proximally-coated ones is much less than expected and, considering the interface motions they inherently provoke, one wonders if they should be applied at all. Somewhat disappointing was the moderate effect of proximal one-third coating relative to full coating on bone loss at the proximal side. The gain is predominantly in the midregion of the stem, because a relatively large share of the load is transferred near the distal edge of the coating. Although this is a gain nevertheless, a more subtle coating configuration might be worth considering. Finally, the effects of flexible, so-called iso-elastic materials were, to us, all but surprising. However, the risks of excessive interface motions and stresses that these materials present can not be emphasized too often, particularly since a number of companies consider them experimental at present.

## REFERENCES

1.   Bauer TW, Geesink RTC, Zimmerman R, McMahon JT. Hydroxyapatite-coated femoral stems. Histological analysis of components retrieved at autopsy. *Journal of Bone and Joint Surgery* 1991;73-A:1439-52
2.   Geesink RGT, de Groot K, Klein CPAT. Bonding of bone to apatite-coated implants. *Journal of Bone and Joint Surgery* 1988;70-B:17-22.
3.   Søballe K, Hansen SE, Rasmussen HB, Jorgensen PH, Bunger C. Tissue ingrowth into titanium and hydroxyapatite-coated implants during stable and unstable mechanical conditions. *Journal of Orthopaedic Research* 1992;10:285-99.
4.   Huiskes R. Biomechanics of artificial-joint fixation. In: Mow VC, Hayes WC, eds. *Basic Orthopaedic Biomechanics*. New York: Raven Press, 1991:375-442.
5.   Huiskes R. The various stress patterns of press-fit, ingrown and cemented femoral stems. *Clinical Orthopaedics* 1990;261:27-38.
6.   Wolff J. *Das Gesetz der Transformation der Knochen*. Berlin: Kirchwald. 1892.(Translated by Maquet P, Furlong R. *The Law of Bone Remodeling*. Berlin: R.Springer-Verlag. 1986).

7.  Roesler H. Some historical remarks on the theory of cancellous bone structure (Wolff's Law). In: Cowin SC, ed. *The biomechanical properties of bone*. New York: The Am Soc Mech Engrs (ASME). 1981; AMD-Vol 45:27-42.
8.  Roesler H. The history of some fundamental concepts in bone biomechanics. *Journal of Biomechanics* 1987;20:1025-34.
9.  Roux W. *Der züchtende Kampf der Teile, oder die 'Teilauslese' im Organismus. (Theorie der 'funktionellen Anpassung')*. Leipzig: Wilhelm Engelmann. 1881.
10. Dibbits JMH. One Century of Wolff's Law. In: Carlson DS, Goldstein SA, eds. *Bone biodynamics in orthodontic and orthopedic treatment*. Ann Arbor, MI: Center for Human Growth and Development. 1992;27:1-15.
11. Cowin SC, Hegedus DH. Bone remodeling I: a theory of adaptive elasticity. *Journal of Elasticity* 1976;6:313-26.
12. Hegedus DH, Cowin SC. Bone remodeling II: small strain adaptive elasticity. *Journal of Elasticity* 1976;6:337-52.
13. Hart RT, Davy DT, Heiple KG. A computational method for stress analysis of adaptive elastic materials with a view toward applications in strain induced bone remodeling. *Journal of Biomechanical Engineering* 1984;106:342-50.
14. Carter DR. Mechanical loading history and skeletal biology. *Journal of Biomechanics* 1987;20:1095-109.
15. Huiskes R, Weinans H, Grootenboer HJ, Dalstra M, Fudala B, Slooff TJ. Adaptive bone-remodeling theory applied to prosthetic-design analysis. *Journal of Biomechanics* 1987;20:1135-150.
16. Cowin SC, Moss-Salentijn L, Moss ML. Candidates for the mechanosensory system in bone. *Journal of Biomechanical Engineering* 1991;113:191-97.
17. Huiskes R, Weinans H, Dalstra M. Adaptive bone remodeling and biomechanical design considerations for noncemented total hip arthroplasty. *Orthopedics* 1989;12:1255-267.
18. Weinans H, Huiskes R, Grootenboer HJ. The behavior of adaptive bone-remodeling simulation models. *Journal of Biomechanics* 1992;25:1425-41.
19. Weinans H, Huiskes R, van Rietbergen B, Sumner DR, Turner TM, Galante JO. Adaptive bone remodeling around bonded noncemented THA: a comparison between animal experiments and computer simulations. *Journal of Orthopaedic Research* 1992;10:in press.
20. Van Rietbergen B, Huiskes R, Weinans H, Sumner DR, Turner TM, Galante JO. The mechanism of bone remodeling and resorption around press-fitted THA stems. *Journal of Biomechanics* 1993; 26:369-82.
21. Van Rietbergen B. and Huiskes R. Predicted effects of reduced stem stiffness on femoral bone resorption, using a strain-adaptive bone-remodeling theory. (*unpublished report*)
22. Huiskes R, Weinans H, van Rietbergen B. The relationship between stress shielding and bone resorption around total hip stems and the effects of flexible materials. *Clinical Orthopaedics* 1992;274:124-34.
23. Frost HM. Vital biomechanics. Proposed general concepts for skeletal adaptations to mechanical usage. *Calcified Tissue International* 1987;42:145-56.
24. Weinans H. *Mechanically induced bone adaptations around orthopaedic implants*. Doctoral Dissertation, University of Nijmegen. 1991.
25. Gruen TA, McNeice GM, Amstutz HC. Modes of failure of cemented stem-type femoral components, a radiographic analysis of loosening. *Clinical Orthopaedics* 1979;141:17-27.
26. Bobyn JD, Mortimer ES, Glassman AH, Engh CA, Miller JE, Brooks CE. Producing and avoiding stress shielding. Laboratory and clinical observations of noncemented total hip arthroplasty. *Clinical Orthopaedics* 1992;274:79-96.
27. Weinans H, Huiskes R, Grootenboer HJ. Effects of material properties of femoral hip components on bone remodeling and interface stresses. *Journal of Orthopaedic Research* 1992;10:845-53.
28. Huiskes R. Some fundamental aspects of human-joint replacement. *Acta Orthopaedica Scandinavica* 1980;Suppl 185.
29. Engh CA, McGovern TF, Bobyn JD, Harris WH. A quantitative evaluation of periprosthetic bone-remodeling after cementless total hip arthroplasty. *Journal of Bone and Joint Surgery* 1992;74-A:1009-20.
30. Steinberg GG, Kearns McCarthy C, Baran DT. Quantification of bone loss of the femur after total hip arthroplasty. *Transactions of the 37th Annual Orthopaedic Research Society* 1991;221.
31. Kiratli BJ, Heiner JP, McNinley N, Wilson MA, McBeath AA. Bone mineral density of the proximal femur after uncemented total hip arthroplasty. *Transactions of the 37th Annual Orthopaedic Research Society* 1991;545.
32. Sumner DR, Galante JO. Determinants of stress shielding: design versus material versus interface. *Clinical Orthopaedics* 1992;274:202-12.

*Hydroxylapatite Coatings in Orthopaedic Surgery,*
edited by R. G. T. Geesink and M. T. Manley.
Raven Press, Ltd., New York, © 1993.

# Process Application of Hydroxylapatite Coatings

## Paul Serekian, M.S.

The structural use of bulk HA is limited by its relatively low tensile properties. The osteoconductive nature of hydroxylapatite (HA) can best be used to advantage by applying a thin layer of HA to the surface of implants in the range of 30 to 100 microns. Coatings in excess of 100 µm thick take on the characteristics of a brittle ceramic and are at particular risk of mechanical failure. Coatings less than 30 microns on "smooth" type surfaces represent a challenge as regards their ability to produce complete HA coating coverage on a substrate.

The clinical success of HA-coated implants is contingent on the degree of coating-substrate integrity as reflected in the coating bond strength to the substrate, and its ability to sustain longterm fatigue loading. Hydroxl-apatite has a rich and complex chemistry that can be influenced by application conditions. There are several methods that can be used to apply HA coatings to smooth and textured surfaces as described in the following text. Although almost all substrates currently being coated are metallic, a number of techniques can be used to coat composite structures; as well.

## PROCESSING

Many methods of applying HA coatings to metallic substrates have been assessed, but the effects of high temperatures can be adverse to either the metal substrate or the HA, causing excessive grain growth or decomposition of the metallic microstructure (13). Also, melting and degradation of the HA to other less stable calcium phosphate compounds have been reported. Coating methods cited by a number of authors include plasma spraying, flame spraying, electrophoresis with or without sintering, ion beam–radio frequency sputtering, dip coating, physical vapor deposition, isostatic compression and frit-slurry enameling. Coating properties are largely dependent upon the coating method used (6, 15, 16).

In their review of several processes utilized to apply HA coatings, Yankee et al. discuss the advantages and disadvantages of the resultant coatings in the biomedical setting (16). HA coatings produced through a slurry coat and sintering method are generated by dipping a dense or porous metallic substrate into a water based slurry of HA particles and an organic binder. The key disadvantage of this method is that the high temperature required in the post-sintering of the HA layer can degrade the metal's strength and compromise the device and/or the hydroxl-apatite. A second method, isostatic compression, is a two-stage process. The first stage involves cold isostatic pressing of HA powder onto a metal substrate; in the second stage, the substrate and coating are encapsulated and hot isostatically pressed at temperatures of 900-1000°C to produce a dense coating. Isostatic pressing has very limited applications due to the complexities of sealing boundaries around complex geometries and the same disadvantages enumerated for the slurry coat and sintering techniques. Electrophoresis, another coating method, relies on the deposition of electrically charged HA particles through a liquid or other medium and is suitable for coating complex-shaped items (i.e., porous-coated surfaces). However, the particle's low energy and the room temperature environment lead to coatings with irregular porosity and generally result in poor binding to the substrate. Additional complications associated with this process are related to electro-deposition of impurities contained in the liquid medium, as well as coating non-uniformity resulting from variable current density. Physical vapor deposition (PVD) is a process that relies on the direction of a beam of energized ions onto the surface of a HA target and subsequent mass transport to the substrate. The atomic nature of the process permits a broad spectrum of substrates to be used, but the process is time intensive since mass transfer takes place on a scale of individual atoms. PVD-produced coatings are significantly thinner (3-5 $\mu$m) than conventionally produced coatings reflecting the extraordinarily low deposition rates associated with the process. Deposition rates associated with this technique are typically 0.2-0.4 $\mu$m per hour. PVD is a line-of-sight technique that is unsuited for complex shapes with undercuts. Yankee et al. conclude that at present, the final method, plasma spraying, continues to be the preferred method of applying HA coatings to devices for clinical use due to the broad base of available technology and equipment, its cost effectiveness, efficiency, and reproducibility. (16)

The technique of choice for HA coating on orthopaedic devices is plasma arc deposition which confirms Yankee's conclusion. Dense, tightly adhered coatings of up to 100 $\mu$m in thickness can be deposited within two minutes. The process involves feeding particulate HA powder through a mechanical transfer apparatus into a high-temperature electric arc- plasma gas atmosphere. An arc is struck between an anode and cathode, with the arc heat causing disassociation of gas to levels attaining temperatures up to 30,000° K. The particulate HA is passed into the plasma arc by a carrier gas such as argon. A schematic depiction of the process at the nozzle is shown in Figure 1. The plasma gas effects surface melting of the HA particulate and acceleration onto the target substrate. The surfaces of the implant to be coated are prepared by a variety of techniques such as grit blasting, shot peening and/or electrochemical milling in order to increase the level of mechanical bonding to the base material. The

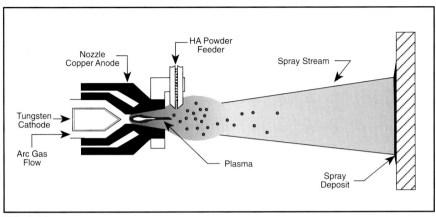

**FIG. 1.** Plasma spray process

integrity of the applied HA coating is usually checked by conducting tensile and shear testing on mechanical specimens processed with the parts to be coated. The quasi-static bond strength under ambient conditions of HA coatings to a titanium (Ti-6Al-4V) alloy substrate are typically 50 MPa in tension and 17 MPa in shear. Among the factors affecting the fatigue strength of HA-coated implants are the roughness of the substrate and coating thickness.

The temperatures associated with the deposition of HA on metal substrates are typically less than 300°C; hence, there is no degradation of the metal's mechanical properties. The very slight decrease in the metal's fatigue properties is more likely due to the surface roughening of the substrate which is necessary to achieve an adequate mechanical bond.

More recently, vacuum plasma spraying of HA and high velocity oxygen fuel (HVOF) coating have been developed as two additional techniques for applying HA coatings. Although enhanced bonding levels and higher purity levels are claimed for the vacuum deposition technique, the clinical performance of vacuum coatings versus conventional air-sprayed coatings remains to be seen. HVOF is a technique by which HA particles are heated to significantly lower temperatures than arc deposition processes, but are applied at higher velocities than conventional arc-deposition. A schematic depiction of the HVOF coating process is shown in Figure 2. The lower temperature and higher velocity associated with the HVOF process have demonstrated higher levels of chemical stability in *in vitro* testing. Sintered and plasma-sprayed apatite surfaces have very similar biological characteristics; however, their mechanical properties are very different due to the density and structure of the base material (16).

## CHEMICAL PROPERTIES OF SURFACE

Collier et al. have indicated that plasma-sprayed tricalcium phosphate can be transformed into HA after immersion in serum, saline or the *in vivo* environment (2). This observation, coupled with the current knowledge of

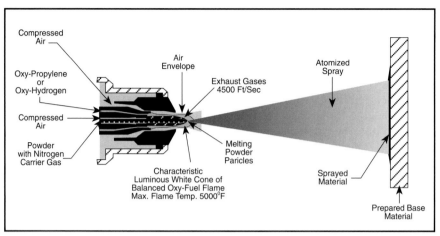

**FIG. 2.** High velocity oxygen fuel (HVOF).

plasma-sprayed high density coatings, underscores the importance of monitoring the crystallographic structure and chemistry of HA before applying the HA surfacing. Ducheyne et al. refer to variations in the deposited material that are characteristic of plasma-sprayed calcium phosphate ceramics. These variations affect the material's dissolution rate and possibly, the bone ingrowth properties of this material (5).

The choice of implant material is critical to the longevity of the device. Titanium and Ti-6Al-4V alloy are used in orthopaedic devices because of their high strength, comparatively low modulus of elasticity,and their corrosion resistance properties (3).

Griffin et al. conducted an *in vitro* study comparing the corrosion rates of HA-coated and uncoated cobalt–chromium alloy specimens (9). This study demonstrated that the corrosion rate of HA-coated cobalt chromium alloy samples measured ten times less than the uncoated specimens at 48 hours. Hayashi et al. observed similar results in their study of HA-coated and uncoated titanium (Ti-6Al-4V) alloy implants, demonstrating their excellent affinity for bone. HA-coated titanium also provides superior corrosion resistance (12).

A similar study performed by Ducheyne et al. analyzed the effects of plasma-sprayed HA coatings on ion release from porous titanium and cobalt chromium alloy implants. In this study, a 20-μm layer of hydroxl-apatite was applied to a porous metal fiber structure containing a pore size of 110 μm. Ion release from these metal substrates was measured by an *in vitro* model, which enhanced ion release and compared results of coated and uncoated specimens. Specimens were immersed for a period of four weeks. Since it is a well established fact that the amount of ion release from orthopaedic implants is minimal, highly sensitive analytical methods were required to measure ion release. A comparison of study results of HA-coated versus uncoated metallic substrates demonstrated that the HA coating on a titanium substrate markedly reduced titanium ion release; HA coating on cobalt–chromium alloy substrate did not. Ducheyne et al. theorize that the energy associated with the plasma-sprayed HA particle may alter the structure and composition of the metal substrate's protective oxide coating (4).

## MECHANICAL PROPERTIES OF SUBSTRATE/SURFACE

Mechanical testing of biomaterials is conducted to calculate their fatigue and quasi-static strengths. Tensile and shear properties are of primary interest in characterizing the quasi-static properties of coatings and substrates. The fatigue strength of orthopaedic materials is very important since in the small incidence where mechanical failure of a prosthesis occurs, it fails through the fatigue mode. The fatigue strength of a material or a coating-substrate interface is its ability to survive cyclic physiologic loading conditions for a defined number of cycles, usually $10^7$ cycles. The drive and interest in developing and manufacturing implants for longer term survivorship will require fatigue data at the 2-3 x $10^7$ cycle level. Shear strength is determined by dividing the push-out force by the total area of contact with the implant. The force needed to loosen an implant is determined by a load displacement curve. As Lemons indicates, calcium phosphate ceramics can fracture under cyclic loading when mechanical stresses are above the material's strength limits (14). Thus, the material needs sufficient mechanical strength to tolerate the compressive, tensile and shear loads to which it is subjected (1). It has been found that the strength limits of calcium phosphate materials differ depending upon whether they are composed of a dense sintered HA or a coating. The strength of the HA coating is dependent upon coating thickness. A compilation of coating strength as a function of thickness on a titanium 6Al-4V alloy substrate is provided below in Table 1:

**TABLE 1.** *Coating Characteristics as a Function of Coating Thickness*

| HA Coating Thickness (μm) | Tensile Strength (MPa) | Fatigue Strength (MPa) at $10^7$ Cycles |
|---|---|---|
| 50 | 50.8 ± 4.0 | 483 |
| 120 | 48.0 ± 4.1 | 483 |
| 240 | 40.0 ± 3.9 | 391 |

Filiaggi et al. evaluated the mechanical properties of HA plasma-sprayed to a titanium alloy substrate utilizing a short bar specimen model. They found that as the surface roughness increased, the interface fracture toughness increased correspondingly. Thus, Filiaggi et al. concluded that, while in their experiments the metal/HA interface represents the weakest link in the coated implant system, the surface roughness of the underlying substrate plays an important role in the interface fracture toughness (7).

The transcortical implant model is a standard *in vivo* model used to evaluate the differences in shear strength and implant attachment at a comparative screening level for various materials, without subjecting the material to physiological loading. A material that performs poorly in the transcortical implant model would be expected to perform poorly, or worse, in functional loading. Another model, the endoprosthesis model, enables direct functional loading of the implant and is more realistic and relevant in design than the transcortical model. Studies, therefore, have evaluated the strength of HA relative to other materials, and the strength of "HA-type" materials relative to one another, utilizing such models. The ability to load the endoprosthesis model provides for more relevant data regarding the integrity of the coating–prosthesis interface as a function of time.

Geesink et al. and de Groot found that a HA coating of approximately 50 microns on a metal substrate enabled apposition to bone while avoiding fatigue failure of the coating ( 8, 10, 11). Each found that the HA-coated plugs studied demonstrated increased shear strength, which approached the shear strength of bone itself when compared to uncoated plugs. These authors found that at the 12-month follow-up, plugs with a 50-$\mu$m coating showed no failure of the HA and direct apposition between the coating and bone without an intervening fibrous tissue seam.

## POST-PROCESSING CONSIDERATIONS

The post-application processing of HA coatings is important because the final cleaned HA surface is the relevant interface with host bone. One of the techniques used to remove loosely bonded plasma-sprayed particles is ultrasonic cleaning in alcohol solutions. Another technique is to process the coated implants through a secondary low-pressure fluid spray chamber. Both methods are effective in removing loosely adhered surface particles and insuring an isolated particle-free surface.

## SUMMARY

Clearly, there are a number of methods that can be used to apply hydroxlapatite coatings to metal substrates achieving bond levels that are clinically acceptable. The majority of the processes are technically cumbersome or cost prohibitive. Plasma spraying remains the most practical technique for coating application. The successful application of plasma-sprayed coating depends upon a chemically and physically consistent source of feedstock coupled with a controlled and consistent spray process.

Although there are a number of studies that suggest plasma-sprayed HA coatings with high levels of crystallinity resorb more slowly than those with lower crystallinity levels, a recent study by Ducheyne et al. suggests that more stable coatings can have intermediate crystallinity levels.

Future studies are planned and underway to determine the influence of cancellous and cortical structures in HA coating resorption.

# REFERENCES

1. Bucholz RW, Carlton A, Holmes R. Interporous hydroxyapatite as a bone graft substitute in tibial plateau fractures. *Clinical Orthopaedics and Related Research.* March 1989; 240: 53-62.
2. Collier JP, Mayor MB, Dwyer KA, Teske DA, Chae J, Surprenant VA. The unsolved problems associated with the use of plasma-sprayed TCP and HA coatings on orthopaedic prostheses. *34th Annual Meeting, Orthopaedic Research Society.* February 1-4, 1988; Atlanta, GA: 51.
3. Cook SD, Thomas KA, Kay JF, Jarcho M. Hydroxyapatite-coated titanium for orthopedic implant applications. *Clinical Orthopaedics and Related Research.* July 1988; 232: 225-243.
4. Ducheyne P, Healy KE. The effect of plasma-sprayed calcium phosphate ceramic coatings of the metal ion release from porous titanium and cobalt chromium alloys. *Journal of Biomedical Materials Research.* 1988; 22: 1137-1163.
5. Ducheyne P, Radin S, Healy K, Cuckler JM. The effect of plasma spraying on the structure and properties of calcium phosphate ceramics. *34th Annual Meeting, Orthopaedic Research Society.* February 1-4, 1988; Atlanta, GA: 50.
6. Ducheyne P, Van Raemdonck W, De Meester P. Physical and material properties of hydroxyl-apatite coatings sintered on titanium. *Second World Congress on Biomaterials: 10th Annual Meeting of the Society for Biomaterials.* April 27-May 1, 1984; Washington, DC: 350.
7. Filiaggi MJ, Coombs NA, Pilliar RM. Characterization of the interface in the plasma-sprayed HA coating/Ti-6Al-4V implant system. *Journal of Biomedical Materials Research.* 1991; 25: 1211-1229.
8. Geesink RGT, de Groot K, Klein CPAT. Chemical implant fixation using hydroxyl-apatite coatings. The development of a human total hip prosthesis for chemical fixation to bone using hydroxyl-apatite coatings on titanium substrates. *Clinical Orthopaedics and Related Research.* December 1987; 225: 147-169.
9. Griffin CD, Kay J, Smith CL. Effect of HA coatings on corrosion of cobalt-chrome alloy. *13th Annual Meeting of the Society for Biomaterials.* June 3-7, 1987; New York, NY: 234.
10. de Groot K. HA coatings for implants in surgery. In: Vincenzini P, ed. *High Tech Ceramics.* Amsterdam, The Netherlands: Elsevier; 1987: 381-386.
11. de Groot K, Geesink R, Klein CPAT, Serekian P. Plasma sprayed coatings of HA. *Journal of Biomedical Materials Research.* 1987; 21: 1375-1381.
12. Hayashi K, Uenoyama K, Matsuguchi N, Sugioka Y. Quantitative analysis of *in vivo* tissue responses to titanium-oxide- and hydroxyapatite-coated titanium alloy. *Journal of Biomedical Materials Research.* 1991; 25: 515-523.
13. Lacefield WR. Hydroxyapatite coatings. *Annals of the New York Academy of Sciences.* 1988; 523: 72-80.
14. Lemons JE. Hydroxyapatite coatings. *Clinical Orthopaedics and Related Research.* October 1988; 235: 220-223.
15. Lemons JE, Bajpai PA, Patka P, Bonel G, Starling LB, Rosenstiel T, Muschler G, Kampner S, Timmermans J. Significance of the porosity and physical chemistry of calcium phosphate ceramics. Orthopaedic uses. *Annals of the New York Academy of Sciences.* 1988; 523: 278-282. Position Paper.
16. Yankee SJ, Pletka BJ, Luckey HA, Johnson WA. Processes for fabricating HA coatings for biomedical applications. *Thermal Spray Research and Applications. Proceedings of the Third National Thermal Spray Conference.* May 20-25, 1990; Long Beach, CA: 433-438.

*Hydroxylapatite Coatings in Orthopaedic Surgery,*
edited by R. G. T. Geesink and M. T. Manley.
Raven Press, Ltd., New York, © 1993.

# Biologic Profile of Calcium-Phosphate Coatings

## John F. Kay, Ph.D., and Stephen D. Cook, Ph.D.

### BONE AND BONE MINERAL

Bone forms the rigid scaffold on which the body is built. The skeleton, accounting for approximately 14% of total body weight, shares many properties with the new composite material structures used in high-performance aircraft and spacecraft. Despite its light composite form, bone is stronger than steel when compared on an ounce-to-ounce basis.

Bone combines the resilience, toughness, and continuity of its organic constituent, collagen, with the stiffness, hardness, and rigidity of an inorganic crystalline ceramic-like material, which is primarily the mineral hydroxylapatite (HA) $(Ca_{10}(PO_4)_6(OH)_2)$ (1–3). These tiny HA crystals (about 250 Å) stiffen the collagen matrix so that, without them, a long bone could be tied into a knot. The crystalline mineral phase of bone represents 60% to 70% of the bone by weight. Bone mineral also has minor amounts of adjunct constituents that vary in their proportions (2, 3). An examination of the nature of biological apatite and the forms of its occurrence has been addressed in a recent compilation (4).

Bone maintenance requires proper nutrient intake, including calcium and phosphorus. Bone also must experience stress to remain vital; otherwise, it atrophies and changes in form, just as unused muscles do. Bone responds to stress by modifying its architecture to best support functional loads through the remodeling process. The cancellous structure of bone that helps support and transfer loads actually looks and acts like a complex truss-and beam-system. The structure of bone is unique in its ability to continuously change its physical structure to accommodate changes in the forces that act on it.

Teeth are lost for a variety of reasons: cavities and decay, periodontal and other diseases, or trauma. Aside from the immediately obvious change in appearance, tooth loss causes other slower changes to occur below the gums in the bone, which can lead to problems with dental appliances. When teeth are lost they can no longer transmit the forces of chewing to the underlying bone; this often causes the bone to change its architectural form and resorb, so that dentures are ill-fitting and painful.

## THE CALCIUM PHOSPHATE BIOMATERIALS

The calcium phosphate family of biomaterials consists of dozens of individual compounds, each of which has potential as an implantable substance. Combinations expand the choices into the hundreds. Despite these choices, two calcium phosphates (Ca-phosphate), hydroxylapatite (HA) and tricalcium phosphate in the ß- crystallographic form (TCP) have, to date, stimulated the largest laboratory and clinical interest. As a result, ASTM Standards were generated for these two forms (5,6). The chemical formulae ($Ca_{10}(PO_4)_6(OH_2$; $Ca_3(PO_4)_2$) reveal an important calcium-to-phosphorus ratio of 1.67 and 1.5, respectively.

The most common method for manufacture of these calcium phosphate ceramics is by aqueous precipitation. Ultrapure starting materials are used for calcium and phosphate ionic sources, and bioceramic forms are prepared by direct filtering/forming or by conventional powder-processing methods after drying, followed by sintering at high temperatures ($900-1200^0C$) (7–13). Physical forms of nearly fully dense, microporous, and macroporous ceramics have been created but have been limited to small particulate or block form since, as ceramics, they are brittle. Other porous forms are possible through processing of naturally occurring substances (coral, bone) to render them to immature forms of HA (12,14–17).

## ANIMAL MODELS FOR MATERIALS SYSTEM EVALUATION

*In vivo* evaluation represents a crucially important phase in the development of new implant materials and designs, yet no single animal model provides all the information to support the use of a materials system, attachment structure, and/or implant design. The canine has been utilized extensively to study hard tissue implants, and therefore provides both a qualitative, and a quantitative basis for comparison. The advent of implants and new biomaterials used for their construction has sparked interest in gross tissue response, histologic evaluation, and bony attachment.

Gross tissue response is derived from the tissue appearance at various times postimplantation, and of the bone–implant complex on uncovering. Postoperative observations of inflammation or in surrounding tissues can be indications of long-term response. Radiographic evidence is more important at longer periods of time, especially in models in which stress shielding effects may arise.

Histologic evaluation provides evidence for the body's response to the implant at the bone contact surface. Over the last 15 years, the techniques, tools, and interpretations of histologic preparations have changed dramatically. Greater definition, preservation of structure, decrease in artifact, and higher magnifications of observation have evolved from early low-magnification decalcified sections. Stained ground sections, scanning and transmission electron microscopy, electron microprobing, and other important observations and innovations now provide much more information at the ultrastructural level. It is important to correlate histologic characteristics with bone–implant mechanical performance.

Innovations in bioactive materials have fostered study of the strength of implant–bone attachment. For over 15 years, the canine transcortical implant model has provided a suitable measure of bone attachment to implant surfaces. Histologic analysis of the bone–implant interface can also be obtained. The advantages of the transcortical model are that multiple samples are obtained, the procedure involves relatively simple surgery with a high degree of precision in the placement, there is a significant pool of data, using the same model, on a variety of materials that provides both a qualitative and a quantitative measure of comparison, and the canine is an accepted species. The disadvantages of the model are that it is a mildly loaded model, the implants are not indicative of any clinical usage, the features of the implant surfaces do not translate well to human devices, and the thin cortices associated with the canine femur do not provide the type of bone contact that is required in human placements. What can be obtained are direct material comparisons of biologic response and measurements of bone adherence. The standard deviations associated with a well-run study are usually in the range of ± 10-15 %. For all the reasons cited, the transcortical model and associated methods of tissue analysis have evolved as a *de facto* standard (18–27).

Loaded functional models, primarily in the canine, have also provided histologic and mechanical testing data on a variety of materials systems. The advantages of loaded functional models, such as hips, knees, or intermedullary rods, are that those implantations, in general, are more indicative of their human use counterparts. Significant functional load are transmitted to the devices, the implants are large, and one can often see the effects of a change in the stress state on the implant and surrounding bone in different areas (stress-shielding or overloading efforts). The disadvantages of the loaded models are that they are not directly applicable to human devices, in that the proportional loads over certain interfaces are many times not equivalent, the surface features are not equivalent to those of equivalent human devices, the loading pattern on the devices, owing to anatomic or loading conditions, is not the same as that experienced by humans, the instrumentation and installation are not always indicative of the type of precision obtained with human devices, and models are usually expensive because fewer implants can be placed in a given animal and observations are made on a limited number of devices.

A combination of a transcortical implant model to study the materials response in a controlled fashion and a loaded model to represent at least some of the aspects of the anticipated loading patterns of the functional human device often provides supporting data for a particular materials system and implant surface design.

## BIOLOGICAL RESPONSE TO THE CALCIUM PHOSPHATES

### Biological Response

The calcium phosphate biomaterials family is probably the most biocompatible materials group available for use in hard tissue sites. The high degree of biocompatibility is a result of the chemical compositions that are significantly close to those of naturally occurring bone mineral (2–4).

## Hydroxylapatite

Synthetic HA, when prepared in pure form without a significant amount of impurities or second phases, exhibits a very high degree of biocompatibility (11-13). It has been shown that this particular material can become bonded strongly to bone at the interface by a natural mechanism without an intervening fibrous tissue layer (28–32). The material serves as a scaffold for bone growth and proliferation. In essence, a natural bone-healing mechanism occurs directly on the surface of the implant material and provides the strong interfacial bond observed between bone and HA implants. This bonding is chemical in nature and has been demonstrated at the ultrastructural level for highly crystalline HA ceramic (28–32). The stability of highly crystalline HA is generally accepted. The higher the crystallinity, the more biostable the form. Low-temperature-sintered HA, precipitated HA and intermediate temperature sintered HA tend to bioresorb at rates indicative of the degree of crystallinity. The lower limit of biostability would be a precipitated, amorphous form of HA, somewhat similar in structure to the amorphous calcium phosphate of immature bone mineral (1,3,4).

## Tricalcium Phosphate

A calcium-phosphate substance of lesser interest, at least as measured by current commercial usage, is tricalcium phosphate (TCP) (8,12,13,16). The earliest reports of investigations involving TCP were attractive but were somewhat softened by observations that the bioresorption characteristics of the material were not predictable. It was thought that TCP would gradually resorb at a rate similar to the rate of bone apposition, and therefore would be replaced by a "creeping substitution" mechanism (16,33–35). Several studies report conflicting data on the bioresorption pattern, including a report that some implants can remain for over five years (36). Nevertheless, TCP has demonstrated excellent biocompatibility, as it is a calcium phosphate that is presumably similar to some of the earlier composition and phases of mineralizing bone. No published work indicates that either material, tested side by side is more attractive from an initial biologic standpoint. The detrimental attributes of TCP lie in the unpredictability of its bioresorption pattern and its difficulty to fabricate in form. Conceptually, HA offers the advantage of crystallographic similarity to natural bone mineral that TCP does not.

## Other Calcium-Phosphate Biomaterials

The biologic profile of other Ca-phosphate materials has been characterized but not published to a great extent. The two exceptions are glassy forms, in the form of Bio-glass and AW glass ceramic(37-42). These materials have extensive animal characterizations that indicate equivalent biocompatibility with both HA and TCP. The bonding characteristics to the surface of these materials are not as well characterized at the ultrastructural level, but for AW glass ceramic, they appear to be significant. The material has the advantage that it can be manufactured as a glass, using a mold or with conventional glass-molding methods, and then can be transformed to a tough glass ceramic by a controlled heat-treatment cycle.

## CALCIUM-PHOSPHATE COATINGS

### Chemical, Physical, and Mechanical Properties of Coatings

Bioactive coatings have been applied to substrates by a variety of techniques, including mechanical capture, plasma-spraying, electrophoresis, dipping, and sputtering (vacuum deposition). All commercially available coatings in use at present are applied by plasma-spraying, a modification of an old thermal-spray technology of the 19th century. (43–45) Because of the high temperatures involved with plasma-spraying, the coating material may be altered during the coating process so that a chemically or structurally different material is the final product. This is particularly true with HA coatings, which are also affected by the composition and purity of the starting powder material and can be altered to differing degrees based on all the operating conditions of the plasma equipment. At least one animal study documented this transformation and disruption phenomenon, with an HA powder transformed into a primarily TCP coating with *in vivo* results equivocal as compared with later investigations (46). The most controversial area associated with contemporary Ca-phosphate coatings is the nature of the chemical and physical properties needed to produce an efficacious coating. There are guidelines for such characterizations from the FDA and ASTM (5,6,47) but, for the most part, these guidelines provide only a listing of the properties that should be characterized and, in all but a few cases, are the exact methods and guideline values already established.

Characterizations of consequence fall into two categories: (a) Physical and chemical characterizations include chemical composition, determination of all phases and relative phase percentages, crystallinity as a percent of the total mass, the levels of impurities in the form of trace elements, infrared spectrum, porosity (or density), thickness and substrate coverage, microstructure as determined by optical cross-section and/or scanning electron microscopy, surface roughness of both the substrate and the coating, the degree of solubility in anticipation of its surface environment, and any other tests a manufacturer or user would deem appropriate to ensure the highest degree of uniformity and consistency. (b) Mechanical characteristics include tensile strength, shear strength, cyclic fatigue performance (both as a material and on the full-scale device), and the effects of conditions expected to be encountered in the service environment.

Before the advent of bioactive materials, such *in vitro* evaluations were definitive enough to properly categorize and screen various implant materials or at least to provide minimal performance standards to which the implants or the materials of construction must conform. Bioactive materials, however, have created a unique problem, in that no *in vitro* evaluation can exactly mimic the environment or performance of the implant once in service. *In vitro* dissolution tests typify such shortcomings. The Ca-phosphate biomaterials experience a net uptake of biologic apatite species from the *in vivo* environment that tend to protect the coating, heal small surface cracks, and generally delay, or bias in a positive fashion, the effects of any dissolution event. A laboratory *in vitro* dissolution test is an entirely negative event throughout the entire test protocol, with the implant experiencing the worst possible degradative effects on a continuous basis. This example, and others, adds support for the correlation of *in vitro* testing of such properties as dissolution to *in vivo* tests with a significant duration to compare the two evaluative methods. This correlation would allow for more valid interpretation of such *in vitro* dissolution tests; otherwise, the data are nearly meaningless.

In the device-manufacturing environment, good manufacturing practices (GMPs) provide guidelines to ensure consistency and uniformity of the coatings and in-process assays to monitor continued adherence to specifications for their manufacture. The quality controls applied to such coatings should characterize and help control the feedstock powder used in the plasma flame-spray process for coating deposition but, perhaps, more important, should provide for definitive testing of the resultant coating based on a series of criteria that can be supported for their acceptance values. Most appropriate would be the establishment of quality acceptance values tied to a set of manufacturing parameters that result in acceptable *in vivo* performance in a longer-term animal evaluation.

## Morphology of Attachment Structures

Three basic types of metallic substrate configurations have been used for the application of Ca-phosphate coatings (48). Smooth or micro-roughened surfaces are used for some dental implant designs but only for a few orthopeadic component designs. These surfaces have no significant surface relief other than the preparatory roughening associated with the application of plasma-sprayed coatings. Macrotextured substrates in the form of grooves, threads or other metal coating depositions such as metal plasma-spray, are used in dental and orthopaedic devices. Such surface features provide additional surface area for osseous deposition and appear to protect the coating from pure shear forces as bone grows and adapts to the more complex surface relief. The third surface structure, used primarily in orthopaedic devices, consists of porous metal coatings in the form of bonded wires, large or small spherical beads, irregular sintered, powdered metallurgical coatings, bonded meshes, or plasma-deposited metal such that interdigitating porosity is created. To date, porous structures have not been applicable to dental implant designs as cleanliness and concerns for bacterial invasion in the event of minor bone resorption have, in theory excluded them from use.

The substrate geometry notwithstanding, uniform coverage by the Ca-phosphate coating material is necessary with few or no uncovered areas, cracks, discontinuities, or flaws. The thickness of the coating should be appropriate for the coating substrate being covered such that the macroscopic surface relief or porosity is not occluded, and the mechanical constraints of a ceramic–metal system will not be violated by application of too thick a coating. A study of coating thickness vs. fatigue properties indicates that coatings of less than 100 μm are suitable. Porous-type coatings require a thickness of 30–50 μm, with macro-textured surfaces requiring a nominal thickness of 50–80 μm.

## BIOLOGIC RESPONSE TO CALCIUM PHOSPHATE COATINGS

HA and HA combined with TCP are the most common Ca-phosphate coatings tested and reported to date. Most coatings have been developed in hopes of the highest possible HA content, as HA has the longest-term established biologic profile and is considered to be more biologically stable than TCP.

The initial interest in development of bioactive coatings for implants was generated by several studies that revealed the direct biologic bonding of synthetic HA to bone tissue; this direct bonding phenomenon has never been established for TCP and, conceptually, would be a different mechanism as the crystallographic registry between bone mineral and synthetic polycrystalline HA is different (1–10). A high level of TCP, even when combined with HA as a minor phase, has been shown to be an unpredictably bioresorbable coating that may compromise the short-term biologic bonding effect seen with HA coatings. A classic example of this effect is a formerly available commercial dental implant system with a high-TCP coating that provoked significant implant exfoliation due to dissolution and separation of the coating (49–51). In this reporting of a series of reported biologic profiles, it is extremely important to remember that all HA coatings are not identical and vary among manufacturers in their composition, crystallinity, density, purity, and structure. Any change in one or more of these properties will significantly affect the coating's bioactivity, biologic response and bioresorption characteristics.(50-51) Therefore, the biological responses summarized below do not apply to all coatings, and one must not generalize or predict the biologic profile of a given coating on the basis of its *in vitro* characteristics.

Likewise, all data in support of one HA-coating, for example, cannot be cited as supportive of any other coating. Another complicating circumstance in reporting or trying to compare *in vivo* data reported by many investigators at a variety of institutions is the difference in test techniques employed. The results reported by Geesink and associates (52–55) are an example of how selected data can fall far outside that expected and observed by other investigators. A later clarification of these particular data stated that the *in vivo* strength originally reported may have been biased erroneously high because the sample was stored in formalin before testing rather than tested fresh immediately after harvesting, as practiced by other investigators (56). It would therefore be appropriate to make comparisons from published literature only among investigations performed and analyzed using similar, if not identical, experimental techniques; several institutions have a long history of using certain animal evaluation models on a variety of biomaterials, and therefore can provide both a qualitative and quantitative comparative database.

Although the coating of smooth metallic substrates with HA does not provide macroscopic surface protection for the coating, many investigators have tested such a system to demonstrate the chemical bonding effects provided by HA when compared with uncoated metal implant materials. Using the transcortical model, several studies have consistently demonstrated the enhanced attachment strength for HA-coated implants, the speed at which the bone adapts to the implant, and its ultimate strength of attachment (18–21,24–27,57–59).

Typically, smooth implant surfaces, roughened to within the range of 4 – 10 um surface roughness, show a four- to eightfold increase in attachment strength as compared with uncoated metallic implants. The microscopic surface roughness of the metallic surfaces was prepared to roughly equate that of the HA-coated surfaces, which have natural micro-undulations. This is important in determining that the effects of HA are not due to the more roughened surface of the implants (26). As previously mentioned, one series of erroneously high push-out test results has been attributed to storing samples in formalin, with more recent data study from this same investigative group reporting values that are much more consistent with other investigators. A study on the effect of formalin, however, introduces controversy because, in this study, no effect of formalin was observed (60). A recent compilation of different coatings, compared using the same model at the same test institution, found that the degree of porosity correlated well with *in vivo* performance; the greater the porosity within the coating, the poorer the push-out test results (61).

Using intermedullary placements, several investigators have reported positive results for HA coatings on smooth substrates as compared with their microtextured, uncoated counterparts (24–26, 53–55, 58,60). An interesting report of the transcortical model on HA-coated/noncoated implants demonstrated that substantial line defects through the coating to the substrate had no significant effect on the biologic response or the performance of the coating up to 32 weeks postimplantation (25). In one study, the short-term (five and ten weeks) effects of intermedullary rod placement showed significant increases in bone attachment (62,63) and, in another study, the long-term effects of HA coating on a smooth intermedullary-like canine hip implant that was sectioned for precision interfacial push-outs revealed a significant effect of HA coating at 18 months postimplantation (64,65). In both studies, high-crystallinity coatings were utilized.

Taking into consideration the physical limitations of contemporary HA coatings, an interesting concept for protecting the coating from pure shear forces and providing a mechanical as well as chemical adaptive mechanism is surface macrotexturing (7,48,66). The benefits of combining surface macrotexturing of the underlying metal with an HA coating applied over it have been confirmed by studies using semicircular and trapezoidal grooved implants, although the enhancement of strength was not as dramatic as for smooth surfaces (24,67). The reason is that the macrotextured uncoated controls themselves increase their amount of bone retention without the effect of HA, although not to the same level of performance (24,59,67,68).

HA increases the early proliferation of new bone on the HA-coated surfaces at very short periods postimplantation, and also increases, albeit to a lesser degree, bone attachment strength. These early observations on macrotextured transcortical implants demonstrated that HA coatings maintained the osteophilic and osteoconductive nature of the material in coating form and allowed the bone to be enticed into areas it would not normally occupy if the implant substrates were not coated. A series of macrotextured implants using the transcortical model, was conducted for periods of up to one year. The macrotextured implants provided the same evidence as the earlier studies, maintained to one year postimplantation at which time the HA coating was shown to be intact and provided enhancement in both strength and histologic profile (59,68). With a high-quality HA coating that maintains its integrity to one year postimplantation, push-out results equivalent to those of fully ingrown porous structures have been achieved. This finding has potentially significant implications for manufacturing technology and the ability to decrease the cost of human femoral implant devices, as application of surface macrotextures is a much less costly process than application of a porous coating to the surface of an implant component.

HA-coated canine hip prostheses have been studied for periods up to 12 months (52–55,64,65,69). Geesink and colleagues (52–55) investigated implants that were designed to mimic a macrotextured human femoral component and reported superior results with the HA-coated devices on the basis of implant fixation and direct bone contact, unlike the fibrous connective tissue layer observed adjacent to the counterpart uncoated implants. Although no functional difference was observed between groups, HA-coated implants did provide a more attractive interfacial structure over periods up to one year.

It may be that with that particular model the functional differences would not be manifested until a longer time postimplantation. In another model comparing a macrotextured surface with and without HA, the coated devices exhibited direct bone apposition at five weeks postimplantation whereas the uncoated textured devices had no direct bone contact for periods up to 10 weeks (69). Again, the HA served as an osteophilic substrate for bone proliferation directly on the surface of the implant device.

In another immediately loaded canine total hip arthroplasty model, another group of investigators compared a grooved proximally filling canine stem and acetabular component with an uncoated metallic porous system (70). The results showed that the coating was unchanged at 13 months postimplantation and that at both six weeks and 13 months, the time periods of observation, the HA-coated macrotextured surfaces provided greater resistance to micromotion when tested in a torque mode, and lysis (around the femoral component) was markedly decreased at both time periods. The results of this study indicate that an HA coating, that does not bioresorb over short time periods, would have the potential for maintaining a proximal seal around the femoral component of a total hip replacement and could perhaps decrease the incidence of particulate-induced lysis around the distal stem. Although this has been demonstrated only in one long-term study and with one coating, the results of long-term clinical evaluations of different stem designs and different HA coatings in the proximal area of various stem designs may demonstrate this to be an added benefit of such coatings.

A third group of studies has focused on the application of Ca-phosphate and HA coatings on porous substrates. Here, it is possible that the composition need not be optimized as HA and a significant proportion of TCP or other phase could be present; in support of this HA/TCP mixture, the theory is that the coating is there only for the earliest response, to entice the bone into the porosity and that afterwards the device design and the ingrown bone/stress transfer contribute to the long-term efficacy of the implant (71,72). Nevertheless, the first report of a primarily TCP coating was produced by a slurry-casting technique and was evaluated on porous, stainless steel intermedullary implants (73). The pull-out strength was compared to uncoated control porous implants for as long as 12 weeks postimplantation. The coating was found to enhance the pull-out strength significantly but approached equivalency at the 12-week time period.

Likewise, another study demonstrated that another plasma-sprayed Ca-phosphate coating applied to a titanium fiber-mesh porous intermedullary implant provided significantly greater attachment strength as compared with the uncoated control for as long as six weeks postimplantation (71). Another study with dipping coating of TCP reported equivalent increases in the short term in yet another intermedullary model (72). An early report of an HA coating on an irregular, porous-structure titanium coating showed early advantages of the HA coating and significant advantage for bone ingrowth, with mechanical equivalence by push-out test demonstrated at approximately 32 weeks (24).

Two other investigators have demonstrated that HA applied to porous, bead-type coatings demonstrates sustained, statistically significant increases to one year postimplantation, based on the presence of a high-quality HA coating on those porous structures as compared with their uncoated controls (57,75). Likewise, the same stable HA when applied to bead porous-coated implants, shows the ability to counteract, to some extent, the presence of a gap between the implant surface and the actual implant placement (57,74–78). This result supports the notion that HA coatings are most beneficial when used in implants where imprecise fits are anticipated, such as total joint revision surgery or placement of dental implants in compromised sites such as fresh tooth extraction sites (50,76,79). Using the transcortical and intermedullary implant models, HA over beaded, porous CoCr, compared with uncoated controls, was carried out for precision press-fit placements and implants placed with gaps between the implant surface and the bone site of 0.5, 1, and 2, for periods up to 52 weeks. HA-coated devices had bone ingrowth at six weeks equivalent to that requiring 12 weeks for the uncoated porous implants for the precision placement. The effect of gaps, in all cases, was to retard the bone adaptation, but the advantage of HA was still significant for gaps as large as 1 mm. The application of HA over porous substrates appears to provide a "belt-and-suspenders" approach towards the use of this new technology.

The results of more than 10 years of study of many Ca-phosphate coatings lead these authors to believe that under optimal conditions, the HA coating will remain for long periods and will provide a continued mechanism for bone enhancement in and around the porous-coated portions of the implant (80,81). In the event that the HA coatings become dissolved long after implantation (after two series of functional remodeling, at a minimum), the coating would have served its function and the device design and the bone that had been enticed into the porosity via the coating would serve as the long-term attachment mechanism of stress transfer medium for the implant. The ability of a nonporous macrotextured surface to serve such a role still remains to be demonstrated in long-term studies.

Many smaller specific studies have been conducted on HA and other Ca-phosphate coatings for specific purposes, to develop a definitive model to study a potential future application or to develop an initial biologic profile. Increasing sections of symposia abstracts attest to the increase in the use of HA coating (82–92). These studies consistently demonstrate the ability of HA to enhance the initial biologic response, regardless of the substrate. One group, however, reports recent studies in which a "hydroxylapatite" coating has been applied and the merits of such coatings as seen by others were not observed (93). The composition or source of the coating is not revealed and points to the necessity for complete characterization of the coating on a comparative basis with those that have been demonstrated to provide significant enhancements.

Table 1 summarizes some of the interfacial shear attachment strengths reported for HA coated implants. It must be emphasized that direct comparisons from published literature are not directly comparable because the experimental conditions under which the tests were performed vary immensely. The results presented in Table 1 were not obtained under identical conditions; in identical models, or on identical implant geometries, and are included only to provide a reference for some of the published data on such coatings.

Many centers have reported a consistent early enhancement of the bone–implant attachment strength resulting from the placement of Ca-phosphate in HA coatings. Early enhancement can be seen with TCP and in HA/TCP combinations, whereas the longer-term *in vivo* data are available only for HA coatings. Implants of smooth, macrotextured, and porous surfaces have been investigated, with significant increases in speed of attachment for the HA vs. uncoated controls.

Enhancements available using HA-coated macrotextures and porosities are roughly equivalent, but it remains to be seen whether the human counterpart devices using macrotextures will withstand the long-term cyclic loading associated with fully ingrown porous devices. Equally as compelling as the increases in mechanical strength associated with HA-coated implants are the histologic findings demonstrating new bone formation directly on the HA-coated surfaces of the device and the elimination or minimization of fibrous tissue on the surface of the implants. The osteoconductive and osteophilic nature of the HA coating has been documented for the coated implants, which may ultimately be their greatest asset because speculation of resorption by natural remodeling mechanisms may be the fate of all coatings.

## SUMMARY AND AREAS FOR FUTURE WORK

### Advantages of Calcium-Phosphate Coatings

At this stage of understanding, HA appears to be the appropriate Ca-phosphate crystalline species for coated implants. Even for porous implants, a longer-lasting "bone magnet" appears to represent the composition of choice. Properly characterized and applied, HA coatings appear to provide an incremental increase in early performance, measured by bone-attachment strength, the speed of this attachment, and by enhanced bone deposition on the surface of the implant. Decreases or elimination of fibrous tissue seams for periods up to 18 months have been observed, and there is the potential for HA-coated implants to counteract, to some degree, the lack of precision associated with contemporary implant installation techniques.

Such HA coatings have been shown to form a direct, chemically-based bond to living bone and offer the potential for true biologic fixation of implants. The advantages observed, however, have been quantitatively reported for experimental studies conducted only in animals. Clearly, the coatings available at present need to be applied to a substrate metal design that provides protection of the coating from pure shear stresses, once bonding occurs, as the attachment mechanisms for coatings to metals are relatively primitive today.

### Questions raised by *In vivo* Studies Conducted To Date

Over the last 10 years, HA coatings have progressed from a laboratory curiosity to early clinical evaluation. What has been learned by the longer-term animal studies and the earliest human clinical evaluations is promising, but there is a tendency by some to overlook some unresolved issues in the excitement of analyzing the early results. The effects of short-term and long-term dissolution, either by solution or cell-mediated means (or combinations thereof), *in vivo* coating separation, and/or fracture are still issues that perhaps only long-term controlled human clinical evaluations and/or widespread human

**TABLE 1** : Selected *In-Vivo* Interfacial Shear Attachment For HA-Coated Implants

| Time Weeks | Cook (26) HA | Uncoated | Thomas (24) HA | Uncoated | Poser (58) Ha | Uncoated |
|---|---|---|---|---|---|---|
| 3 | — | — | 6.05 (1.94) | 4.43 (1.32) | 6.04 (3.02) | 1.31 (0.69) |
| 5 | 6.96 (3.22) | 0.93 (0.57) | 9.56 (3.55) | 4.88 (1.01) | — | — |
| 6 | — | — | — | — | 8.75 (1.99) | 2.80 (1.16) |
| 10 | 7.27 (2.08) | 0.98 (0.73) | 14.17 (4.87) | 10.53 (3.29) | — | — |
| 12 | — | — | — | — | 8.17 (1.09) | 2.84 (0.46) |
| 26 | — | — | 12.12 (2.43) | — | — | — |
| 32 | 6.07 (1.29) | 1.21 (0.77) | — | — | — | — |
| 52 | — | — | — | — | 11.06 (2.72) | 5.51 (1.66) |
| Implant description | CP-Ti uncoated grit blasted | | CP-Ti grooved uncoated grit blasted | | Ti6Al4V uncoated grit blasted | |
| Animal model | Canine femoral TC pushout | | Canine femoral TC pushout | | Canine femoral TC pushout | |

| Time Weeks | Poser (97) HA | Uncoated | Cook (74) HA | Uncoated | Dalton (74,78) HA | Uncoated |
|---|---|---|---|---|---|---|
| 2 | — | — | 5.04 (1.79) | 3.11 (1.60) | — | — |
| 3 | 9.38 (1.67) | 7.01 (1.00) | — | : | — | — |
| 4 | — | — | 9.17 (4.20) | 6.95 (2.17) | 1.83 (0.98) | 1.18 (1.22) |
| 6 | 11.10 (2.31) | 6.55 (1.67) | 12.80 (2.30) | 10.50 (2.08) | — | — |
| 8 | — | — | 12.60 (2.72) | 10.52 (2.26) | 5.37 (2.42) | 2.81 (1.81) |
| 12 | 13.61 (2.86) | 8.92 (2.99) | 15.73 (2.36) | 11.10 (1.46) | 9.11 (5.43) | 3.70 (1.96) |
| 18 | — | — | 23.15 (3.64) | 17.58 (3.10) | — | — |
| 24 | — | — | — | — | 9.60 (4.55) | 5.57 (3.24) |
| 26 | 18.09 (3.35) | 14.80 (3.13) | 27.06 (2.36) | 22.08 (3.88) | — | — |
| 52 | 18.49 (3.77) | 13.05 (4.23) | 21.21 (3.80) | 18.71 (3.74) | 11.44 (5.82) | 4.71 (2.68) |
| Implant description | Ti6Al4V grooved uncoated grit blasted | | Co-Cr-Mo spherical beads porous | | Ti6Al4V spherical beads porous | |
| Animal model | Canine femur TC pushout | | Canine femur TC pushout | | Canine femur IM pushout | |

clinical experience can totally determine.

The subject of coating stability (or lack thereof) is a controversial issue that is still not well understood. The if, when, and consequences of coating resorption are not understood at all, and the factors that may affect such behavior are being debated. Causes could be related to coating chemistry, structure, porosity, (surface area), or a combination thereof (49–51,65,68,94–97). The ultimate fate of all Ca-phosphate coatings may be physiologic resorption by natural mechanisms, as part of the bone remodeling process (95–97).

After all, the coatings available today represent our best effort to mimic naturally occurring bone mineral. This controversy is an extension of one debated several years earlier on the permanence and ultimate fate of various forms of particulate Ca-phosphates (4,11–13,36,98). It is clear that all HA and Ca-phosphate coatings available today are not equivalent; coatings can differ in chemical, physical, and structural values and in their index of biologic activity. There exists a meaningful concern regarding the standards and analytical techniques to be employed by manufacturers who apply coatings. Techniques may yet need to be developed that unequivocally establish guidelines for obtaining proper analysis, with quality standards based on these techniques to follow.

The data presented in this short summary of the biologic responses observed to date are based on animal evaluations that, at first blush, appear extremely attractive. The direct correlation to responses, time frames and effects in human beings is only speculative, although based on reasonable expectations of similarities based on the generic nature of bone response. In addition, the implants and stresses imparted from the animal implants used in the preclinical evaluations summarized do not translate directly to the scale and magnitude of surface features experienced by implants installed in human beings.

Finally, any new technology has its proponents and skeptics. The true value of any material or technique delivered to the hard tissue implant marketplace has always been an average of the most enthusiastic and the most pessimistic viewpoints of the technology at a time such as this in the development of the bioactive coatings. It has been said that these coatings represent an incremental increase in performance over uncoated metallic implants, but the magnitude of this incremental increase has yet to be firmly established. Until long-term human implantation data are available from controlled, prospectively defined studies, reports regarding HA coatings must be viewed in a somewhat critical light and compared to the responses of other technologies at equivalent points in their developmental timeframe.

## Areas for Future Development

Based on the responses and perceived weaknesses summarized in this work, areas for the immediate future coating development would be the establishment of analytical techniques and standards by which the application of the coatings could be controlled in a more uniform fashion. The attachment of the coatings to the substrate metal, no matter what its form, is clearly an area that could well be perceived as being the area of greatest attention. As advances in each of these and other areas progress, the predictability and perhaps the clinical efficacy of the use of HA coatings will increase such that the incremental step in performance is a significant one.

# REFERENCES

1. Brown WE, Smith JP, Lehr JR, et al., Crystallo-graphic nature and chemical relations between octacalcium phosphate and hydroxylapatite, *Nature*, 1962: 196-1050.
2. McConnell D, *Apatite*, New York: Springer-Verlag, 1973.
3. Posner AS, Betts F, Synthetic amorphous calcium phosphate and its relation to bone mineral structure, *Accounts in Chemical Research*, 1975; 8:273.
4. LeGeros RZ, *Calcium phosphate in oral biology and medicine*, New York: Karger, publ., 1991.
5. Standard specification for ceramic hydroxylapatite for surgical implants; ASTM, F-1185-89.
6. Standard specifications for tricalcium phosphate for surgical implants; ASTM, F-1088-87.
7. Jarcho M, Bolen CH, Thomas MB, et al., Hydroxyl-apatite synthesis and characterization in dense poly-crystalline form. *Journal of Material Science*, 1976;11:2027.
8. Jarcho M, Salsbury RI, Thomas MB, et al., Synthesis and fabrication of beta-tricalcium phosphate ceramics for potential prosthetic applications. *Journal of Material Science*, 1979; 14:142,.
9. Eanes ED, Thermochemical studies on amorphous calcium phosphate, *Calcified Tissue Response*, 1970;5:133.
10. Eanes ED, Gillessen IH, Posner AS, Intermediate states in the precipitation of hydroxylapatite, *Nature*, 1965; 208:365.
11. deGroot K, Bioceramics consisting of calcium phosphate salts, *Biomaterials*, 1980;1:47.
12. Jarcho M.: Biomaterial aspects of calcium phosphates, *Dental Clinics of North America*, 1980; 30:25.
13. Jarcho M., Calcium phosphate ceramics as hard tissue prosthetics, *Clinical Orthopaedics*, 1981;157:259.
14. Roy DM, Linnehan SK, Hydroxylapatite formed from coral skeletal carbonate by hydrothermal exchange, *Nature*, 1974; 247:220.
15. Rejda BV, Peelen JGJ, deGroot K, Tricalcium phosphate as a bone substitute, *Journal of Bioengineering*, 1977;1:93.
16. Hassler CR, McCoy LG, Rotaru JH. Long-term implants of solid tricalcium phosphate, *Proceedings of 27th Annual Conference of Engineering Medicine and Biology*,1974;16:488.
17. Sayler K, Holmes R, Johns D. Replamineform porous hydroxylapatite as bone substitute in craniofacial osseous reconstruction. *Journal of Dental Research*, 1977;56B:173.
18. Anderson RC, Cook SD, Weinstein AM, Haddad RJ. An evaluation of skeletal attachment to LTI pyrolytic carbon, porous titanium, and carbon-coated porous titanium implants, *Clinical Orthopaedics*, 1984; 182:242.
19. Cook SD, Walsh KA, Haddad RJ. Interface mechanics and bone growth into porous Co-Cr-Mo alloy implants, *Clinical Orthopaedics*, 1985;193:271.
20. Thomas KA, Cook SD. An evaluation of variables influencing implant fixation by direct bone apposition, *Journal of Biomedical Materials Research*, 1985; 19:875.
21. Thomas KA, Cook SD, Renz EA, Anderson RC, Haddad RJ, Haubold AD, Yapp R. The effect of surface treatments on the interface mechanics on LTI pyrolytic carbon implants, *Journal of Biomedical Materials Research*, 1985; 19:145.
22. Jowsey J, Kelley PJ, Riggs BL, Bianco AJ, Scholz DS, Gershon-Cohen, J.: Quantitative microradiographic studies of normal and osteoporotic bone, *Journal of Bone and Joint Surgery*, 1965; 47A:758.
23. Klawitter JJ, Hulbert SF. Applications of porous ceramics for the attachment of load bearing internal orthopedic applications, *Journal of Biomedical Materials Research Symposium*, 1971; 2(1):161.
24. Thomas KA, Kay JF, Cook SD, et al. The effect of surface macrotexture and hydroxylapatite coatings on the mechanical strengths and histological profiles of titanium implant materials, *Journal of Biomedical Materials Research*,1987; 21:1395.

25.    Cook SD. Experimental Coating Defects in hydroxylapatite-coated implants, *Clinical Orthopaedics*,1991; 265:80.

26.    Cook SD, Kay JF, Thomas K, et al. Interface mechanics and histology of titanium and hydroxylapatite coated titanium for dental implant applications, *Journal of Oral Maxillofacial Implants*, 1987; 2:15.

27.    Cook SD, Kay JF, Thomas K, et al. Hydroxylapatite coated porous titanium for use as an orthopaedic biological attachment system, *Clinical Orthopaedics*,1988;230-303.

28.    Kay JF. *Physiological acceptance of a ceramic bone implant determined by electron microscopic analysis.* Doctorate thesis, Rensselaer Polytechnic Institute, Troy, New York, 1977.

29.    Jarcho M, Kay JF, Gumaer K, et al. Tissue, cellular and subcellular events at a bone-ceramic hydroxylapatite interface, *Journal of Bioengineering*, 1977; 1:79.

30.    Kay JF, Doremus R, Jarcho M. Ion micromilling of bone-implant interfaces. *Procedures of 4th Annual Meeting Society for Biomaterials*, 1978; San Antonio, 154.

31.    Tracy B, Doremus R. Director electron microscopy; studies of the bone hydroxylapatite interface, *Journal of Biomedical Materials Research*, 1984; 18:719.

32.    Ogiso M. Basic research on apatite ceramics and clinical application to dental implants. *Quintessence* 1985; 4:61.

33.    Hubbard W. *Physiological calcium phosphates as orthopaedic biomaterials,* Ph.D. Thesis, Marquette University, 1974.

34.    Driskell TD, Hassler CB, McCoy LR. The significance of resorbable bioceramics in the repair of bone defects, *Procedures of the 26th Annual Conference of English Medical Biologists* 1973;15:199.

35.    Driskell TD, Hassler CR, Tennery VJ, McCoy LR, Clarke WJ. Calcium phosphate resorbable ceramics: A potential alternative to bone grafting, *Journal of Dental Research*, 1973; 52:123.

36.    Lemons JE. Response of combined electrical stimulation and applied laboratory and clinical studies on biodegradable ceramic, *U.S. Army Medical Reserve Development Commission*, DAMD, 1983;17.79.C9173.

37.    Hench L, Paschall HA, Allen WC, Piotrowski G. *An investigation of bonding mechanisms at the interface of a prosthetic material.* Report No. 4, Contract No. DADA 17-70-C-0001, 1978.

38.    Hench L. Development of a new biomaterial-prosthetic device: In Ghista DH, Roaf R. eds., *Orthopedic Mechanics: Procedures and Devices*, London, Academic Press, 1978; 287.

39.    Hench L, Ethridge EC. B*iomaterials: An interfacial approach*, Academic Press, New York, NY, 1982.

40.    Kokubo T, Ito S, Shigematsu M, Sakka S, Yamamuro T. Mechanical property of a new type of apatite-containing glass ceramic for prosthetic application. *Journal of Material Science,* 1985; 20:2001-4.

41.    Nakamura T, Yamamuro T, Higashi S. A new glass-ceramic for bone replacement: evaluation of its bonding to bone tissue. *Journal of Biomedical Materials Research*, 1985; 19:685-98.

42.    Yamamuro T, Shikata J, Kakutani Y, Yoshii S, Kitsugi T, Ono K. *Novel methods for clinical applications of bioactive ceramics in bioceramics: material characteristics versus in vivo behavior:* Ducheyne, Lemons, eds., NY Academy of Science Press, 1988.

43.    Herman H. Advances in thermal spray technology, *Advanced Materials and Processes,* 1990; 137:(No.4) 41-5.

44.    Kulkarni KM, Anand V. Metal powders used for hardsurfacing, *In: Metals Handbook, 9th Ed., Vol.7, Powder Metallurgy,* American Society for Metals, Metals Park, OH, 1984; 832-6.

45.    d'Angelo C, El Joundi H. Reliable coatings via plasma arc spraying, *Advanced Materials and Processes,*1988;134(No.6):414.

46.    Rivero DP, Fox J, Skipor AK, Urban RM, Galante JO. Calcium phosphate-coated porous titanium implants for enhanced skeletal fixation, *Journal of Biomedical Materials Research*, 1988; 22:191-201.

47.    FDA Draft document for metallic, surface treatment, orthopaedic implant guidance Document, March 13, 1992.

48.    Kay JF. Designing to counteract the effects of initial device instability: materials and engineering, *Journal of Biomedical Materials Research,*1988; 22:1127.

49.    Kay J. Bioactive Surface Coatings for Hard Tissue Biomaterials, In: Yamamuro, M., Hench L., Wilson, J., eds., *Handbook of Bioactive Ceramics*, ed. 3, Boca Raton, FL, CRC Press, 1990; 111:122.

50.   Kay JF. Bioactive Surface Coatings: Cause for Encouragement and Concern, *Journal of Oral Implants,*1988; 14:43.
51.   Kay JF. Calcium Phosphate coatings for dental implants: current status and future potential, *Dental Clinics of North America,* 1992; 36:1-18.
52.   Geesink RGT. *Hydroxylapatite coated hip implants,* Doctoral Dissertation, State University of Limburg, Maastricht, Netherlands, 1988.
53.   Geesink RGT, deGroot K, Klein CPAT. Chemical implant fixation using hydroxylapatite coatings, *Clinical Orthopedics and Related Research,* 1987; 225:147-70.
54.   deGroot K, Geesink R, Klein CPAT, Serekian P. Plasma sprayed coatings and hydroxylapatite, *Journal of Biomedical Materials Research,* 1987; 21:1375-81.
55.   Geesink RGT, deGroot K, Klein CPAT. Bonding of bone to apatite-coated implants, *Journal of Bone and Joint Surgery,* 1988; 70-b:17-22.
56.   deGroot K, Thomas KA. Letter to editor and reply, *Journal of Biomedical Materials Research,* 1989; 23:1367-71.
57.   Cook SS, Thomas KA, Dalton JE, Volkman TK, Whitecloud TS, Kay JF. Hydroxylapatite coating of porous implants improves bone ingrowth and interface attachment strength. *Journal of Biomedical Materials Research,* 1992; 26:989-1001.
58.   Poser RD, Magee FP, Kay JF, Hedley AK. *In vivo* characterization of an hydroxylapatite coating, *Transcripts of the Society of Biomaterials,* 1990; 16:170.
59.   Poser RD, May TC, Kay JF, Emmanual J, Werner ME. Hydroxylapatite coated macrotextured titanium interface study, *Transcripts of the Society of Biomaterials,*1991; 17:171.
60.   Van DeWyngaerde D, Magee FP, Kay JF. Effects of speciman handling on transcortical orthopaedic implants. *Procedures of the Academy of Surgical Research,* 5th Annual Meeting, Atlanta, GA, 1989.
61.   Cook SD, Dalton JE. Biocompatibility and biofunctionality materials: tissue response to implanted materials. *In: Endosseous Implants for Maxillofacial Reconstruction,* M. Block, ed., in Press, 1992.
62.   Manley MT, Kay JF, Uratsuji M, Stern LS, Stulberg BN. Hydroxylapatite coatings applied to implants subjected to functional loads. *Transcripts of the Society of Biomaterials,* 1987; 13:210.
63.   Manley MT, Kay JF, Yoshiya S, Stern LS, Stulberg BN. Accelerated fixation of weight bearing implants by hydroxylapatite coatings. *Transcripts of the Orthopaedic Research Society,*1987; 12:214.
64.   Poser RD, Magee FP, Kay JF, Toal TR, Hedley AK. Biomechanical and histologic assessment of HA enhanced long-term fixation in a unique loaded canine implant. *Fourth World Biomaterials Congress,* Berlin, Germany, April 24-28, 1992.
65.   Poser RD, Kay JF, Magee FP, Hedley AK. Pre- clinical evaluation of the effect of hydroxylapatite on the comprehensive bone-implant interface. ASTM, *STP characterization and performance of calcium phosphate coatings for implants.* Parr J, Horowitz E. eds., In Press, 1992.
66.   Kay JF. A new concept for noncement fixation of orthopaedic devices. *Techniques in Orthopaedics,* 1987; 2:1.
67.   Poser RD, May TC, Kay JF, Emmanuel J, Werner ME. Enhancement of macrotextured titanium interface stress by hydroxylapatite. *Transcripts of Combined Meeting of Orthopedic Research Society of USA, Japan and Canada,* 1991, in Press.
68.   Poser RD, May TC, Kay JF, Emmanual J, Koeneman JB, Hedley AK. Long-term performance and load sharing effects of HA coated macrotextured titanium. *Fourth World Biomaterials Congress,* Berlin, Germany, April 24-28, 1992.
69.   Thomas KA, Cook SD, Haddad RJ, Kay JF, Jarcho M. Biologic Response to hydroxyapatite-coated titanium hips. *Journal of Arthroplasty,* 1989; 4:143.
70.   Taylor JK, Bargar WB, Kay JF et al. *Effect of hydroxylapatite coating on proximal bone adaptation and mechanical stability.* Accepted for Presentation, 60th Mtg, American Academy of Orthopedic Surgeons, San Francisco, CA 1993.
71.   Rivero DP, Fox J, Skipor AK, Urban RM, Galante JO. Calcium phosphate-coated porous titanium implants for enhanced skeletal gixation. *Journal of Biomedical Materials Research,* 1988; 22:191-201.
72.   Berry JL, Geiger JM, Moran JM, Skraba JS, Greenwald AS. Use of tricalcium phosphate or electrical stimulation to enhance the bone-porous implant interface. *Journal of Biomedical Materials Research,* 1986; 20:65.

73.     Ducheyne P, Hench L, Kagan A, Martens M, Bursens A, Mulier J. Effect of hydroxyapatite impregnation on skeletal bonding of porous coated implants. *Journal of Biomedical Materials Research,* 1980; 14:225-37.

74.     Cook SD, Thomas KA, Dalton JE, Kay JF. Enhanced bone ingrowth and fixation strength with hydroxylapatite-coated porous implants. *Seminars in Arthroplasty,* 1991; 2:4:268.

75.     Cook SD, Thomas KA, Dalton JE, Volkman T, Kay JF. Enhancement of bone ingrowth and fixation strength by hydroxylapatite coating porous implants, *Transcripts of the 37th Meeting of the Orthopedic Research Society,* 1991;16:550.

76.     Kay JF. Hydroxylapatite coatings for non-precision implant placements. *Proceedings of the HARC Symposium,* 49, 1992.

77.     Thomas KA, Cook SD, Dalton JE, Baffes JC, Halvorson TL, Kay JF. The effects of surgical fit and hydroxylapatite coating upon the biologic and mechanical response to porous implants, *Transcripts of the 17th American Meeting of the Society of Biomaterials,* 1991; 14:172.

78.     Dalton JE. *Effects of surgical fit and hydroxylapatite coatings on the mechanical and biological response to porous implants,* Masters Thesis, Tulane Univ, New Orleans, LA, 1991.

79.     Kay JF. Hydroxylapatite coatings for non-precision implant placements, A*STM Special Technical Publication Calcium Phosphate Coatings,* In Press, 1992.

80.     Søballe K, Stender Hansen ES, Brockstedt-Rassmussen HB, Pedersen CM, Bünger C. Hydroxyapatite coating enhances fixation of porous coated implants, *Acta Orthopaedica Scandinavica,* 1990;61(4):299,.

81.     Søballe K, Hansen ES, Brockstedt-Rassmussen H, Juhl GI, Pedersen CM, Knudsen V, Huid I, Bunger C. Enhancement of Osteopenic and normal bone ingrowth into porous coated implants by hydroxyapatite coating, *Transcripts of the Orthopedic Research Society,* 1989: 14:554.

82.     *Transcript 37th Meeting Orthopedic Research Society,* 1991; Vol 16.

83.     *Transcript 36th Meeting Orthopedic Research Society,* 1990; Vol 15.

84.     *Transcript 35th Meeting Orthopedic Research Society,* 1989; Vol 14.

85.     *Transcript 34th Meeting Orthopedic Research Society,* 1988; Vol 13.

86.     *Transcript 33th Meeting Orthopedic Research Society,* 1987; Vol 12.

87.     *Transcript 18th Annual Meeting Society Biomaterials,* 1992; Vol 15.

88.     *Transcript 17th Annual Meeting Society Biomaterials,* 1991; Vol 14..

89.     *Transcript 16th Annual Meeting Society Biomaterials,* 1990; Vol 13.

90.     *Transcript 15th Annual Meeting Society Biomaterials,* 1989; Vol 12.

91.     *Transcript 14th Annual Meeting Society Biomaterials,* 1988; Vol 11.

92.     *Transcript 13th Annual Meeting Society Biomaterials,* 1987; Vol 10.

93.     Gottlander M, Albrektsson T. Histomorphometric analysis of hydroxylapatite coated and uncoated titanium implants. *Clinical Oral Implant Research,* 1992; 3:71-6.

94.     Søballe K, Gotfredsen K, Brockstedt-Rasmussen H, Nielsen PT, Rechnagel K. Histological analysis of a retrieved hydroxylapatite coated femoral prosthesis, *Clinical Orthopaedics,* 1991; 268.

95.     Bloebaum PD, Merrell M, Gustke K, Simmons M. Retrieval analysis of a hydroxylapatite coated hip prosthesis, *Clinical Orthopaedics,* 1991;267:97-102.

96.     Bauer TW, Geesink RGT, Zimmerman RC, McMahon JT: Histologic analysis of HA coated human femoral stems, *Transcript 17th Annual Meeting Society Biomaterials,* 1991; 14, 174.

97.     Poser RD. *The Bone-implant interface: The role of hydroxylapatite in optimizing long-term fixation.* Osteonics Corporation-Bio-Interfaces, Inc. Technical Publication, #LSA11,1992.

98.     Ducheyne P, Lemons J. B*ioceramics: Material characteristics versus in vivo behavior,* New York: NY Academy of Science Press, 1988.

Hydroxylapatite Coatings in Orthopaedic Surgery,
edited by R. G. T. Geesink and M. T. Manley.
Raven Press, Ltd., New York, © 1993.

# The Effects of Osteoporosis, Bone Deficiency, Bone Grafting, and Micromotion on Fixation of Porous-Coated Versus Hydroxylapatite-Coated Implants

Kjeld Søballe, M.D., Ebbe S. Hansen, M.D.,
Helle B. Rasmussen, M.D., and Cody Bünger, M.D., Ph.D.

The number of revisions that must be performed because of mechanical loosening after total hip replacement has been predicted to increase steadily from year to year (1). The results after revision arthroplasty are clearly inferior to those of primary arthroplasty with an eight-year survival rate of 75% (2) and even worse results after re-revision (3).

Indeed, great demands are placed on total joint replacements. The load transmitted on hip and knee prostheses may be up to six times body weight and, especially in younger active patients, the conventional prostheses do not live up to expectations. Younger active patients usually outlive the fixation of the prosthesis, and there is widespread concern about the considerable risk of failure in these patients, especially because of the subsequent need for even more difficult operative treatment with less beneficial results (2-5). Patients with diseased bone, such as those with rheumatoid arthritis, are also at increased risk for early mechanical loosening (1). These facts have led to increased interest in other principles for implant fixation, primarily by means of biologic fixation to the bone without the use of bone cement (6).

Different types and designs of noncemented prostheses are now available, but thus far no evidence suggests that noncemented joint replacements perform better than cemented prostheses. Clinical retrieval studies of noncemented metal porous-coated hip and knee prostheses have revealed that many of the components were fixed to the skeleton by fibrous tissue ingrowth instead of bony ingrowth (7-11). Therefore, great efforts have been concentrated on enhancement of bony ingrowth into the noncemented prosthetic surface. Special interest has focused on hydroxylapatite (HA), which recently has been demonstrated to be successfully coated on a metal surface by a plasma-spray technique (12-14).

This chapter describes a series of experimental studies performed to systematically evaluate potential improvements of bone implant fixation with an HA coating when implants were subjected to pathologic and mechanical conditions mimicking the clinical situation (15-23).

## CLINICAL BACKGROUND AND PURPOSE OF PRESENT STUDIES

In the clinical situation, initial direct apposition of implant to bone is often limited to relatively small areas (24), and most of the porous-coated area of femoral components has been demonstrated to lack osseous contact (25). Anatomic variations in the bone (26), deficient implant design, and poor surgical technique are factors responsible for gaps between the implant surface and surrounding bone. The first step in the series of studies on implant fixation therefore focused on enhancement of bone ingrowth across a gap between bone and implant by HA coating, compared with implants inserted in press-fit.

Most studies on bone ingrowth have been performed on healthy young animals, where bone ingrowth has been found in high percentages. Because many patients with joint disease have deficient bone stock (e.g. with osteoporosis, prolonged steroid treatment, and rheumatoid arthritis), the next challenge in this series of studies called for a new experimental model of osteopenia, because few quantitative data are available on the ingrowth capability of osteopenic bone (27-29). A reproducible experimental model of unilateral arthritis (30) was adapted after a study on juxtaarticular bone loss in experimental arthritis of the knee (16). This model of osteopenia was applied to study the influence of osteopenia of the host bone bed on the fixation of Ti- and HA-coated implants (17). In addition, the effect of HA coating on the healing capacity of osteopenic bone ingrowth into porous-coated implants when surrounded by a gap was studied (18).

The use of bone bank allografts in endoprosthetic surgery has recently gained increasing importance, particularly in cementless reconstruction of failed arthroplasties in which direct fit to host bone cannot be obtained because of loss of bone stock around the loose implant (31-36). Furthermore, disease states of the bone resulting in increased resorption activity, as seen in rheumatoid arthritis (37), may affect the strength of biologic fixation (38) and often require bone grafting for stabilization of cementless prostheses. No previous studies have investigated the combined effect of bone grafting and HA coating. We therefore created a new model to study bone graft incorporation into porous-coated implants and analyzed the incorporation of allogeneic bone graft into Ti- and HA-coated implants as compared with implants without bone graft (19). In addition, the influence of arthritic host bone changes on the incorporation of allogeneic bone graft was studied.

An important cause of inferior bone implant fixation might be the presence of relative motion between implant and bone. Experimental studies of cementless hip and knee prosthetic components implanted into cadaver bone have shown micromotion ranging between 100 and 500 μm (39-44). In clinical studies, inducible displacement of noncemented tibial trays in total knee replacements has been demonstrated to be in the range of 400-1300 μm one year postoperatively (45). These movements might be responsible for fibrous fixation of retrieved noncemented hip and knee prostheses from humans (7-11). Because the degree of micromotion and its effect on bone tissue is difficult to assess in clinical practice, we found it important to create a dynamic system to study the significance of controlled micromotion between bone and implant. In this model we analyzed the host tissue response around porous-coated Ti- and HA-coated implants subjected to controlled relative movements between implant and bone. The implants were subjected to 500 μm movements and 150 μm movements during each gait cycle (20, 21). Both studies revealed interesting findings in motion-induced membrane formation around implants after short-term observation. Several unanswered questions arose concerning the long-term course of the fibrous membrane. We therefore performed one last experiment to study the further course of a motion-induced fibrous membrane around Ti- and HA-coated implants subjected to continuous load (22). Finally, the effect of immobilization of fibrous anchored implants was investigated (22).

## EXPERIMENTAL DESIGN

### Animals

An animal model is advantageous because it is possible to separate the more complex clinical situation into different well-defined elements that can be controlled, enabling us to study isolated problems.

Studies of orthopaedic implants require a certain size of experimental animal. The mature Labrador dog has the appropriate size and its bone structure is close to that of humans (46, 47). Furthermore, this breed is often used for studies on bone ingrowth and has previously been used in our research group for studies on experimentally-induced arthritis (30), which were also applied in the initial studies to investigate bone ingrowth from an osteopenic bone bed. Labrador dogs with known birthdates were delivered in litters (up to seven dogs in each litter), which was advantageous to minimize interindividual variation. The animals were bred for scientific purposes, and the care and use of these laboratory animals complied with the Danish law on animal experimentation.

### Implants

The two types of implant coatings used were plasma-sprayed HA and plasma-sprayed Ti alloy. The cylindrical Ti- and HA-coated plugs were 6 mm in diameter with an overall length of 10 mm, fabricated with a precision of ±0.05 mm. Ti implants consisted of a solid Ti-6A1-4V alloy core with a coating of Ti-6A1-4V deposited by plasma-spray technique resulting in a mean pore size of 300 μm (Fig. 1A).

The HA-coated implants consisted of analogous Ti porous-coated implants on which a layer of spray-dried synthetic HA was deposited by plasma-spraying (Fig. 1B). According to the manufacturer, the strength of attachment between the HA and the substrate, as determined by ASTM standard C-633 for cohesive strength of coatings to metal, revealed minimum tensile strength of 34.5 MPa and a minimum shear strength of 20.7 MPa. Results from x-ray diffraction analysis of the ceramic coating are given in Table 1 including the crystallinity, Ca/P ratio, and coating thickness.

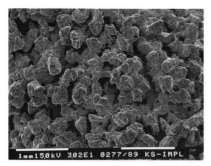 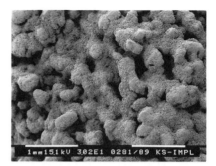

**FIG. 1. (A)** Scanning electron microscopy of titanium (**A**) and hydroxylapatite (**B**) coating. Note the porous structure of titanium coating (A) and the preservation of pores after coating with HA. X 50.  bar = 1 mm. (From ref .22.)

**TABLE 1.** *Characteristics of HA Coatings Used in Different Series.*

| Reference | HA | TCP | Crystallinity | Ca/P | Thicknes |
|---|---|---|---|---|---|
| 15-19 | Yes | Trace (10%) | Mixture of amorphous and crystalline HA | 1.65 | 150-200 μm |
| 20-22 | Yes | No | 75% | 1.64-1.70 | 50-75 μm |

## Models for Implantation

The site for implantation was selected to mimic the clinical patient findings, including presence of a cancellous bone bed. We therefore chose the distal femoral epiphysis as the implantation site because it contains cancellous bone and is affected by arthritic joint changes (30).

Two basically different models were used. In the first five studies an unloaded model was used and in the last three studies a loaded model was used. The unloaded model was employed to study the amount of bone apposition onto HA and Ti implant surfaces under standardized conditions without possible variations in load pattern of the implant.

A gap model was developed in which the holes were drilled 2 mm larger in diameter than the diameter of the implant, permitting a 1 mm gap surrounding the implants. The implants were centralized by two titanium spacers fixed at each end of the implant (Fig. 2). In addition, a bone graft model was developed in which 2 mm overreaming was conducted to study incorporation of bone graft around implants. The graft was added until the canal was filled and a Ti washer was mounted to keep the graft in place and to superficially centralize the implant (Fig. 3).

Finally, a micromotion device was constructed. This model consisted of an

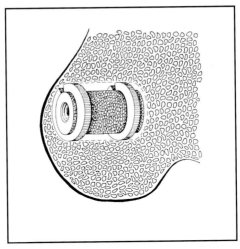

**FIG. 2.** Schematic drawing showing an implant which is centralized in the drill hole by two titanium spacers fixed at each end of the implant, permitting a 1 mm gap around the implant.

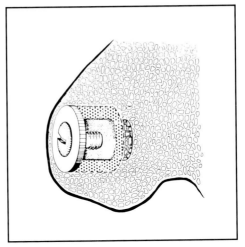

**FIG. 3.** Schematic drawing illustrating the implant centralized in the overreamed canal, surrounded by a 2 mm gap that allows bone graft to be packed around the implant. The deep part of the implant is fixed in the bone by press-fit. A Ti washer keeps the graft in place and centralizes the implant superficially. Dotted area illustrates bone graft. (From ref. 19.)

implantable dynamic device (Fig. 4) that was inserted into the knee joint as illustrated in Fig. 5. The system was adjusted preoperatively to a stiffness of approximately 14 N/mm with a preload of 0.5 N, the total displacement force being 10 N. The maximal movements in the axial direction could be predetermined and limited to the desired amount owing to the design of the device. Movements of 500 μm and 150 μm were used.

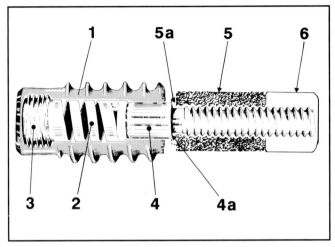

**FIG. 4**  The unstable device consists of seven components all manufactured from titanium alloy (Ti-6A1-4V) as the porous-coated Ti implant.  A hollow Ti cylinder (1) with self tapping threads ensures firm fixation in the bone.  A spring (2) is placed inside the cylinder and held in place by a screw (3) at one end. In the other end a Ti piston (4) can move freely in the axial direction. When mounted, the platform (4a) on the piston projects exactly 500 µm over the end of the Ti cylinder. When the implant (5) is screwed onto the threads of the piston and axial load is applied on the polyethylene plug (6), the implant will move until it is stopped by reaching the Ti cylinder and the movement is limited to 500 µm.  To prevent rotation of the piston, one end of the spring is fixed to the piston (4) and the other to the screw (3), which is locked into the Ti cylinder by a small polyethylene plug inserted into the threads of the screw.  A hole through the piston and the polyethylene plug connects the compartment in the Ti cylinder with the knee joint.  The coating is removed at the distal end of the implant (5a) to prevent bony ingrowth in this area. (From ref. 20.)

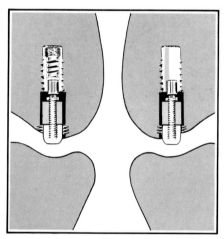

**FIG. 5.**  The dynamic system consists of an implantable device manufactured from titanium alloy (Ti-6A1-4V) which is inserted into the weight-bearing part of the medial femoral condyle (see Fig. 2). Details of the dynamic device are shown in Fig. 4. The polyethylene plug projects above the femoral articular cartilage.  A Ti ring is mounted subchondrally and serves as a bearing and centralizer for the polyethylene plug.   When the knee is loaded during gait, load transfer from the tibial part of the knee will displace the polyethylene and the implant in axial direction and tighten the spring. When the leg later is  unloaded, the tightened spring will move the implant back to the initial position.  Thus, a controlled movement (predetermined to 500 µm or 150 µm ) will occur during each gait cycle. (From refs. 20 and 21.)

## General Postoperative Registration

The dogs were regularly inspected, with special attention to wound healing and weight bearing. All animals were allowed immediate postoperative weight bearing. They stayed in individual cages that measured 1.5 x 2.5 m with outdoor training for three hours a day (1.5 x 3.5 m).

Seventy mature dogs were used in the study and 224 implants were inserted and analyzed. There were no complications related to the operative procedure, and all dogs were sacrificed according to the original time schedule. No clinical infections were encountered.

## Evaluation

After sacrifice, the distal femora were prepared. Standardized sections were cut at a right angle to the long axis of the implant. One section was used for UV fluorescence microscopy, another for histomorphometric and morphologic evaluation on ground-stained specimens, and one for mechanical testing (Fig. 6). In addition, some results were evaluated by polarized light microscopy, collagen analysis, and transmission electron microscopy with microanalysis (EDAX) (Fig. 7).

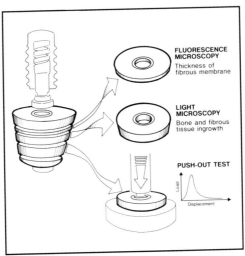

**FIG. 6.** Sections were cut at a right angle to the long axis of the implant. One section was used for measurement of membrane thickness, one section for quantitative analysis of bony ingrowth, and one section for mechanical push-out test.

# EXPERIMENTAL STUDIES ON HYDROXYLAPATITE COATING

## Effect of a Gap Between Bone and Implant

The quantity of bone ingrowth into porous-coated implants depends on available bone stock and the degree of interference obtained between the

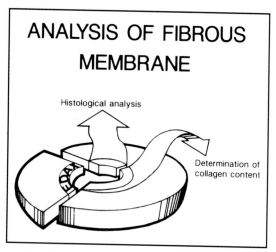

**FIG. 7.** Schematic drawing of standardized biopsies of the membrane for histologic analysis, collagen determination and elemental analysis (EDAX). (From ref. 21.)

implant and the surrounding bone (48-52).

In our laboratory, the effect of HA was investigated when implants were surrounded by a gap compared with press-fit implants (15). The observation period was four weeks and six mature dogs comprised the material.

The initial 1 mm gaps surrounding the Ti implants (Fig. 8A) were bridged by very limited amounts of immature woven bone, whereas a great amount of newly formed bone filled the gap around the HA-coated implants (Fig. 8B). Bone tissue was observed on the HA implant surface, with no interposed fibrous tissue layer present. In some areas a thin fibrous layer separated the Ti implant surfaces from the ingrown bone, but in other areas direct apposition of bone was noted (Fig. 8A).

**A**                                                                                     **B**

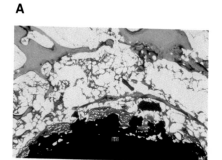
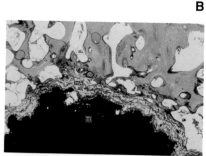

**FIG. 8 (A).** Microphotograph from a Ti-coated implant initially surrounded by a 1 mm gap. Note the limited amounts of bone (*green*) bridging the gap and fibrous tissue (*red*) separating the implant from the newly formed bone. **(B)** Microphotograph from HA-coated specimen initially surrounded by a 1 mm gap. Note the large amount of newly formed bone bridging the initial gap, compared with the Ti-coated implant in *A*. Basic fuchsin and light green, X 25.

The gap around the Ti-coated implants led to a 65% reduction in fixation as compared with the press-fit implants. In contrast, no differences were found between the "gap" and press-fit implants when an HA coating was used. Surrounded by a gap, the fixation of HA-coated implants was 120% increased as compared with Ti implants. The corresponding value for shear stiffness was 425%. No effect of HA coating was obtained when implants were inserted in press-fit (Fig. 9).

The greatest amount of bone ingrowth was found with the press-fit, HA-coated implants. This was increased compared with HA-coated implants surrounded by a gap which, again, was greater than Ti implants in press-fit. The smallest amount of bone ingrowth was found at Ti implants surrounded by an initial gap.

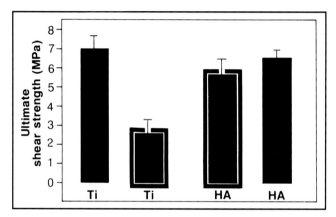

**FIG. 9.** Results from push-out test. The line around the two bars in the middle illustrate implants surrounded by an initial gap. The two other bars represent implants inserted in press-fit. Mean ±SEM, n=6.

For noncemented tibial components, the cutting procedure has been demonstrated to result in lack of optimal flatness after bone cutting (53, 54). In that study, it was calculated that the prosthesis would rest on only 1-2% of the surface area immediately after insertion. Other authors have emphasized lack of direct apposition of implant to bone in the clinical situation (24, 55, 56). We demonstrated that the quantity of bone ingrowth into porous-coated implants depends on the interference fit obtained with the surrounding bone and that gaps resulted in inferior bone ingrowth when Ti implants were used (15). However, the need for improved surgical technique appeared to be less when HA coating was used. In our study, HA coating eliminated the negative influence of a gap between the bone and implant and provided stable mechanical conditions. The high speed of gap healing might increase the chance for improved stabilization of the prosthesis and allow earlier weight-bearing.

## Effect of Osteopenia on Implant Fixation

The biologic response to the implant depends, among other factors, on the status of the host bone bed at the time of implantation. The bone bed can be osteopenic because of disuse, arthritis, or osteoporosis. Few quantitative data are available on the ingrowth capability of osteopenic bone (27-29).

We used an experimental model with arthritis-induced bone changes resulting in osteopenia (16). Implants were inserted with tight press-fit in the distal femoral condyles for four weeks (17). Twelve mature dogs comprised the material. Before surgery, CT scanning had verified reduced bone density at the implantation site in the arthritic bone as compared with control bone, amounting to 21% (16). After sacrifice, the mechanical properties were verified to be weaker at the arthritic bone by indentation test, and the trabecular bone volume was also shown by histomorphometry to be reduced.

At the time of sacrifice, gross capsule thickening, slight chronic synovial effusion, severe synovial thickening and muscle atrophy were observed in the arthritic knees. The articular cartilage was pale and fibrillated, and in areas of the patellofemoral groove and the tibial plateaus the articular surfaces were denuded of cartilage. Ti implants displayed several areas without direct bone-implant apposition, whereas bone tissue was in direct contact with the HA-coated implants, with an interposed fibrous tissue layer present only sporadically.

The anchorage of Ti-coated implants in osteopenic bone was significantly reduced compared with the control bone ($p<0.01$). However, with HA-coated implants, no differences between the osteopenic and control bone were found. In the control bone, the ultimate shear strength of the Ti implants was significantly higher as compared to that of the HA implants ($p<0.01$), whereas no difference was found between HA and Ti implants in osteopenic bone (Table 2).

The weakened fixation of Ti implants in osteopenic bone suggests that the quality of the bone can be a limiting factor for biological fixation. These results are in agreement with two other experimental studies using ovariectomized dogs (27) and old dogs (28) but do not agree with a steroid-induced osteopenic model in rabbits, in which bone ingrowth was not reduced (29).

A clinical study on osseointegration of pure Ti screws implanted in patients with rheumatoid arthritis (57) showed inferior bone contact with most screws as compared with that in osteoarthritic patients with good bone quality.

**TABLE 2.** *Push-out values for Ti and HA-coated implants after four weeks in osteopenic and control bone (n=6)*

| Ultimate Shear strength (MPa) | Osteopenic Bone (mean ± SEM) | Control Bone (mean ± SEM) |
|---|---|---|
| Titanium Implants | 7.4 (0.22) | 10.1 (0.6) |
| Hydroxylapatite Implants | 7.7 (0.6) | 7.5 (0.1) |

If the results mentioned above can extrapolate to weight bearing human joint prostheses, they suggest inferior results with metal porous-coated, noncemented prostheses in patients with an osteopenic host bone bed.

### Effect of Bone Grafting on Implant Fixation

Incorporation of autogenous and allogenic bone grafts has been studied by several investigators (58-63). Both non-weight-bearing and weight-bearing models have demonstrated a positive effect of autogenous and allogenic bone grafts. Autologous bone has a higher degree of osteogenic capacity and undergoes more rapid revascularization compared with allograft (60,63,64). However, diminished osteogenic potential does not seem to impair the incorporation of allogenic bone graft into porous-coated implants. McDonald et al. (65) found only slightly increased fixation of revised femoral components in dogs, using autograft compared with fresh-frozen allograft, after 12 weeks. This is in agreement with Lewis et al. (66) who found equivalent strength and bony ingrowth using autograft and fresh-frozen allograft in an unloaded dog model after four, eight, and 16 weeks of implantation. However, a recent study demonstrated no effect of freeze-dried allograft in a non-weight-bearing model (67). One weight-bearing study using autogenous bone graft has even shown inhibition of bone ingrowth compared with a negative untreated control (68). Recently, Turner et al. (69) demonstrated advantages of a two-stage procedure in bone grafting of noncemented total hip replacement in dogs.

A new model was created in our laboratory (Fig. 3) to study cancellous allogenic bone graft incorporation into Ti- and HA-coated implants with and without bone graft. The observation time was six weeks and 12 mature dogs were used. The cancellous bone graft was taken from the proximal humerus from 12 other dogs, stored in sterile containers at -80°C, and milled into a homogeneous graft.

This study demonstrated a 400% enhanced fixation of grafted Ti-coated implants compared with that of the overreamed controls (Fig. 10). However, HA coating used without bone graft was capable of enhancing the fixation to nearly the same degree. Only minor improvement was obtained when bone graft was used together with HA. Since both components are known to increase bony ingrowth when used separately, this lack of a measurable additive effect of adding bone graft to HA-coated implants might be explained by the presence of bone graft packed around the implant, which probably eliminated the osteoconductive effect of HA.

### Effect of Micromotion on Implant Fixation

Obtaining rigid initial stability appears to be one of the major problems in noncemented endoprosthetic surgery and is initially dependent on the strength of the mechanical interlock achieved between implant and bone during implantation. Several studies have investigated the stability of hip and knee prostheses immediately after implantation, and there is agreement that relative movement

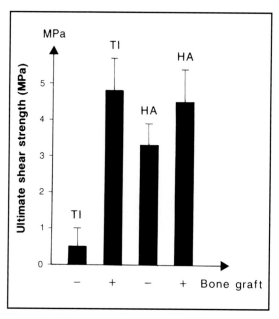

**FIG. 10.** Results from push-out test. Use of bone graft filled in the defect is illustrated by +, - indicates that bone graft was not used, leaving the implant surrounded by a 2 mm gap. Mean ±SEM, n=7.

between implant and bone occurs in the range of 100-600 μm (39-44). Even when rigid fixation with screws and pegs is used, differences in elasticity between bone and the metallic porous material have been shown to result in tangential displacement of 150 μm at the periphery of tibial trays (70). More-over, macroscopic motion has been demonstrated at tibial interfaces (71). In contrast, cemented prostheses have been shown to be more stable (45).

Because the degree of micromotion and its effect on bone tissue are difficult to assess in clinical practice, we found it important to create a dynamic system to study the significance of controlled micromovements between bone and implant (Fig. 4, Fig. 5).

In the first study (20) movements of 500 μm were studied, and in the next study (21) 150 μm movements were investigated. Mechanically stable implants served as controls and the observation period was four weeks. In both studies, micromotion resulted in formation of a fibrous membrane (Fig. 11), whereas variable amounts of bone ingrowth were obtained in mechanically stable implants (Fig. 12). Both studies also demonstrated development of fibrocartilage around unstable HA-coated implants (Fig. 13), whereas the membrane con-sisted predominantly of connective tissue around unstable Ti implants (Fig. 14). Results from histomorphometric analysis of the presence of fibrocartilage in the membrane are shown in Table 3.

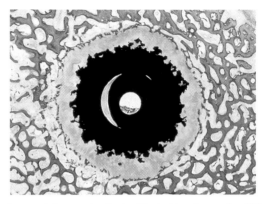

**FIG. 11.** Photomicrograph from an implant subjected to micromotion (150 μm) showing fibrous tissue (red) around HA-coated implant. Light green, Basic Fuchsin, grounded section, X6. (From ref. 21.)

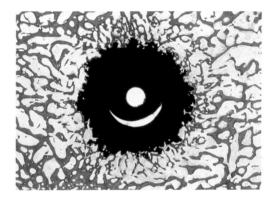

**FIG. 12.** Photomicrograph from a stable HA-coated implant showing bone ingrowth (green) across the initial gap and bone apposition on the implant. Light green, Basic Fuchsin, grounded section. (From ref. 21.)

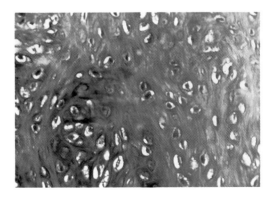

**FIG. 13.** Membrane from the unstable HA-coated implant showing islands of fibrocartilage with chondrocytes in lacunae. Toluidine blue at pH 5, x250. (From ref. 20.)

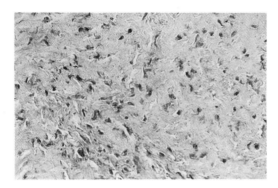

**FIG. 14.** Membrane from the unstable Ti-coated implant showing fibrous connective tissue. Toluidine blue at pH 5, x250. (From ref. 20.)

**TABLE 3.** *Results from quantitative analysis of presence of fibrocartrilage in membranes around Ti and HA-coated implants (n=7)*

| Fibrocartilage | 500 µm movement (20) (mean ± SEM) | 150 µm movement (21) (mean ± SEM) |
|---|---|---|
| Titanium Implants | 1.7 (1.2)% | 5 (2.7)% |
| Hydroxylapatite Implants | 52 (21.5)% | 53 (11.5)% |

### 500 µm Movements

Seven mature dogs were used. Push-out test showed that the shear strength of unstable Ti and HA implants was significantly reduced as compared with the corresponding mechanically stable implants ($p<0.01$). However, shear strength values of unstable HA-coated implants were significantly greater than those of unstable Ti implants ($p<0.01$) and were comparable to those of stable Ti implants. The greatest shear strength was obtained with stable HA-coated implants, which was increased threefold as compared with the stable Ti implants ($p<0.001$) (Fig. 15). Quantitative determination of bony ingrowth confirmed the mechanical test, except for the stronger anchorage of unstable HA implants as compared with unstable Ti implants, in which no difference in bony ingrowth was found. Collagen concentration was significantly higher in membranes around HA-coated implants as compared with membranes around Ti implants.

### 150 µm Movements

This study comprised 14 mature dogs. Results from the 500 µm study were reproduced in this study regarding the presence of fibrocartilage around unstable HA-coated implants (Table 3), whereas fibrous connective tissue

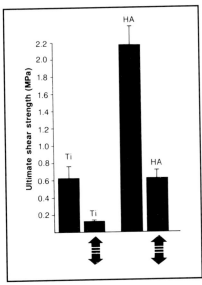

**FIG. 15.** Results from mechanical test from the 500 μm study. Arrows indicate unstable implants; the two other bars represent stable implants. (From ref. 20.)

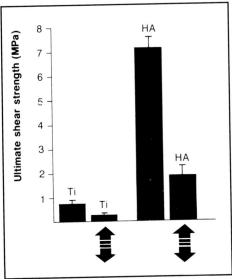

**FIG. 16.** Results from mechanical test from the 150 μm study. Arrows indicate unstable implants; the two other bars represent stable implants. (From ref. 21.)

characterized the membrane around unstable Ti implants. In addition, this study revealed a thinner membrane around unstable HA implants compared with unstable Ti implants. A radial orientation of collagen fibers was found in the membrane around unstable HA-coated implants, whereas a more random orientation was found in most membranes around Ti implants. The shear strength of unstable HA-coated implants was significantly greater than that of unstable Ti implants ($p<0.001$) but also than that of stable Ti implants ($p<0.05$). The greatest shear strength obtained by stable HA-coated implants was tenfold higher than that of stable Ti implants ($p<1 \times 10^{-8}$) (Fig. 16). No significant difference was demonstrated between the amount of bone apposition on the unstable HA and stable Ti implants. The gap-healing capacity around stable HA-coated implants increased toward the HA surface and was significantly greater than that of Ti implants (Fig. 17A, B).

In conclusion, initial stability of the implant was shown to be a prerequisite for achieving bone ingrowth (20-22) which is supported by other studies (72-82). However, HA coating seemed to be capable of modifying the fibrous membrane, resulting in a stronger fibrous anchorage when subjected to relative motion between bone and implant.

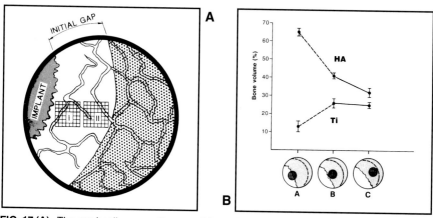

**FIG. 17 (A).** The gap healing capacity around the stable implants was quantitatively assessed in two well-defined zones from the implant surface. Zone I; 1-6 intersections (i.e. 37-225 μm) from implant surface; Zone II; 6-11 intersections (i.e. 225-412 μm) from implant surface. Measurements were made on successive adjacent fields along the entire implant circumference. **(B)** Results from quantitative evaluation of the gap healing capacity around stable implants in two well-defined areas from the implant surface. For location of Zones I and II see **A**.. A, bone apposition on implant surface; B, new bone formation in the initial gap in Zone I; C, new bone formation in the initial gap in Zone II. Note the positive gradient of newly formed bone toward the HA-coated surface which was not found toward the Ti coating. (From ref. 21.)

## Magnitude of Motion

The threshold of implant motion that allows bone ingrowth is still unknown. A recent dog study showed bone ingrowth and remodeling into cementless THA femoral components, despite the initial implant motion, to be as high as 56 μm (83). Burke et al. (84) supported our results using another model with controlled movements of 150 μm for 8 h/day that prevented bone ingrowth and led to a dense fibrous tissue layer surrounding the implants. Similar implants with 20 μm movements achieved bone ingrowth, indicating that the threshold for bone ingrowth is between 20 and 150 μm movement. These findings seem to be in agreement with those of Sumner et al. (70), who showed that bone ingrowth occurred close to the fixation pegs in Ti-fiber, metal-coated tibial components, whereas minor amounts of bone ingrowth were obtained at more peripheral sites of the prosthesis. This was probably due to tangential displacement in the range of 150 μm at the periphery of the tibial tray (85,86).

There appears to be a relationship between the magnitude of bone-implant motion and the type of interfacial tissue developed. It is therefore interesting to look at the effect of differing amounts of movement on implant fixation in our studies (Table 4). An increased fixation strength was obtained with decreased range of motion (500 - 150 μm) by both HA and Ti implants and a further increase in fixation when the observation time was extended from four weeks to 16 weeks (20-22). Comparing the fixation strength of continuously loaded Ti implants with 16 weeks of observation time (1.8 MPa) with those from the four weeks study with HA coating (1.85 MPa) indicates that the fixation of fibrous anchored HA implants is obtained in one-quarter of the time required for the equal fixation of implants without HA coating.

## Fibrous Anchorage

It has been suggested that ingrowth of fibrous tissue could be beneficial for energy absorption by providing better distribution of stresses (87-89). In a recent study, Longo et al. (90) demonstrated a stable fibrous tissue interface around press-fit carbon composite femoral stems in dogs. After a one-year observation period these clinical results are comparable with those of HA-coated stems that were anchored by bone apposition. These authors concluded that bone bonding of the implant is not essential for implant success. These suggestions are supported by clinical experience showing that fibrous tissue anchorage is often present in clinically satisfactory prostheses (10). The observation by Ryd (45), who showed significant displacement of clinically stable tibia plateaus in total knee replacements, confirms these *in vivo* observations in dogs.

According to our results, after four weeks of implantation (20,21) the fibrous membrane around Ti-coated implants had almost no capacity of fixation. However, the fibrocartilaginous membrane around unstable HA-coated implants was found to be significantly stronger and might be sufficient to dissipate stresses in total joint arthroplasties.

**TABLE 4.** *Ultimate shear strength (MPa) of unstable Ti and HA-coated implants with different observation time and range of motion. Mean (SEM).*

| Obs. time | 4 weeks (20) | 4 weeks (21) | 16 weeks (22) |
|---|---|---|---|
| Range of Motion | 500 μm | 150 μm | 150 μm |
| Titanium | 0.12 (0.01)[a] | 0.26 (0.07)[a] | 1.8 (0.8)[a] |
| Hydroxylapatite | 0.63 (0.1)[a] | 1.85 (0.4)[a] | 4.6 (1.0)[a] |

a = Mean ± SEM.

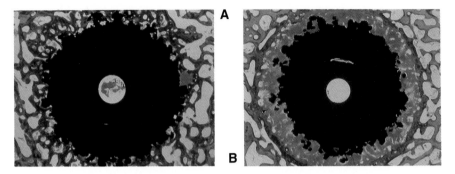

**FIG. 18** Photomicrograph of continuously loaded implants. **A**: HA-coated implant, **B**: Ti-coated implant. Note that bone has filled the gap between bone and HA-coated implant (A), whereas a fibrous membrane is still present around the Ti implant **(B)**. Around the periphery of the fibrous membrane (B), a plate of condensed lamellar bone was found concentric to the implant surface. Light microscopy, light green and Basic Fuchsin, x 8. (From ref. 22.)

### Effect of Continuous Load on Fibrous-Anchored Implants

In the two previous studies (20,21), a fibrocartilaginous membrane was demonstrated around HA-coated implants subjected to micromotion for four weeks, whereas fibrous connective tissue predominated around Ti implants. In the present study (22), 14 dogs were used and the long-term course of continuous load on fibrous-anchored Ti- and HA-coated implants was studied. All implants were subjected to 150 μm movements and were allowed continuous load for 16 weeks.

Histologic analysis of implants with continuous load for 16 weeks showed a fibrous membrane around Ti implants (Fig. 18B), whereas the membrane around HA-coated implants was replaced by bone (Fig. 18A). The push-out test showed inferior fixation of Ti implants as compared with HA-coated implants ($p<0.001$). Bone ingrowth was increased sevenfold in continuously loaded HA implants compared with continuously loaded Ti implants ($p<1$ x $10^2$) (Fig. 19).

### Further Course of Fibrous Membrane

Although ingrowth of fibrous tissue into porous implants has been shown to provide adequate mechanical support for weight-bearing in dogs (78, 90) and humans (10), the long term course of fibrous anchorage of loaded implants is still unknown. Ryd and Linder (91) reported recently on three stable, fixed Marmor (cemented) knee arthroplasties revised five to seven years after insertion for reasons other than mechanical loosening. These authors found fibrocartilage at the central part of the supporting tissue and suggested that the presence of fibrocartilage around the prosthesis provided adequate mechanical support for a successful clinical course. However, our study (22) revealed that the motion-induced membrane around HA-coated implants was replaced by

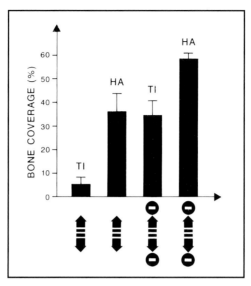

**FIG. 19.** Results from histomorphometry on bony ingrowth 16 weeks post implantation. *Arrows* indicate unstable implants subjected to continuous load. Stop marks indicate implants immobilized after four weeks of micromotion. Mean ±SEM, n=7. (From ref.22.)

bone after three months despite application of continuous load (Fig. 18A). The membrane around similar implants without HA coating, however, was still present after three months (Fig. 18B). This suggests that in addition to the well-known osteoconductive effect demonstrated in stable implants with initial contact with surrounding bone (14,92-4), HA also seems to have the capacity to change the further course of the membrane by inducing new bone formation even under loaded conditions.

The reasons for conversion of fibrous membrane to bone around HA-coated implants (22) are multifactorial. In theory, it can be explained by the presence of fibrocartilaginous tissue around HA-coated implants as found at four weeks, which may prepare the gap around the implant mechanically and biologically for later bony anchorage of the implant by endochondrial ossification. This explanation seems to be in agreement with the interfragmentary strain theory (95), which states that the initial presence of fibrous tissue in fracture healing may reduce the strain between the fracture fragments to a level at which cartilage can be formed. The presence of fibrocartilage may further reduce the strain to a level at which bone can be formed.

A similar presence of bone ingrowth around HA-coated implants and fibrous tissue around Ti implants (22) after a longer observation period has been demonstrated in other studies. In a loaded model, Manley et al. (96) demonstrated that HA-coated intramedullary implants were anchored in bone and that Ti alloy implants were surrounded by fibrous tissue after 10 weeks. Another weight-bearing model with femoral hemiarthroplasty in dogs (97) showed bone apposition on HA-coated, grooved macrotextured prostheses, whereas fibrous connective tissue surrounded uncoated control implants after

10 weeks. Geesink et al. (12) reported on total hip replacements with HA coating in dogs and found similar differences after observation periods as long as 12 months. In a recent study on hemiarthroplasties in dogs, the interface shear strength of HA-coated prostheses 18 months after surgery (98) was superior to those without HA coating. Therefore, HA coating also appears to be efficacious in a more clinically relevant situation, when the implant is subjected to loaded conditions during the entire observation period.

The radiating orientation of collagen fibers and higher collagen content might also contribute to a more steady mechanical milieu around HA-coated implants. The radiating fiber orientation might be similar to those described in other studies in which oblique fiber orientation to the implant surface was found in membranes from a loaded CoCr-Mo intramedullary model (78) and porous-coated Ti segmental prosthesis (80). One possible explanation for the radiating orientation of fibers is that the collagen fibers might be integrated into the HA-coated surface (99). When the implant moves, load transfer is reflected by the collagen fibers, which results in radiating orientation of the fibers. In contrast, the integration between collagen fibers and Ti surface might be weaker, leaving minor load transfer in the membrane and thus a more random fiber orientation. It should be emphasized, however, that a radiating orientation was also observed in membranes around some Ti-coated implants.

Studies on bioactive glasses have shown that collagen is structurally integrated within the crystalized apatite (99). If the collagen fibers are similarly embedded and bonded within the surface of the bioactive HA used in the present study, the stronger fibrous anchorage of unstable HA-coated implants compared which those of stable and unstable Ti implants could be explained by a stronger bonding capacity of collagen to HA.

### Implant Loosening

The further course of a persistent fibrous membrane could lead to loosening of the prosthesis due to bone resorption caused by the presence of macrophages in the membrane. According to Goldring et al. (100), the membrane might be transformed to a "macrophage" membrane initiated by continuous movement between implant and bone. Such "macrophage" membranes have been described around cemented prostheses (100,101) to contain $PGE_2$ and collagenase. The presence of these substances may explain the progressive lysis of bone around both cemented and noncemented prostheses. In the present studies (20-22), macrophages were particularly present around Ti implants, which suggests that these membranes can produce $PGE_2$ and collagenase. However, these substances were not quantitated because of lack of sufficient membrane material.

### The Effect of Immobilization of Fibrous-Anchored Implants

In this study (22), HA and Ti implants initially subjected to 150 μm movements were immobilized after four weeks (when a fibrous membrane was developed around the implants) to prevent further micromotion. The total observation time was 16 weeks, and 14 dogs comprised the material. All immobilized implants were surrounded by various amounts of bone tissue up to the implant surfaces irrespective of type of coating.

Immobilization of Ti implants resulted in 330% stronger fixation compared with continuously loaded Ti implants ($p < 0.01$). Immobilization of HA implants increased the fixation by 40% (NS). The anchorage of immobilized Ti implants was 20% stronger than that of HA-coated implants (NS). HA-coated implants had a significantly greater amount of bone ingrowth as compared with Ti-coated implants (Fig. 19).

The finding that the fibrous membrane around the porous-coated implant was replaced by bone due to immobilization seems interesting. This result is partly in agreement with observations by Uhthoff and Garmain (73), who showed that immobilization of an unstable fracture with screws surrounded by fibrous tissue resulted in some new bone formation around the screws after four weeks. However, a narrow layer of fibrous tissue was still interposed between the screw and bone. These authors concluded that the "beginning of loosening around screws can be reversed by addition of simple external immobilization." Our result (VIII) is also partly in agreement with that of Eschenroeder et al. (81), who presented a model with gross movement between proximal tibial trabecular bone and implant and who showed that immobilization of a motion-induced fibrous membrane resulted in bone formation around and up to a porous-coated CoCr surface. However, most of the implant surface was surrounded by fibrous tissue.

## The Effect of Load Versus Stress Shielding on Stable Implants

A striking finding in the present studies was that the dynamic load on HA-coated implants increased the amount of bone ingrowth and implant fixation, which was threefold greater compared with completely unloaded implants (20,21) (Fig. 20). According to these studies (20,21), the fixation seems to be related to the loading conditions. Differences were found between the stable and unloaded situation, the stable but loaded situation, and the unstable situation in which the interlock cannot resist the load applied, resulting in relative movements between bone and implant.

The best anchorage and the greatest amount of bone ingrowth was obtained in the *loaded* but stable situation when the implant was coated with HA (20,21). In other words, some kind of weight-bearing enhances bony anchorage of the implant as compared with the completely unloaded situation. On the other hand, too much weight-bearing induces a negative effect on implant fixation, as the amount of micromotion surpasses the limit compatible with bone ingrowth (20, 21). The limit between enhancement of bone ingrowth by load and development of fibrous formation is still unknown but is definitely less than 150 μm.

One explanation for the lacking effect of weight-bearing on stable Ti implants (Fig. 20) might be delayed gap healing as compared with that observed

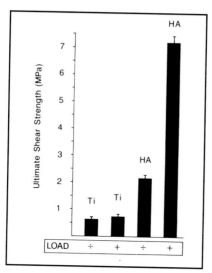

**FIG. 20.** Ultimate shear strength of stable HA-and Ti-coated implants, with and without weight-bearing, after four weeks. Mean ±SEM, n=7. (From refs. 20 and 21,)

in HA implants. This delay in bone ingrowth means that only minor amounts of bone are present at the time of weight-bearing and therefore there is no bone to respond to the mechanical stress applied on the implant. In other words, a positive effect of early weight-bearing is obtainable only when continuity between surrounding bone and implant is achieved early after implantation. Another explanation might be that applied stress on HA-coated implants results in increased dissolution of HA which, according to Beight et al. (102), would stimulate additional bone ingrowth.

The stronger fixation of loaded HA implants is in agreement with the findings of Turner et al. (103), who suggested that underloading (stress shielding) results in inferior bone ingrowth and cortical resorption around the implant. Jasty and Harris (104) also showed the importance of loads on rigidly fixed acetabular components, as unloaded components showed inferior bone ingrowth compared with loaded components. This is in agreement with Wolff's law stating that bone adapts to functional demands by remodeling to reflect the distribution of effective stresses (105).

## Effect of HA Coating on Implant Fixation

The effect of calcium-phosphate coating has been studied extensively in recent years. Some studies have failed to demonstrate enhanced fixation of calcium-phosphate coatings. Berry et al. (106) studied the effect of a coating consisting of a slurry of fresh blood and TCP without any demonstrable effect on implant fixation after one and five weeks of observation time. In another non-weight-bearing press-fit study (107), the authors also failed to demonstrate any effect of HA coating compared to porous-coated Ti implants, which is in agreement with a clinical study on unloaded conical implants (108). In general, for these studies the implants were inserted in tight press-fit.

The effect of HA coating depends of course on the surface morphology of the control implant. The effect of HA has not failed when HA has been coated on smooth or bead-blasted metal substrate used as control (12, 92, 109).

Another series of experimental non-weight-bearing studies has demonstrated a positive but transient effect of calcium-phosphate coatings (93,94), since the demonstrated stimulatory effect of HA at early time periods (four weeks) diminished with time and the fixation approximated those without HA coating at six and 12 weeks, respectively. The transient effect might be explained by insufficient coating techniques, as the HA powder used by Ducheyne et al. (93) was deposited by dipping the implants into a water slurry, followed by drying at 80° C. This method is not sufficient for bonding between the HA and metal substrate. Rivero et al. (94) used a plasma-flame technique for application of HA powder. However, the HA powder used was transformed to TCP during the coating procedure, which might explain the relatively poor effect of the coating. Only 24% increased fixation was obtained at four weeks and no effect was obtained at the other time periods tested (one, two and six weeks). One study using HA coating in goats showed the same tendency, since the enhanced fixation decreased after six weeks of implantation to reach values obtained without HA coating after 12 weeks (110).

A major group of non-weight-bearing models with pure HA coating have demonstrated enhanced fixation for longer time periods from three to 12 weeks (14,111,112), 32 weeks (92,113), and 52 weeks (114) after implantation compared with identical implants without HA coating.

In our studies (16,18-21) the gap healing capacity of bone was increased by HA coating compared with Ti coating, even at a relatively great distance from the HA surface. This indicates that the osteoconductive effect of HA is not limited to the bone forming capacity on the surface of the implant. HA also activates bone formation at some distance from the surface (Fig. 17B). The positive gradient of bone demonstrated towards the HA surface indicates that the osteoconductive effect of HA is more pronounced close to the surface under stable conditions (21). We found no comparable studies demonstrating this phenomenon, but the finding may support those of Beight et al. (102), who suggested that calcium phosphate coating acts by providing a local source of Ca and $PO_4$ ions essential for mineralization of the surrounding tissue. The same explanation can be applied to the thinner membrane found around unstable HA implants, probably caused by activation of newly formed bone at the border of the drill hole. An interesting finding was the presence of bone growing directly on the surface of HA-coated implants even when subjected to micromovements (21).

Several weight-bearing models have confirmed the positive effects on implant fixation of HA coating (12,96-98,115,116). Manley et al. (96) used HA-coated intramedullary implants which were demonstrated to be anchored in bone, whereas Ti alloy implants were surrounded by fibrous tissue after 10 weeks. In another weight-bearing model with femoral hemiarthroplasty in dogs, Thomas et al. (97) showed bone apposition on HA-coated grooved macrotextured prostheses, whereas fibrous connective tissue surrounded uncoated control implants after 10 weeks. Geesink et al. (12) reported on total hip replacements with HA coating in dogs and found similar differences after observation periods up to 12 months. The longest observation time on an HA-coated hip prosthesis known to the present author is 18 months (98). In that study Poser et al. (98) reported greater interference shear strength at all levels of the HA-coated prosthesis as compared with grit-blasted Ti-alloy implants.

In conclusion, most experimental studies have shown strong bonding of HA-coated implants. Variations in results may be ascribed to differences in the composition of calcium phosphate after coating and also by different testing conditions and surface characteristics of the control implant.

## SUMMARY

The success of bone ingrowth into porous-coated implants depends on several factors (48,117) which can be separated into four main groups: status of host bone bed; implant related factors; mechanical stabilization and loading conditions applied on the implant; and adjuvant therapies. The present series of studies was performed to investigate the effect of HA coating on bone ingrowth into porous-coated implants subjected to pathologic and mechanical conditions mimicking the clinical situation. The studies particularly focused on the effect of osteoporosis, bone deficiency, bone grafting, and micromotion on implant fixation.

Host bone-related factors were studied in the first four experiments. First, the significance of a gap between bone and implant was studied and compared with press-fit insertion. The HA coating yielded a superior effect on bone ingrowth compared with Ti in situations where the implant was surrounded by a gap. No effect was found in the press-fit situation. Gaps of 1 mm and 2 mm around the implant were bridged by bone around HA implants, whereas significantly smaller amounts of bone filled the gap around Ti implants. To investigate the significance of arthritic bone changes (osteopenia) on fixation of porous-coated implants, we adopted the carrageenan-induced gonarthritis model, resulting in significant bone loss as determined by CT scanning. In experimental arthritic bone the anchorage of Ti implants was weakened compared with control bone; this weakening did not occur when HA coating was used. HA coating was shown to accelerate the rate of bone ingrowth in the presence of an initial gap between bone and implant, even in the presence of osteopenic host bone bed.

To study the effect of adjuvant therapies, a bone graft model was developed to investigate bone graft material in combination with Ti- and HA-coated implants. Allogeneic bone graft packed around the implant enhanced the anchorage of Ti implants, but HA coating alone without bone graft offered almost the same improvement in anchorage in 2 mm defects. Only minor improvement was obtained when bone graft was used together with HA.

The last three experiments focused on the significance of mechanical stabilization and loading conditions of the implant immediately after surgery.

Micromotion between bone and implant prevented bony ingrowth and resulted in development of a fibrous membrane. HA coating was shown to modify this fibrous membrane, as evidenced by presence of fibrocartilage, higher collagen concentration, radiating orientation of collagen fibers, and a thinner membrane as compared with Ti-coated implants. In a long-term study (16 weeks), the membrane around HA implants was demonstrated to be replaced by bone even when subjected to continuous load, whereas the membrane around Ti implants persisted after 16 weeks.

Great amounts of bone ingrowth into loaded but stable HA-coated implants were demonstrated even in the presence of an initial gap around the implant. Dynamic load was even demonstrated to increase the amount of bone ingrowth into HA-coated implants, which was threefold greater compared with completely unloaded implants. This effect of dynamic load was not demonstrated on Ti implants. The best anchorage and the greatest amount of bone ingrowth were obtained in the loaded stable situation when the implant was coated with HA.

Increased fibrous fixation was obtained with decreased range of motion (from 500 μm to 150 μm) by both HA and Ti implants, and a further increase in fixation was obtained when the observation time was extended from four weeks to 16 weeks. From these studies it could also be demonstrated that the fixation of fibrous-anchored HA implants was obtained in one quarter of the time required for the equal fixation of implants without HA coating.

The consequence of immobilization of a motion-induced fibrous-anchored implant was complete replacement of the membrane by bone, irrespective of the type of coating.

## CONCLUSION

From the results presented, it can be concluded that HA coating has a positive effect on bone-implant fixation under stable unloaded conditions, stable loaded conditions, and unstable mechanical conditions. HA coating yielded no effect when implants were inserted in optimal press-fit in normal bone. The most striking effects of HA were its enhancement of bone growth across a gap around the implant during both stable and unstable mechanical conditions, and its ability to convert a motion-induced fibrous membrane to bony anchorage.

## ACKNOWLEDGEMENTS

This chapter is based on the work of several researchers in our laboratory, including Dr. Vibeke E. Hjortdal, Dr. Ivan Hvid, Dr. Gitte I. Juhl, Dr. Jørgen Jørgensen, Dr. Peter H. Jørgenson, Professor Flemming Melsen, Dr. Anders Odgaard, and Dr. Claus Möger Pedersen, whose contributions should be acknowledged. The studies were supported by The Danish Rheumatism Association, The Danish Medical Research Council, The Institute of Experimental Clinical Research, University of Aarthus, The Aarhus University

Research Foundation, The Danish Foundation for the Advancement of Medical Science, Biomet, Inc,, Direktor Madsen og hustru Olga Madsens Fond, Ferd. og Ellen Hindsgauls Fond, Svend Fældings Fond, and Kong Kristian Den Tiendes Fond. Biomet Inc., USA, kindly delivered the implants used in the studies.

# REFERENCES

1. Ahlfelt I, Herberts P, Malchau H, Anderson GBJ. Prognosis of total hip replacement.   A swedish multicenter study of 4,664 revisions. *Acta Orthopaedica Scandinavica* 1990; 61:238.
2. Strömberg CN, Herberts P, Palmertz B - Cemented revision hip arthroplasty. A multicenter 5-9 year study of 204 first revisions for loosening. *Acta Orthopaedica Scandinavica* 1992;63 (2):111-19.
3. Retpen JB, Varmarken J-E, Röck ND, Jensen JS. Unsatisfactory results after repeated revision of hip arthroplasty. 61 cases followed for 5(1-10) years. *Acta Orthopaedica Scandinavica* 1992;63(2):120-7
4. Chandler HP, Reineck FT, Wixson RL, McCarthy JC. Total hip replacement in patients younger than thirty years old. *Journal of Bone and Joint Surgery* 1981;63-A:1426-34.
5. Halley DK, Wroblewski BM. Long-term results of low-friction arthroplasty in patients 30 years of age or younger. *Clinical Orthopaedics* 1986;211:43-50.
6. Galante JO, Rostoker W, Lueck R, Ray RD. Sintered fiber metal composites as a basis for attachment of implants to bone. *Journal of Bone and Joint Surgery* 1971;53-A:101-8.
7. Bobyn JD, Engh CA, Glassman, AH. Histological analysis of a retrieved microporouscoated femoral prosthesis. *Clinical Orthopaedics* 1987;224:303-10.
8. Collier JP, Mayor MB, Chae JC, et al. Macroscopic and microscopic evidence of prosthetic fixation with porous-coated materials. *Clinical Orthopaedics* 1988;235:173-80.
9. Cook SD, Barrack RL, Thomas KA, Haddad RJ. Quantitative analysis of tissue growth into human porous total hip components. *Journal of Arthroplasty* 1988;3:249-62.
10. Cook, SD, Thomas KA, Haddad RJ. Histological analysis of retrieved human porous-coated total joint components. *Clinical Orthopaedics* 1988;234:90-101.
11. Engh CA, Bobyn JD, Petersen TL. Radiographic and histologic study of porous- coated tibial component fixation in cementless total knee arthroplasty. *Orthopedics* 1988;11:725-31.
12. Geesink RGT, de Groot K, Klein CPAT. Chemical implant fixation using hydroxylapatite coatings. *Clinical Orthopaedics* 1987; 225:147-70.
13. de Groot K, Geesink RGT, Klein CPAT, Serekian P. Plasma sprayed coatings o hydroxylapatite. *Journal of Biomedical Materials Research* 1987; 21:1375-81.
14. Thomas KA, Kay JF, Cook SD, Jarcho M. The effect of surface macro texture and hydroxyapatiite coating on the mechanical strengths and histological profiles of titanium implant materials. *Journal of Biomedical Materials Research* 1987;21:1395-414.
15. Søballe K, Hansen ES, B-Rasmussen H, Pedersen CM, Bünger C. Hydroxyapatite coating enhances fixation of porous coated implants. A comparison between press fit and non-interference fit. *Acta Orthopaedica Scandinavica* 1990;60(4):299-306.
16. Søballe K, Pedersen CM, Odgaard A, et al. Physical bone changes in Carragheenin-induced arthritis evaluated by quantitative computed tomography. *Skeletal Radiology* 1991;20:345-52.
17. Søballe K, Hansen ES, Rasmussen HB, et al. Fixation of titanium and hydroxyapatite coated implants in osteopenia. *Journal of Arthroplasty* 1991;6(4):307-16.
18. Søballe K, Hansen ES, B-Rasmussen H, et al. Gap healing enhanced by hydroxyapatite coating in dogs. *Clinical Orthopaedics* 1991;272:300-07;
19. Søballe K, Hansen ES, B-Rasmussen H, Pedersen CM, Bünger C. Bone graft incorporation around titanium-alloy and hydroxyapatite coated implants in dogs. *Clinical Orthopaedics* 1992;274:282-93.
20. Søballe K, Hansen ES, B- Rasmussen H, Bünger C. Tissue ingrowth into titanium and hydroxyapatite coated implants during stable and unstable mechanical conditions. *Journal of Orthopaedic Research* 1992;10:285-99.

21. Søballe K, B-Rasmussen H, Hansen ES, Bünger C. Hydroxyapatite coating modifies implant membrane formation. Controlled micromotion studied in dogs. *Acta Orthopaedica Scandinavica* 1992;63(2):128-40.
22. Søballe K, Hansen ES, B-Rasmussen H, Bünger C. Hydroxyapatite coating converts fibrous tissue to bone around loaded implants; *Journal of Bone and Joint Surgery.* 1993, 75B:270.
23. Søballe K, Toksvig-Larsen S, Gelineck J, et al. Hydroxylapatite coating in total hip arthroplasty. *Journal of Bone and Joint Surgery (Br)*, September 1993, in press.
24. Schimmel J-W, Huiskes R. Primary fit of the Lord cementless total hip. A geometric study in cadavers. *Acta Orthopaedica Scandinavica* 1988;59:638-42.
25. Noble PC, Alexander JW, Granberry MI, Granberry WM, Maltry JA, Tullos HS. The myth of "press-fit: in the proximal femur. *Scientific Exhibit 55th Annual Meeting American Academy of Orthopaedic Surgeons* 1988.
26. Noble PC, Alexander JW, Lindahl IJ, Yew DT, Granberry WM, Tullos HS. The anatomical basis of femoral component design. *Clinical Orthopaedics* 1988;235:148-65.
27. Martin RB, Paul HA, Bargar WL, Dannucci GA, Sharkey NA. Effects of estrogen deficiency on the growth of tissue into porous titanium implants. *Journal of Bone and Joint Surgery* 1988;70-A:540-7.
28. Nakajima I, Dai KR, Kelly PJ, Chao EYS. The effect of age on bone ingrowth into titanium fibermetal segmental prosthesis: an experimental study. *Transactions of 31st Annual Meeting Orthopaedic Research Society* 1985;9:296.
29. Rønningen H, Urban RM, Galante JO. Bone ingrowth in a fiber metal implant in rabbits with steroid induced osteopenia. *Transactions of 29th Annual Meeting of Orthopaedic Research Society* 1983;8:134.
30. Bünger C. Hemodynamics of the juvenile knee. *Acta Orthopaedica Scandinavica*, Ph.D. Thesis, Suppl 222 1987; vol. 58.
31. Gustilo RB, Pasternak HS. Revision total hip arthroplasty with titanium ingrowth prosthesis and bone grafting for failed cemented femoral component loosening. *Clinical Orthopaedics* 1988; 235:111-19.
32. Head WC, Malinin TI, Berklacich F. Freeze-dried proximal femur allografts in revision total hip arthroplasty. *Clinical Orthopaedics* 1987; 215:109-21.
33. Hungerford DS, Jones LC .The rationale for cementless revision of cemented arthroplasty failures. *Clinical Orthopaedics* 1988;235:12-24.
34. McGann WA, Welch RB, Picetti GD. Acetabular preparation in cementless revision total hip arthroplasty. *Clinical Orthopaedics* 1988; 235:35-46.
35. Samuelson KM. Bone grafting and noncemented revision arthroplasty of the knee. *Clinical Orthopaedics* 1988; 226:93-101.
36. Turner TM, Urban RM, Sumner DR, Galante JO. Bone ingrowth in cementless revision of an aseptically loosened canine THA model. *Transactions of 35th Annual Meeting Orthopaedic Research Society* 1989; 14:551.
37. Kennedy AC, Lindsay R. Bone involvement in rheumatoid arthritis. *Clinical Rheumatoid Diseases* 1977; 3:403-20.
38. Spector M . Factors augmenting/inhibiting biological fixation of porous-coated noncemented prostheses. *Orthopaedic Transactions of the Hip Society* 1986; 10 (3):547-8.
39. Branson PJ, Steege JW, Wixson RL, Lewis J, Stulberg SD. Rigidity of internal fixation with uncemented tibial knee implants. *Journal of Arthroplasty* 1989;4:21-6.
40. Burke DW, O'Connor DA, Zalenski EB, Jasty M, Harris WH. Micromotion of cemented and uncemented femoral components. *Journal of Bone and Joint Surgery* 1991; 73B:33-7.
41. Shimagaki H, Bechtold JE AU. Sherman R, Gustilo RB. Initial stability of tibial components in cementless total knee arthroplasty. *Transactions of 34th Annual Meeting Orthopaedic Research Society* 1988; 13:477.
42. Strickland AB, Chan KH, Andriacchi TP, Miller J. The initial fixation of porous coated tibial commponents evaluated by the study of rigid body motion under static load. *Transactions of 34th Annual Meeting Orthopaedic Research Society* 1988; 13:476.
43. Vanderby R, Manley PA, Kohles SS, Belloli DM, McBeath AA. A micromotion comparison of cemented and porous ingrowth total hip replacements in a canine model. *Transactions 35th Annual Meeting, Orthopaedic Research Society,* 1989, 14:577.
44. Volz RG, Nisbet JK, Lee RW, McMurtry MG. The mechanical stability of various noncemented tibial components. *Clinical Orthopaedics* 1988;226:38-42.
45. Ryd L. Micromotion in knee arthroplasty. *Acta Orthopaedica Scandinavica.* Ph.D. Thesis, Suppl 220, vol 57; 1986.
46. Frost HM. *Intermediary organization of the skeleton,* vol I, Boca Raton, Florida: CRC Press, Inc. 1986: 50-52.

47. Eitel F, Klapp F, Jacobsen W Schweiberer L. Bone regeneration in animals and in man. A contribution to understanding the relative value of animal experiments to human pathophysiology. *Archives of Orthopaedic Traumatic Surgery* 1981;99:59-64.
48. Albrektsson T, Albrektsson B. Osseointegration of bone implants. A review of bone implant fixation, *Acta Orthopaedica Scandinavica* 1987;58:567-77.
49. Cameron HU, Pilliar RM, Macnab I. The rate of bone ingrowth into porous metal. *Journal of Biomedical Materials Research* 1976; 10:295-302.
50. Carlsson L, Röstlund T, Albrektsson B, Albrektsson T. Implant fixation improved by close fit. *Acta Orthopaedica Scandinavica* 1988;59 (3):272-5.
51. Harris WH, White RE, McCarthy JC, Walker PS, Weinberg EH. Bony ingrowth fixation of the acetabular component in canine hip joint arthroplasty. *Clinical Orthopaedics* 1983;176:7-11.
52. Sandborn PM, Cook SD, Spires WP, Kester MA. Tissue response to porous-coated implants lacking initial bone apposition. *Journal of Arthroplasty* 1988;3:337-46.
53. Toksvig-Larsen S. Ryd L. Surface flatness after bone cutting. A cadaver study of tibial condyles. *Acta Orthopaedica Scandinavica* 1991;62 (2):15-18.
54. Toksvig-Larsen S - On bone cutting. *Ph D Thesis, Lund, Sweden* 1992;
55. Bobyn JD, Engh CA. Human histology of the bone- porous metal implant interface. *Orthopaedics* 1984; 7:1410
56. Engh CA, Bobyn JD, Glassman A . Porous-coated hip replacement. *Journal of Bone and Joint Surgery* 1987; 69-B:45-55.
57. Linder L, Carlsson Å, Marsal L, Bjursten LM, Brånemark P-I. Clinical aspects of osseointegration in joint replacement. *Journal of Bone and Joint Surgery* 1988;70-B:550-5.
58. Albrektsson T. Healing of bone grafts. *Thesis. Gothenburg*, 1979.
59. Burchardt H, Jones H, Glowczewskie F, Rudner C ,Enneking WF. Freeze-dried allogenic segmental cortical-bone grafts in dogs. *Journal of Bone and Joint Surgery 1978;60-A:* 1082-90.
60. Burchardt H. The biology of bone graft repair. *Clinical Orthopaedics* 1983;174:28-42.
61. Goldberg VM, Powell A, Zika J, Bos GD, Heiple KG. Bone grafting: role of histocompatibility in transplantation. *Journal of Orthopaedic Research* 1985; 3:389-404.
62. Friedlaender GE. Current concepts review. Bone grafting. *Journal of Bone and Joint Surgery* 1987,69-A:786-9.
63. Heiple KG, Chase SW, Herndon CH. A comparative study of the healing process following different types of bone transplantation. *Journal of Bone and Joint Surgery 1963;45-A: 1593-616.*
64. Goldberg VM, Stevenson S. Natural history of autografts and allografts. *Clinical Orthopaedics* 1987;225:7-16.
65. McDonald DJ, Fitzgerald RH, Chao EYS. The enhancement of fixation of a porous-coated femoral component by autograft and allograft in the dog. *Journal of Bone and Joint Surgery* 1988;70-A: 728-37.
66. Lewis CG, Jones LC, Connor KM, Lennox DW, Hungerford DS. An evaluation of grafting materials in cementless arthroplasty. *Transactions 33rd Annual Meeting, Orthopaedic Research Society* 1987; 12:319.
67. Kienapfel H, Sumner DR, Turner, TM, Urban RM, Galante JO. Efficacy of autograft and freedze-dried allograft to enhance fixation of porous coated implants in the presence of interface gaps. *Journal of Orthopaedic Research* 1992; 10:423-33.
68. Kang JD, McKerman DJ, Kruger M, Mutschler T, Thompson WH, Rubash HE. Defect filling and bone ingrowth: a comparative study in a canine fiber metal total hip model. *Transactions of 35th Annual Meeting Orthopaedic Research Society* 1989;14:552.
69. Turner TM, Urban RM, Sumner DR, Galante JO. Enhancement of bone ingrowth in cementless revision THA using a two stage procedure. *Transactions of 38th Annual Meeting of Orthopaedic Research Society* 1992;17:369.
70. Sumner DR, Jacobs JJ, Turner TM, Urban RM, Galante JO. The amount and distribution of bone ingrowth in tibial components retrieved from human patients. *Transactions of 35th Annual Meeting Orthopaedic Research Society* 1989;14:375.
71. Stulberg BN, Watson JT, Stulberg SD, Bauer TW, Manley MT. A new model to assess tibial fixation. II. Concurrent histologic and biomechanical observation. *Clinical Orthopaedics* 1991;263:303-309.
72. Schatzker J, Horne JG, Sumner-Smith G. The effect of movement on the holding power of screws in bone. *Clinical Orthopaedics* 1975;111:257-62.
73. Uhthoff HK Germain J-P. The reversal of tissue differentiation around screws. *Clinical Orthopaedics* 1977;123:248-52.
74. Uhthoff HK. Mechanical factors influencing the holding power of screws in compact bone. *Journal of Bone and Joint Surgery* 1973;55-B:633-9.

75. Cameron HU. The effect of movement on the bonding of porous metal on bone *Journal of Biomedical Materials Research* 1973;7:301-311.

76. Cameron HU, Macnab I, Pilliar RM. Porous surfaced vitallium staples. *South African Journal of Surgery* 1972;10:63-70.

77. Pilliar RM, Lee JM, Maniatopoulos C. Observations on the effect of movement on bone ingrowth into porous-surfaced implants. *Clinical Orthopaedics* 1986;208:108-13.

78. Pilliar RM, Cameron HU, Welsh RP, Binnington AG. Radiographical and morphological studies of load-bearing porous surfaced structured implants. *Clinical Orthopaedics* 1981;156:249-57.

79. Ducheyne P, DeMeester P, Aernoudt E, Martens M, Mulier C. Influence of a functional dynamic loading on bone ingrowth into surface pores of orthopaedic implants. *Journal of Biomedical Materials Research* 1977;11:811-38.

80. Heck DA, Nakajima I, Kelly PJ, Chao EYS . The effect of load alteration on the biological and biomechanical performance of a titanium fiber-metal segmental prosthesis *Journal of Bone and Joint Surgery* 1986;698-A:118-26.

81. Eschenroeder HC, Jones LC, Hungerford DS. Biological ingrowth into a porous metal surface following established fibrous reaction.*Transactions of Orthopaedic Research Society* 1988;13:333.

82. Aspenberg P, Goodman S, Toksvig-Larsen S, Ryd L, Albrektsson T. Intermitent micromotion inhibits bone ingrowth. Titanium implants in rabbits. *Acta Orthopaedica Scandinavica* 1992;63(2):141-5.

83. Zalenski EB, Jasty M, O'Connor DO, et al. Micromotion of porous-surfaced, cementless prostheses following 6 months of in vivo bone ingrowth in a canine model. *Transactions of 35th Annual Meeting Orthopaedic Research Society* 1989;14:377.

84. Burke DW, Bragdon CR, O'Connor DO, Jasty M, Haire T, Harris WH . Dynamic measurement of interface mechanics in vivo and the effect of micromotion on bone ingrowth into a porous surface device under controlled loads in vivo. *Transactions of 37th Annual Meeting Orthopaedic Research Society* 1991;16:103.

85. Natarajan R, Andriacchi TP. The influence of displacement in compatibilities on bone ingrowth in porous tibial components. *Transactions of 34th Annual Meeting Orthopaedic Research Society* 1988;13:331.

86. Yang A, Sumner DR, Choi S, Natarajan R, Andriacchi TP. Direct measurement of micromotion at the bone-implant interface: The tibial component in a canine model. *Transactions of 36th Annual Meeting Orthopaedic Research Society* 1990;15:233.

87. Hori RY, Lewis JL. Mechanical properties of the fibrous tissue found at the bone- cement interface following total joint replacement. *Journal of Biomedical Materials Research* 1982; 16:911-27.

88. Tibrewal SO, Grant KA, Goodfellow JW. The radiolucent line beneath the tibial components of the Oxford meniscal knee. *Journal of Bone and Joint Surgery* 1984;66- B:523-8.

89. Walker PS, Onchi K, Kurosawa H, Rodger RF. Approaches to the interface problem in total joint arthroplasty. *Clinical Orthopaedics* 1984;182:99-108.

90. Longo JA, Magee FP, Mather SE, Yapp RA, Koeneman JB, Weinstein AM. Comparison of HA and non-HA coated carbon composite femoral stems. *Transactions of 35th Annual Meeting Orthopaedic Research Society* 1989;14:384.

91. Ryd L, Linder L. On the correlation between micromotion and histology of the bone-cement interface. *Journal of Arthroplasty* 1989;4:303-9.

92. Cook SD, Thomas KA, Kay JF, Jarcho M . Hydroxylapatite-coated titanium for orthopaedic implant application. *Clinical Orthopaedics* 1988;232:225-43.

93. Ducheyne P, Hench LL, Kagan A, Martens M, Bursens A, Mulier C . Effect of hydroxyapatite impregnation on skeletal bonding of porous coated implants. *Journal of Biomedical Materials Research* 1980;14:225-37.

94. Rivero DP, Fox J, Skipor AK, Urban RM, Galante JO. Calcium phosphate-coated porous titanium implants for enhanced skeletal fixation. *Journal of Biomedical Materials Research* 1988;22:191-201.

95. Perren SM . Physical and biological aspects of fracture healing with special reference to internal fixation. *Clinical Orthopaedics* 1979;138:175-96.

96. Manley MT, Kay JF, Yoshiya S, Stern LS, Stulberg BN . Accelerated fixation of weight bearing implants by hydroxyapatite coatings. *Transactions of 33rd Annual Meeting Orthopaedic Research Society* 1987;12:214.

97. Thomas KA, Cook SD, Haddad RJ, Kay JF, Jarcho M. Biological response to hydroxylapatite-coated titanium hips. *Journal of Arthroplasty* 1989;4:43-53.

98. Poser RD, Magee FP, Kay JF, Toal TR, Hedley AK. Biomechanical and histologic assessment of HA enhanced long-term fixation in a unique loaded canine implant. *Fourth World Biomaterials Congress* 1992.

99. Hench LL . Bioactive ceramics. *In Bioceramics: material characteristics versus in vivo behavior.* (Eds: Ducheyne P and Lemons JE). Ann NY Acad Sci vol 523 part II 1988: 54-71.

100. Goldring SR, Schiller AL, Roelke M, Rourke CM, O'Niell DA, Harris WH . The synovial-like membrane at the bone cement interface in loose total hip replacements and its proposed role in bone lysis. *Journal of Bone and Joint Surgery* 1983;65-A:575-84.

101. Goldring SR, Jasty M, Roelke MS, Rourke CM, Bringhurst FR, Harris WH. Formation of a synovial-like membrane at the bone-cement interface. *Arthritis and Rheumatism* 1986;29:836-842.

102. Beight J, Radin S, Cuckler J, Ducheyne P. Effect of solubility of calcium phosphate coatings on mechanical fixation of porous ingrown implants. *Transactions of 35th Annual Meeting Orthopaedic Research Society* 1989;14:334.

103. Turner TM, Sumner DR, Urban RM, Rivero DP, Galante JO. A comparative study of porous coatings in a weight-bearing total hip arthroplasty model. *Journal of Bone and Joint Surgery* 1986;68-A:1396-409.

104. Jasty M, Harris WH. Observations on factors controlling bony ingrowth into weight-bearing, porous, canine total hip replacements. *In non-cemented total hip replacement.* (Ed R Fitzgerald Jr.) Raven Press, Ltd., New York 1988:175-89.

105. Wolff J. *Das Gesetz der Transformation der Knochen,* Qvarto, Berlin, 1892.

106. Berry JL, Geiger JM, Moran JM, Skraba JS ,Greenwald AS. Use of tricalcium phosphate or electrical stimulation to enhance the bone-porous implant interface. *Journal of Biomedical Materials Research* 1986;20:65-77.

107. Cook SD, Thomas KA, Kay JF, Jarcho M. Hydroxyapatite-coated porous titanium for use in an orthopaedic biologic attachment system. *Clinical Orthopaedics* 1988;230:303-12.

108. Carlsson L, Regnér L, Johansson C, Gottlander M, Herberts P. Histomorphometrical comparison of titanium and hydroxyapatite-coated implants in the human arthritic knee. *Transactions of 38th Annual Meeting Orthopaedic Research Society* 1992;17:267.

109. Cook SD, Thomas KA, Dalton JE, Kay JF. Enhanced bone ingrowth and fixation strength with hydroxyapatite-coated porous implants. *Seminars in Arthroplasty* 1991;2(4):268-79.

110. Oonishi H, Yamamoto M, Tsuji E, Kushitani S, Aono M, Ukon Y. The effect of hydroxyapatite coating on bone growth into porous coated titanium alloy implants. *Journal of Bone and Joint Surgery* 1989;71-B:213-16.

111. Boone PS, Zimmerman MC, Gutteling E, Lee CK, Parsons JR. Bone attachment to hydroxyapatite coated polymers. *Journal of Biomedical Materials Research* 1989;23:183-99.

112. Stephenson PK, Freeman MAR, Revell PA, Germain J, Tuke M , Pirie CJ . The effect of hydroxyapatite coating on ingrowth of bone into cavities in an implant. *Journal of Arthroplasty* 1991;6(1):51-8.

113. Cook SD, Kay JF, Thomas KA , Jarcho M. Interface mechanics and histology of titanium and hydroxyapatite coated titanium for dental implant application. *International Journal of Oral Maxillofacial Surgery* 1987;2:15-22.

114. Geesink RGT, de Groot K, Klein CPAT. Bonding of bone to apatite-coated implants. *Journal of Bone and Joint Surgery* 1988;70-B:17-23.

115. Stulberg BN, Watson JT, Bauer TW , Kambic H . Hydroxyapatite vs. titanium mesh coating for uncemented tibial fixation in the canine knee. *Transactions of 38th Annual Meeting Orthopaedic Research Society* 1992;17:381.

116. Berger RA, Klein AH, Rodosky MW, Seel MJ, Anderson G, Rubash HE. The mechanical and histological effects of plasma sprayed hydroxyapatite coating in a canine femoral endoprosthesis model. *Transactions of 38th Annual Meeting Orthopaedic Research Society* 1992;17:401.

117. Spector M - Current concepts of bone ingrowth and remodeling. In Fitzgerald RH. ed. *Non-cemented total hip arthroplasty.* Raven Press, Arizona, 1987:69.

*Hydroxylapatite Coatings in Orthopaedic Surgery,*
edited by R. G. T. Geesink and M. T. Manley.
Raven Press, Ltd., New York, © 1993.

# Preclinical Evaluation of the Effect of Hydroxylapatite on the "Comprehensive" Bone Implant Interface

Robert D. Poser, D.V.M., John F. Kay, Ph.D.,
Frank P. Magee, D.V.M., and
Anthony K. Hedley, M.D., F.R.C.S.

Optimization of the interfacial environment between endoprostheses and host bone is of paramount importance. Factors affecting the bone-implant interface and therefore the stability of cementless endoprostheses are numerous. They include surgical technique (1,23,33,38,41,42), initial appositional fit (13), motion at the interface (3,12,49), quality and metabolic status of host bone (35,57,61,62), biocompatability of implant material (10,25,28,29,32,44,64,67), and bioactivity of the implant surface and coating (1,9,17,18,21,22,24,30,31,39,46, 47,50,52,60,63,66). Optimizing these factors enhances fixation by creating a biomechanical interface environment conducive to early osseointegration of the implant (1,2,41,42). This maximizes initial implant stability, essential for good long term clinical performance.

Many investigations have demonstrated that thin hydroxylapatite (HA) coatings, a biocompatable osteoconductive calcium phosphate ceramic, enhances implant-bone attachment (18,19,21,22,26,30,31,34,39,43,46,47,50-52, 54,55,58,60,61,63,65,66,69). Others report insignificant or only transient increases in attachment strength of various HA-coated macrotextured surfaces (20,23,59). Under ideal interface conditions (i.e., tight interference fit, minimal motion at the interface, no direct loading of the implant) HA significantly enhances host tissue adaptation and initial implant fixation (18,22-24,26,30,31,34,50,51,54,66,69). However, ideal interface conditions are not always attainable at the time of surgery. Of greater clinical importance is the significant improvement in host tissue adaptation to HA-coated implants in suboptimal and clinically more realistic interface conditions. These include better implant fixation in osteoporotic bone (57,58,61), noninterference fit (19,58-61,63), and excessive motion at the implant-bone interface (60).

The application of HA coatings to orthopaedic and dental implants remains the topic of much research (36,40). Efforts to increase bone ingrowth of cementless orthopaedic prostheses, shown in humans to be primarily by fibrous tissue ingrowth (6-8,14-16,27,68), has led to the application of thin HA coatings to porous, grooved, and plasma-sprayed macrotextured surfaces. Certain reports document focal areas of thinning and loss of HA coatings from metal endoprostheses after different periods of implantation (4,23,34,55,56).

Despite clinical reports of infrequent radiolucency at the bone/HA-coated surface interface (21) and significant reduction in implant subsidence (39), isolated retrieval studies of HA-coated human femoral prostheses report various degrees of bone apposition to HA -coated prostheses (4,5,48,57).

This chapter addresses three important issues in the potential *long-term* clinical performance of HA-coated, load-bearing prostheses: the load-sharing effect of HA-coated macrotextured implants, the concept of a "comprehensive" HA-bone interface, and the long term fate/requirement of HA coatings on orthopaedic implants.

## MATERIAL AND METHODS

### Grooved Transcortical Implant Study

Host tissue adaptation to implants manufactured from Ti-6Al-4V with multiple circumferential grooves (Fig. 1) was evaluated as a function of time (54). HA-coated and uncoated Ti implants were examined. Uncoated implants were grit-blasted to approximate the surface roughness of the coated implants. HA coating (Bio-Interfaces, San Diego,CA) was applied by a plasma-spray process to a thickness of $60 \pm 10 \mu m$. Employing a standard transcortical model, three pellets were placed in the coronal (medial/lateral) plane across the femoral diaphysis. Implants were harvested at 3, 6, 12, 26, and 52 weeks postoperatively. Interfacial attachment strength was measured by a standard mechanical test (50) that loads the bone-implant interface to failure. Statistical analysis was done by Students *t*-test and one-way analysis of variance. Both tested and intact specimens from each animal and time period were processed for histologic and electron microscopic analysis.

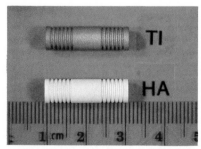

**FIG. 1.** Macrotextured, grooved transcortical implants. Hydroxylapatite-coated (HA),grit blasted Ti-6Al-4V (Ti).

## Weight-Bearing Modular Canine Femoral Implant Study

Long-term performance of an HA-coated femoral prosthesis was evaluated in skeletally mature greyhound dogs (55). Host tissue adaptation and ultimate bone–implant interface attachment strength were analyzed. Femoral prostheses were manufactured from Ti-6Al-4V in a unique modular design (Fig. 2) (45). Intramedullary (IM) stem components were either coated with HA (Bio-Interfaces, San Diego, CA) or grit-blasted to approximate surface roughness of the coated stems along their entire length (Fig. 3). All implanted femurs were harvested 18 months postoperatively and contact radiographs were taken. After removal of the head and neck, self-aligning fixtures permitted standardized sectioning and analysis along the entire length of the treated IM portion of the prosthesis (Fig. 4). Evaluation of interfacial attachment strength by modified pushout test and histologic analysis of HA-coated and uncoated Ti prostheses were performed at each level.

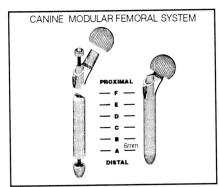

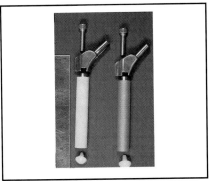

**FIG. 2.** Harrington Canine Modular Hip. Implanted as a femoral prosthesis, components include a femoral head, neck, and shoulder, gun-bored intramedullary rod, articulating screw, and distal polyethylene plug.

**FIG. 3.** Harrington Canine Modular Hip. IM rods are treated separately. Prostheses are then assembled and sterilized before surgery.

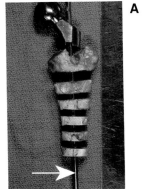

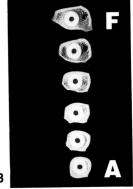

**FIG. 4 (A)** Recovered 18-month femur after sectioning. **(B)** Contact radiographs of serial sections of implanted femur (A-distal, F-proximal). Alignment pin ( →) used for standardized processing coincides with central canal seen in radiographs.

**RESULTS**

**Grooved Transcortical Implant Study**

The HA-coated specimens had significantly stronger interface strengths than the uncoated specimens at *all* time periods ($p<0.05$) (Fig. 5). HA-coated implants attained attachment to periprosthetic bone at an accelerated rate. The 3-week HA specimens had similar attachment strengths to the 12-week uncoated specimens. HA specimens had increased attachment strength at each successive time period up to 26 weeks. No increase was noted between 26 and 52 weeks.

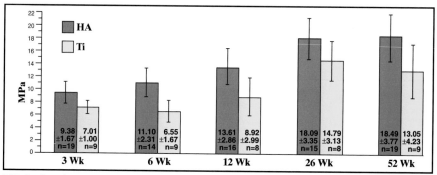

**FIG. 5.** Interface attachment strengths of grooved implants in MPa, standard deviation (±), and specimen number (n). *p*<0.05.

Histologic processing of both intact and tested specimens allowed analysis of the host tissue biologic response and mechanism of interface failure. Bone was in direct apposition to all HA-coated surfaces at all time periods (Fig. 6). Initially, linear deposition of osseous tissue was present along all HA-coated surfaces. This tissue later mineralized and bone was found in direct apposition to all HA-coated surfaces. Although intermittent bone apposition was noted in uncoated specimens, intervening fibrous tissue between implant and host bone was noted in a high percentage of uncoated specimens at each time period. Qualitatively, greater amounts of bone were noted in HA-coated vs. uncoated grooves at 3, 6, and 12 weeks. By 26 weeks the amount of mineralized bone present within the grooves of coated and uncoated implants appeared similar. At no time period was an adverse host tissue response noted at the bone implant interface.

Histologic analysis of mechanically tested specimens revealed that interface failure occurred through the ingrown tissue at the level of the groove crest. Ingrown bone in HA-coated grooves remained undisturbed with the HA-bone interface intact, whereas bone in uncoated grooves was more consistently displaced (Fig. 7). At the groove crests, failure predominated at the HA-bone interface during early time periods (less than 12 weeks) and at the HA-Ti substrate interface during later periods.

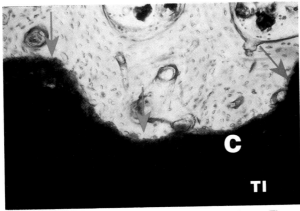

**FIG. 6.** Light micrograph of 26 week HA-coated grooved specimen. The groove has been fully ingrown with bone. Bone is in direct apposition (->) to the HA coating (C). Bone is seen in direct apposition (->) to the titanium (Ti) substrate with no adverse tissue response in an area devoid of coating.

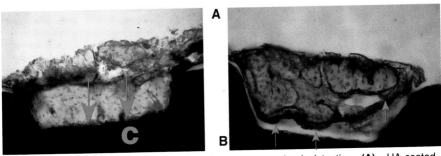

**FIG. 7.** Light micrographs of grooved implants after mechanical testing. **(A)** HA-coated specimen with undisturbed bone in direct apposition (->) to coated surface (C). **(B)** Uncoated specimen with intervening fibrous tissue ( ->). Ingrown bone has been displaced at testing.

## Weight-bearing Modular Canine Femoral Implant Study

All femoral components were clinically functional until animal sacrifice at 18 months. A consistent radiographic finding was increased density at the most proximal and distal levels of these fully HA-coated femoral components as compared with the uncoated stems (Fig. 8). Mechanical test results are summarized in Fig. 9. Interfacial attachment strengths of HA-coated stems were significantly greater than those of the uncoated Ti stems at all levels.

On histologic analysis, mineralized bone was seen in direct apposition to the HA-coated stems (Fig. 10) in all but a few areas. These areas had well-oriented intervening fibrous tissue between the HA-coated stems and periprosthetic bone. The uncoated Ti stems were surrounded by comparatively thick, moderately oriented fibrous tissue (Fig. 11). HA coatings remained intact and well-adherent to the underlying Ti substrate in all but a few focal areas. Certain of these appeared to be focal areas of resorption and exhibited bone or marrow

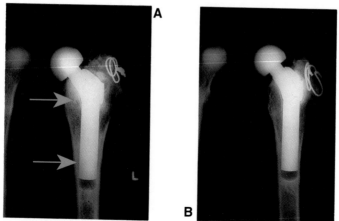

**FIG. 8.** 18-month postoperative contact radiographs of HA-coated **(A)** and uncoated Ti **(B)** modular stems. Areas of increased density (->), representing those most likely to transfer load, are at more proximal and distal levels of HA-coated IM rod.

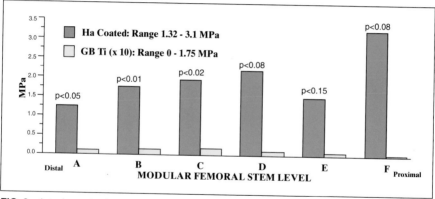

**FIG. 9.** Interface attachment strengths of canine modular stems by level. Individual *p* values represent the significance between interface strengths of the HA-coated and uncoated stems at that level.

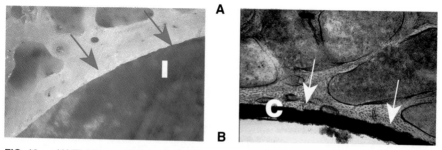

**FIG. 10.** **(A)** Eighteen-month HA-coated femoral stem, post-pushout specimen. Macroscopic view of bone in direct apposition ($\rightarrow$) to the HA coated stem (I) with no intervening fibrous tissue. **(B)** Light micrograph of bone in direct apposition ($\rightarrow$) to the intact HA coating (C). Circumferential layer of densified bone was a common finding.

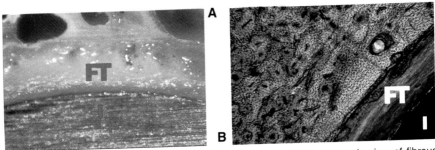

**FIG. 11.** Eighteen-month uncoated titanium femoral stem. **(A)** Macroscopic view of fibrous tissue (FT) at the bone-implant interface. **(B)** Light micrograph of intervening fibrous tissue (FT) between bone and implant (I).

space in direct apposition to the underlying Ti substrate (Fig. 12). In other isolated areas the coating was intact but delaminated from the underlying substrate. These areas consistently had thin, extremely well-oriented fibrous tissue between and adherent to both the coating and the substrate metal.

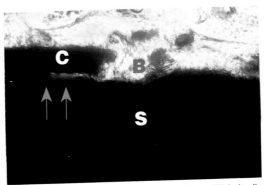

**FIG. 12.** Light micrograph of area devoid of HA coating. Bone (B) is in direct apposition to the exposed metal substrate (S). A thin, well-oriented fibrous tissue (→) beneath the delaminated coating (C) appears adherent to both coating and substrate metal.

## DISCUSSION

The grooved transcortical study demonstrated that HA coating of grooved implants significantly improves early postoperative bone apposition and interface attachment strengths at 3, 6, and 12 weeks, confirming previous studies by Thomas et al. (66) and Stephensen et al. (63). Our data, however, demonstrated enhanced interface strength in HA-coated grooved implants still present at 26 and 52 weeks. These findings were unexpected (66) because bone ingrowth into all implants should be complete by 26 weeks and would be expected to govern long-term attachment strength. The attachment strength resulting from ingrowth at this time was expected to overshadow any early osteoconductive effect of an HA coating. Equivalent interface strengths of HA-coated implants at 26 and 52 weeks probably represent a steady state in interfacial bone remodeling. These data demonstrated for the first time that HA coating of a macrotextured grooved surface enhances attachment strength after the bone–implant interface has achieved a relative steady remodeling state.

Load sharing between the ongrowth (crest) and ingrowth (recess) surfaces of this macrotextured geometry creates a "comprehensive" interface. This offers a theoretical explanation for this improved long-term attachment strength of the HA-coated specimens at 26 and 52 weeks. Individually, osseointegration and bone ingrowth each result in improved attachment strength. Grooved HA-coated surfaces provide both accelerated osseointegration and bone ingrowth of the implant surface. Smooth ongrowth surfaces, represented by the groove crest, have inherently weaker interface characteristics than those ingrown with bone. Such ongrowth areas, initially in direct contact with host bone, are osseointegrated more rapidly in HA-coated implants (18,26,47,50). This enhances early attachment strength. At later time periods, direct apposition of bone to the HA-coated grooves increases overall interface stiffness (66). The relative fraction of the load carried by the groove as compared with the crest is therefore greater in the HA-coated implants. The fibrous interface on the uncoated grooves decreases interface stiffness, causing a greater fraction of the total load to be carried by the outer, inherently weaker, uncoated crest surface. The load-sharing biomechanics of the grooved surface geometry therefore appear enhanced by the osteoconductive properties of an HA coating and significantly improves the "comprehensive" interface environment.

The modular hip study permitted histologic *and* mechanical evaluation of an HA-coated metal prosthesis in the clinically significant corticocancellous bone of the proximal femur, under weight-bearing conditions. Enhanced host-tissue adaptation to HA-coated modular hips compared with uncoated hips was consistent with experimental transcortical and transmetaphyseal implants (17,18,23,24,26,30,34,50,51,58–61,63,66), of functionally loaded HA-coated endoprosthesis (19,43,46,47,65) and with HA-coated human implant retrieval (4,5,48,57) studies.

The most significant difference in attachment strength between coated and uncoated modular stems was at the more proximal and distal levels where load transfer would be expected to be greatest (37). This coincides with areas of greatest proliferation of periprosthetic bone. Bauer et al. (4) reported similar results, with periprosthetic bone most prominent in areas of predicted load transfer, in retrievals of HA-coated human femoral stems. Both findings are consistent with Wolff's law.

At 18 months postoperatively, small focal areas devoid of HA coating were present in this modular femoral stem. Bauer et al. (4) described similar findings in human implant retrievals. He noted remodeling canals with osteoclasts close to some areas of focal resorption of the HA coating. He suggested, however, that this may simply represent osteoclastic resorption of the available periprosthetic calcium phosphate (present in both the host bone matrix and HA coating). Such resorption is necessary in the normal bone remodeling process (and often preceeds bone formation) in areas of load transfer (11). Lack of adverse host tissue response in areas devoid of HA in the modular hip was consistent with the canine transcortical studies of Cook et al. (17) and the human implant retrieval results of Bauer et al. (4). Localized areas, in fact, had bone in direct apposition to the exposed metal substrate of this modular stem (Fig. 12).

In addition, areas devoid of HA coating at 18 months comprised only a small fraction of the overall interface surface area. Given the report of Cook et al. (17) that small, experimentally-created HA coating defects did not significantly decrease transcortical implant attachment strengths, and the findings of Bauer et al. (4), these modular hip histologic and mechanical test results suggest that focal loss of HA coatings may not significantly affect the long term comprehensive attachment strength of weight-bearing prostheses.

Careful consideration of those areas totally devoid or minimally delaminated of HA coatings is required. Søballe et al. (60) demonstrated in the immediate postoperative period (four weeks) that the osteoconductive effect of HA-coated metal implants causes modification of adjacent fibrous tissue in initially unstable condylar plugs. This resulted in more functional, stronger fibrous anchorage. Modified fibrous tissue morphology combined with increased interface strengths of the 18-month HA-coated modular hips supports this concept in longer-term weight-bearing implants.

The "comprehensive" interface in these weight-bearing implants includes both the coated and focally exposed metal substrate surfaces. Enhancement of the overall bone-implant interface condition of HA-coated implants improves the local interface condition. This creates a conducive environment for host tissue adaptation to subsequently exposed metal substrate. In addition, increasing macroscopic implant surface texture significantly increases direct apposition of bone and interface strength (64). Roughening of the substrate metal surface (a standard procedure before coating that maximizes HA substrate bonding) could improve the host tissue response to substrate subsequently exposed *in vivo*.

## CONCLUSIONS

Evaluation of an indirectly loaded implant model demonstrated that a macrotextured, grooved surface shared load between bone grown into the groove recesses and that grown onto the outer crest. The cumulative effect of this load sharing resulted in improved "comprehensive" interface conditions. Application of HA coatings further enhanced these conditions, improving both immediate and longer-term biomechanical fixation. HA coatings applied to weight-bearing metal implants improved the interface environment in the early postoperative period. This early improvement in interfacial environment allowed favorable longer-term host tissue adaptation.

Methods of maximizing the osteoconductive, load-sharing effects of HA, while limiting the load-bearing requirements of the ceramic coating, remain important goals in long-term utilization of HA coatings in weight-bearing prostheses. These results indicate that an HA-coated, grooved, macrotextured surface may offer a promising alternative for achieving these requirements. However, these data raise an important question: Is long term maintenance of the HA coating necessary for successful implant performance? The improved host tissue adaptation to coated prostheses in the early postoperative period significantly improved implant attachment. Despite focal loss of HA, improvement in the "comprehensive" interface characteristics and load sharing occur over the longer term. Enhancement of the overall bone-implant interface environment by HA appears important in optimizing conditions required for host bone to gradually integrate with areas of exposed metal substrate. A slow "physiologic" resorption of calcium phosphate coatings that permits gradual osseointegration of underlying metal might prove crucial to the long-term stability and success of coated prostheses.

Enhancement of interfacial attachment strength remains encouraging. However, significant issues that may affect the focal bone-implant interface as well as the adjoining intra-articular bearing surface remain for future consideration. These include rate and mechanism of resorption/degradation, installation and in-service delamination, potential particulate-induced periprosthetic osteolysis, and the efficiency of the host tissue response in processing these coatings.

Specific prosthetic designs may require particular interface conditions for optimal long term clinical results (36,43,53). The application of HA coatings to orthopaedic prostheses must not be considered a panacea. The performance of all calcium phosphate coatings is device, material, fabrication, and application dependent (40). Future analyses of retrieved human HA-coated prostheses and animal research at more extended time periods are required to address prosthesis-specific long term performance of HA coatings.

## ACKNOWLEDGEMENTS

The authors gratefully acknowledge the support of the Olin Foundation and Bio-Interfaces, Inc., as well as the collaborative efforts of Dr. James Koeneman, Dr. Joseph Longo, Dr. Stephen Gilson, Dr. David Van de Wyngaerde, Dr. Thomas Toal, Dr. Mark Werner, Mr. Thomas May, Mr. Janson Emmanual, Ms. Becky Reinke, and Ms. Barbara Capwell. This work was performed at the Harrington Arthritis Research Center.

## REFERENCES

1.  Albrektsson T, Branemark P I, Hansson H A, and Lindstrom J. Osseo-integrated titanium implants. Requirement for ensuring a long-lasting, direct bone-to-implant anchorage in man. *Acta Orthopaedica Scandinavica* 1981, 15:155.
2.  Albrektsson T, Jansson T, and Lekholm V. Osseointegrated dental implants. *Dental Clinics of North America* 1986, 30:151.

3.  Aspenberg P, Goodman S, Toksvig-Larsen, S, Ryd L, and Albrektsso n T. Intermittent micromotion inhibits bone ingrowth. *Acta Orthopaedica Scandinavica* 1992, 63(2):141.
4.  Bauer TW, Geesink RGT, Zimmerman R, and McMahon JT. Hydroxyapatite-coated femoral stems. *Journal of Bone and Joint Surgery* 1991,73-A:10:1439.
5.  Bloebaum RD, Merrell M, Gustke K, Simmons M. Retrieval analysis of a hydroxypatite-coated hip prosthesis. *Clinical Orthopaedics* 1991, 267:97.
6.  Bobyn JD, Engh CA, Glassman AH. Histologic analysis of a retrieved microporous coated femoral prosthesis: A seven year case report. *Clinical Orthopaedics* 1987, 224:303.
7.  Bobyn JD, Engh CA. Human histology of the bone-porous metal implant interface. *Orthopedics* 1984, 7:1410.
8.  Bobyn JD, Pilliar RM, Cameron HU, Weatherly GC. The optimum pore size for the fixation of porous-surfaced metal implants by the ingrowth of bone. *Clinical Orthopaedics* 1980, 150:263.
9.  Boone PS, Zimmerman MC, Gutteling E, Lee CK, Parsons JR, Langrana N. Bone attachment to hydroxylapatite coated polymers. *Journal of Biomedical Materials Research* 1989, 23 (A2):18
10. Brown SA, Merritt K, Farnsworth LJ, Crowe TD. Biological significance of metal ion release. In Lemons, JE (ed.): *Quantitative characterization and performance of porous implants for hard tissue applications,* ASTM STP 953. Philadelphia: American Society for Testing and Materials, 1987:163-81.
11. Burr DB, Schoffler MB, Yang KH, Wu DD, Lukoschek M, Kandzari D, SivaneriN, Blaha JD, Radin EL. The effect of altered strain environments on bone tissue knetics. *Bone* 1989, 10:215.
12. Cameron HV, Pilliar RM, and Macnab I. The effect of movement on the bonding of porous metal on bone. *Journal Biomedical Materials Research* 1973, 7:301.
13. Carlsson L, Rostlund T, Albrektsson B, Albrektsson T. Implant fixation improved by close fit. Cylindrical implant bone interface studied in rabbits. *Acta Orthopaedica Scandinavica* 1988, 59(3):272.
14. Collier JP, Mayer MB, Chae JC, Surprenant VA, Surprenant HP, Dauphinais LA. Macroscopic and microscopic evidence of prosthetic fixation with porous-coated materials. *Clinical Orthopaedics* 1988, 235:173.
15. Cook SD, Barrack RC, Thomas KA, Haddad RJ. Quantitative analysis of tissue growth into human porous total hip components. *Journal of Arthroplasty* 1988, 3:249.
16. Cook SD, Thomas KA, Haddad RJ. Histologic analysis of retrieved porous-coated total joint components. *Clinical Orthopaedics* 1988, 234:90.
17. Cook SD, Thomas KA, Kay JF. Experimental coating defects in hydroxylapatite-coated implants. *Clinical Orthopaedics* 1991, 265:280.
18. Cook SD, Thomas KA, Kay JF, Jarcho M. Hydroxyapatite-coated titanium for orthopedic mplant applications. *Clinical Orthopaedics* 1988, 232:225.
19. Cook SD, Thomas KA, Dalton JE, and Kay JF. Enhanced bone ingrowth and fixation strength with hydroxyapatite-coated porous implants. *Seminars in Arthroplasty* 1991, 2:268.
20. Cook SD, Thomas KA, Kay JF, Jarcho M. Hydroxyapatite- coated porous titanium for use as an orthopaedic biologic attachment system. *Clinical Orthopaedics* 1988, 230:303.
21. D'Antonio JA, Capello WN, Crothers OD, Jaffe WL, Manley MT. Early clinical experience with hydroxyapatite-coated femoral implants. *Journal of Bone and Joint Surgery* 1992, 74-A:7:995.
22. deGroot K, Geesink RGT, Klein CPAT, Serekian P. Plasma sprayed coatings of hydroxylapatite. *Journal of Biomedical Materials Research.* 1987, 21:1375.
23. Dhert WJA, Klein CPAT, Wolke JGC, van der Lubbe HBM, deGroot K, Rozing PM. A transcortical implant study of fluoroapatite magnesiumwhitlockite, and hydroxylapatite plasma-sprayed coatings in goats. *Transactions of the Society for Biomaterials* 1991, 17:168.
24. Ducheyne P, Hench LL, Kagan A, Martens M, Burssens A, Mulier JC. The effect of hydroxylapatite impregnation on skeletal bonding of porous coated implants. *Journal of Biomedical Materials Research* 1980, 14:225.
25. Ducheyne P, Healy KE. The effect of plasma sprayed calcium phosphate ceramic coatings on the metal ion release from porous titanium and cobalt chromium alloys. *Journal of Biomedical Materials Research* 1988, 22:1137.
26. Edwards B, Aberman HM, Dichiara JF, Higham P, Cantwell H, Gillis P, Weber W. *In vivo* performance of a hydroxylapatite coating system deposited by low pressure plasma spraying. *Transactions of the Society for Biomaterials* 1991, 17:173.
27. Engh GA, Bobyn JD, Petersen TL. Radiographic and histologic study of porous coated tibial component fixation in cementless total knee arthroplasty. *Orthopedics* 1988, 11:725.

28. French HG, Cook SD, Haddad RJ. Correlation of tissue reaction to corrosion in osteosynthetic devices. *Journal of Biomedical Materials Research* 1984, 18:817.
29. Galante JO, Lemons J, Spector M, Wilson PD, Wright TM. The biologic effects of implant materials. *Journal of Orthopaedic Research* 1991, 9:5:760.
30. Geesink RGT, deGroot K, Klein CPAT. Chemical implant fixation using hydroxyl-apatite coatings. *Clinical Orthopaedics* 1987, 225:147.
31. Geesink RGT, deGroot K, Klein CPAT. Bonding of bone to apatite-coated implants. *Journal of Bone and Joint Surgery* 1988, 70B:17.
32. Goldring SR, Flannery MS, Petrison KK, Evins AE, Jasty MJ, Goldring MB. *In vitro* model for characterization of the biochemical and cellular responses to orthopaedic implant materials. *Transactions of the Orthopaedic Research Society* 1989, 14:495.
33. Huiskes R. Some fundamental aspects of human joint replacement. Analyses of stresses and heat conduction in bone-prosthesis structures. *Acta Orthopaedica Scandinavica (Suppl)* 1979, 185:36.
34. Jansen JA, van de Waerden JPCM, Wolke JGC, deGroot K. Histologic evaluation of the osseous adaptation to titanium and hydroxyapatite-coated titanium implants. *Journal of Biomedical Materials Research* 1991, 25:973.
35. Kennedy AC, Lindsay R. Bone involvement in rheumatoid arthritis. *Clinics in Rheumatic Diseases* 1977, 3:403.
36. Koeneman JB, Lemons J, Ducheyne P, Lacefield W, Magee F, Calahan T, Kay J. Workshop on characterization of calcium phosphate materials. *Journal of Applied Biomaterials* 1990, 1:79.
37. Koeneman JB. Fundamental aspects of load transfer and load sharing. In; Lemons, J E. (ed.): *Quantitative characterization and performance of porous implants for hard tissue applications.* ASTM STP 953. Philadelphia: American Society for Testing and Materials, 1987, 241-8.
38. Krause WR, Bradbury DW, Kelly JE, Lunceford E M. Temperature evaluations in orthopaedic cutting operations. *Journal of Biomechanics* 1982, 15:267.
39. Kroon PO, Freeman MAR. Hydroxyapatite coating of hip prostheses: Effect on migration into the femur. *Journal of Bone and Joint Surgery* 1992, 74B:518.
40. Lemons JE. Hydroxyapatite coatings. *Clinical Orthopaedics* 1988, 235:220.
41. Linder L. Osseointegration of metallic implants. I.Light microscopy in the rabbit. *Acta Orthopaedia Scandinavica* 1989, 60(2):129.
42. Ling RSM. Observations on the fixation of implants to the bony skeleton. *Clinical Orthopaedics* 1986, 210:80.
43. Longo JA, Magee FP, Mather SE, Yapp RA, Koeneman JB, Weinstein AM. Comparison of HA and non-HA coated carbon femoral stems. *Transactions of the Orthopaedic Research Society* 1989, 14:384.
44. Lucas LC, Lemons JE, Lee T, Dale P. *In vitro* corrosion of porous alloys. In Lemons JE. (ed.): *Quantitiative characterization and performance of porous implants for hard tissue applications,* ASTM STP 953. Philadelphia: American Society for Testing and Materials, 1987, 241-8.
45. Magee FP, Kay J, Hedley AK. Canine modular femoral component. *7th Annual Scientific Session of the Academy of Surgical Research,* Scottsdale, Arizona, September 26-27, 1991.
46. Manley MT, Kay JF, Uratsuji M, Stern LS, Stulberg BN. Hydroxylapatite coatings applied to implants subjected to functional loads. *Transactions of the Society for Biomaterials* 1987, 13:210.
47. Manley MT, Kay JF, Yoshiya S, Stern LS, Stulberg BN. Accelerated fixation of weight bearing implants by hydroxylapatite coatings. *Transactions of the Orthopaedic Research Society* 1987,12:214.
48. Osborn J. The biological behavior of the hydroxyapatite ceramic coating on a titanium stem of a hip prosthesis: The first histological evaluation of human specimens. *Biomedical Technology (Berlin)* 1987, 32:177.
49. Pilliar RM, Lee JM, Maniatopoulos C. Observations on the effect of movement on bone ingrowth into porous-surfaced implants. *Clinical Orthopaedics* 1986, 208:108.
50. Poser RD, Magee FP, Kay JF, Hedley AK. *In vivo* characterization of a hydroxylapatite coating. *Transactions of the Society for Biomaterials* 1990, 16:170.
51. Poser RD, May TC, Kay JF, Emmanual J, Werner ME. Hydroxylapatite coated macrotextured titanium interface study. *Transactions of the Society for Biomaterials* 1991, 17:171.
52. Poser RD, Magee FP, Kay JF, Van de Wyngaerde DG, Toal TR, Hedley AK. HA enhanced osseointegration in a loaded canine implant model. *7th Annual Scientific Session of the Academy of Surgical Research,* Scottsdale, Arizona, September 26-27, 1991.

53. Poser RD, Magee FP, Longo JA, Koeneman JB, Emmanual J, Hedley AK. *In-vivo* evaluation of four stem interface conditions in a canine hemiarthroplasty. *Transactions of the Orthopaedic Research Society* 1992, 17:385.

54. Poser RD, May TM, Kay JF, Emmanual J, Koeneman JB, Hedley AK. Long-term performance and load sharing effects of HA coated macrotextured titanium. *Transactions of the World Biomaterials Congress* 1992, 4:500.

55. Poser RD, Magee FP, Kay JF, Toal TR, Hedley AK. Utilization of a unique canine modular femoral component to assess long term performance of an HA coating. *ASTM Symposium on characterization and performance of calcium phosphate coatings for implants.* Miami, Florida. November 17, 1992.

56. Shen W, Chung K, Wang G, McLaughlin RE. Mechanical failure of hydroxyapatite and polysulfone-coated titanium rods in a weight-bearing canine model. *Journal of Arthroplasty* 1992, 7:1:43.

57. Søballe K, Gotfredsen K, Brockstedt-Rasmussen H, Nielsen PT, Rechnagel K. Histologic analysis of a retrieved hydroxyapatite coated femoral prosthesis. *Clinical Orthopaedics* 1992 272:252.

58. Søballe K, Stender Hansen ES, Brockstedt-Rasmussen H, Hjortdal VE, Juhl GI, Pedersen CM, Hvid I, Bunger C. Gap healing enhanced by hydroxyapatite coating in dogs. *Clinical Orthopaedics* 1991, 272:300.

59. Søballe K, Stender Hansen ES, Brockstedt-Rasmussen HB, Pedersen CM, Bunger C. Hydroxyapatite coating enhances fixation of porous coated implants. *Acta Orthopaedica Scandinavica* 1990, 61(4):299.

60. Søballe K, Brockstedt-Rasmussen H, Stender Hansen E, Bunger C. Hydroxyapatite coating modifies implant membrane formation. *Acta Orthopaedica Scandinavica* 1992,63(2):128.

61. Søballe K, Hansen E, Brockstedt-Rasmussen H, Juhl GI, Pedersen CM, Knudsen V, Huid I, Bunger C. Enhancement of osteopenic and normal bone Iingrowth into porous coated implants by hydroxyapatite coating. *Transactions of the Orthopaedic Research Society* 1989, 14:554.

62. Spector M. Factors augmenting/inhibiting biological fixation of porous-coated noncemented prosthesis. *Orthopaedic Transactions of the Hip Society* 1986, 10:547.

63. Stephensen PK, Freeman MAR, Revell PA, Germain J, Tuke M, Pirie CJ. The effect of hydroxyapatite coating on ingrowth of bone into cavities in an implant. *Journal of Arthroplasty* 1991, 6:51.

64. Thomas KA, Cook SD. An evaluation of variables influencing implant fixation by direct bone apposition. *Journal of Biomedical Materials Research* 1985, 19:875.

65. Thomas KA, Cook SD, Haddad RJ, Kay JF, Jarcho M. Biologic response to hydroxylapatite-coated titanium hips. *Journal of Arthroplasty* 1989,4:1:43.

66. Thomas KA, Kay JF, Cook SD, Jarcho M. The effect of surface macrotexture and hydroxylapatite coating on the mechanical strengths and histologic profiles of titanium implants materials. *Journal Biomedical Materials Research* 1987, 21:1395.

67. Thomas KA, Cook SD, Harding AF, Haddad RJ. Tissue reaction to implant corrosion in 38 internal fixation devices. *Orthopedics* 1988, 11:441.

68. Thomas KA, Cook SD, Thomas KL, Haddad RJ. Tissue growth into retrieved noncemented human hip and knee components. In Saha, S. (ed.): *Biomedical Engineering V, Recent Developments.* New York, Pergamon Press, 1986, 198-203.

69. Zimmerman MC, Scalzo H, Parsons JR. The attachment of hydroxylapatite coated polysulfone to bone. *Journal of Applied Biomaterials* 1990, 1:295.

*Hydroxylapatite Coatings in Orthopaedic Surgery,*
edited by R. G. T. Geesink and M. T. Manley.
Raven Press, Ltd., New York, © 1993.

# Hydroxylapatite-Coated Hip Implants: Experimental Studies

## Rudolph G.T. Geesink, M.D., Ph.D.

## EXPERIMENTAL STUDIES

The application of hydroxylapatite (HA) coatings for orthopaedic implants is one of the accomplishments of the last decade. Therefore, knowledge concerning its behavior with bone is still limited. Although there are many analogies with sintered HA, some aspects are new. The mechanical characteristics of HA coatings deserve special attention, because they differ markedly from sintered HA ceramics. The biological characteristics should, at least theoretically, not differ too much from sintered HA. Only the surface characteristics are relevant in this aspect because the HA coating has a dense structure. Nevertheless, it appears necessary to repeat some of the experiments that have been carried out with solid sintered HA implants with HA-coated implants. In addition, *in vivo* testing of HA-coated implants appears more suitable for the determination of the ultimate mechanical strength of the coating. This chapter will deal with two experimental studies to validate the use of HA coatings for orthopaedic implants.

## PLUG STUDY

This section describes the determination of elementary biologic and mechanical interface characteristics of HA bone coatings. A simple plug design serves this purpose. Although the reliability of push-out tests for establishing interface strength values is in itself questionable, its use can still improve understanding of the principles involved. The absolute values to be obtained are very dependent on the experimental design, and should therefore not be taken too literally. The plugs in our study were implanted into dog femora. After follow-up, a mechanical, radiologic and histologic evaluation was performed.

## MATERIALS AND METHODS

Cylindrical rods of standard Ti-6Al-4V titanium alloy were prepared, measuring 4.5 by 6 mm (Fig. 1). An HA coating of 50 μm thick was applied using the standard plasma-spray technique. The characteristics of the coating are described in Table 1. Using sterile surgical techniques, the plugs were inserted into predrilled holes in the lateral cortex of adult canine (labrador retriever) femora. To study exclusively the bone bonding properties of the material, the holes were slightly oversized (4.7 mm). This allowed the plugs to move in and out but without undue laxity. The initial plug–bone interface strength therefore is zero. A total of 48 HA-coated plugs were inserted into the femora of eight dogs (three plugs per femur). There were no surgical complications. After follow-up periods of six weeks, three, six, 12, and 24 months, the dogs were sacrificed. After explant radiography, the femora were used for histologic examination and mechanical push-out testing. One implant from each femur was selected at random and left intact for histological examination.

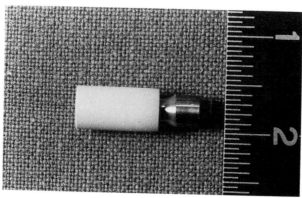

**FIG. 1.** Plug implant.

Histology was reviewed with regard to the following objectives: character of coating–bone interface; response with cortical and trabecular bone; quality and quantity of new bone formation; response of bone-marrow (biocompatibility); and condition of HA coating.

**TABLE 1.** Characteristics of HA coating

| | |
|---|---|
| Thickness (μm) | 50 (45 – 65) |
| Porosity | < 2% |
| HA content after spraying | ≥ 95% |
| HA crystalline phase after spraying | ≥ 70% |
| Tensile bond strength | ≥ 65 MPa |
| Fatigue life | |
| Tensile/Tensile at 8.3 MPa | > $10^7$ cycles |

## RESULTS

### Visual Inspection

All coated plug implants appeared well-incorporated into the bone. Upgrowth of bone was invariably visible along the protruding part of the plug up to the external ending of the HA coating. The trabecular bone around the intramedullary part of an HA-coated plug often displayed densification to bone of cortical nature (Fig. 2). There were no macroscopically loose implants at any follow-up period.

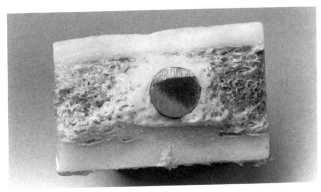

**FIG. 2.** Femoral cross-section of plug explant at two years. Note circumferential dense bone.

### Explant Radiography

All coated implants exhibited proliferation of bone along the protruding periosteal and endosteal part of the implant. This was already visible at six weeks and became more prominent at longer follow-up periods. After three months of follow-up, the entire endosteal and periosteal part of the plug was invariably completely covered with bone (Fig. 3).

A

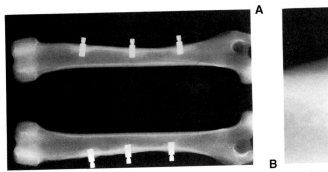
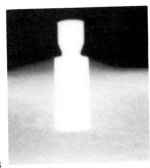

B

**FIG. 3.** Femur explant radiographs. *A*: Overview of femoral plug implants at two years; *B*: radiographic detail of transcortical plug explant at six weeks of follow-up.

## Mechanical Testing

The push-out data are summarized in Table 2. After six weeks there was already a mean interface shear strength of 48.5 MPa. A mean implant bone interface shear strength of 54 MPa was achieved after three months. Up to two years follow-up, the implant–bone interface shear strength remained at this level with plugs in conventionally prepared bone.

**TABLE 2.** *Average Plug–bone Interface Strength With Time (MPa)*

| Follow-up (weeks) | Number of Plugs (n) | Force (Newton ± SD) | Shear strength (MPa) |
|---|---|---|---|
| 6 | 8 | 1270 ± 60 | 49.5 |
| 12 | 8 | 1360 ± 70 | 55.1 |
| 25 | 8 | 1540 ± 50 | 62.1 |
| 52 | 3 | 1440 ± 40 | 58.6 |
| 104 | 4 | 1380 ± 60 | 56.3 |
| 104 | 4 Fresh | 720 ± 70 | 29.7 |

On the basis of paired $t$ test calculations, the differences in values obtained after three months and two years are not statistically significant at the $P < 0.05$ significance level, although the numbers are probably too small to provide hard proof of any differences. The average of values obtained after the third month was therefore 58 MPa. With fresh bone, an average plug–bone shear strength value of 29.7 MPa was obtained after two years of follow-up. Values for plug–bone interface shear strength, measured directly after sacrifice, thus proved to be approximately half of those obtained somewhat longer after sacrifice, when time delay and/or preparation artifacts can distort results.

## Failure Mode

The failure at the implant bone interface was predominantly within the HA coating itself (about 70% of surface area) and over the remainder of the surface area at the metal–coating interface. After dislodging the implant, there was still approximately 60% to 70% of the maximal force necessary to further move the implants out of their holes.

## Histology

Histologic sections make it clear that defects in both the periosteum and bone around the implant fill with bone within six weeks (Fig. 4). In addition, the periosteal tissue shows excellent adaptation to the HA coating. Periosteal and endosteal bone proliferate along the protruding ends of the plugs in and out of the femur. In the cortical area, bone is in very close contact with the implant, without any interposition of fibrous tissue. The bone shows remodeling, with many active osteoblasts and osteoclasts along the lacunae. Not only mature osteocytes but also many young osteoblasts and complete Haversian systems are seen in direct contact with the HA coating. Their osteoid is directly deposited on the coating.

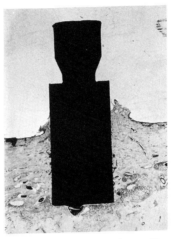

**FIG. 4.** Histologic cross-section of transcortical plug in femoral bone, showing bone proliferation around HA-coated plug (basic fuchsin, six weeks, x1).

## Condition of HA Coating

In the microscopic sections after one and two years, the HA coating is still discernible as such (Fig. 5). It has a smooth and dense appearance with a sharp transition from remaining coating to bone. There is no fragmentation of ceramic particles and there are no persisting surface irregularities. The thickness of the coating can be determined with the aid of a micrometer. A remaining thickness of 10–30 μm can regularly be observed. However, the recorded values are not very precise, because there is no guarantee that the measurements are perpendicular to the implant surface. In addition, initial coating thickness was somewhat variable and was not precisely known for each location. Although some degradation of the HA coating is therefore certainly possible, the major part of the coating appears intact. There were no areas with complete loss of HA coating on any plug.

## Microradiography

Microradiography of microscopic sections gives insight into the extent of mineralization of newly formed bone. In the first six postoperative weeks, there

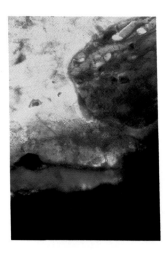

**FIG. 5.** HA coating to interface bone. Plug implant at two years (basic fuchsin, two years, x500). Coating thickness 30μm.

is already abundant calcification in the transition area between the implant with HA coating and bone. The newly formed bone has a woven and lamellar structure. After three months or more, the bone becomes much denser and assumes the characteristics of dense cortical bone. There is an increase in radiodensity of bone toward the implant with HA coating. This means that there is an increase in the calcium content of bone in close contact with the coating.

### Scanning Electron Analysis of Implant–Bone Interface

On a few sections, electron probing was performed to establish the Ca:P ratio of the bone in contact with the coating. The obtained values indicate a Ca:P ratio of nearly 10:6. This means that the bone in contact with the HA coating has a normal composition and calcification.

### DISCUSSION

The average plug–bone push-out force was 1440 Newtons after the third month of follow-up. Because the plugs were initially completely loose, with a push-out force of zero, the occurrence of plug–bone bonding to this extent is indeed significant. The mean plug–bone interface shear strength with the first series of HA-coated implants was 59 MPa. Based on paired **t** test calculations, there proves to be no statistical difference at the $P < 0.05$ significance level between values of shear strength after the three-month or one- and two-year interval. The mechanism of implant–bone bonding is thought to be both chemical and biologic. Evidence supporting the chemical bonding concept comes from the histologic results. Many osteoblasts are in direct contact with the HA coating, without any interposition of fibrous tissue. The osteoblasts deposit their osteoid directly on the coating. The bone quality in the coating–bone transition area is very good, and there is an increase in calcium content of bone toward the coating.

Biocompatibility, as measured in the bone marrow, is good. Initially there are many polymorphonuclear leukocytes. This is probably caused by the surgical trauma of implantation.

After follow-up of three months and longer, the bone marrow reassumes its usual appearance, consisting of a mixed population of lymphocytes, plasma cells, and a few other cell lines.

In contrast to the coated implants, noncoated titanium implants do not show any bone-bonding properties (1). The highest value obtained for interface shear strength was 0.6 MPa. The rate of improvement in bone bonding by HA coatings is therfore almost fiftyfold. In this study, we obtained a mean interface shear strength of approximately 30 MPa by means of chemical bonding between implant and bone using HA coatings and bone. Although the absolute magnitude of the obtained plug–bone interface strength rates is subject to interpretation errors, the relative increase in plug–bone bonding from zero to the obtained high values is certainly significant. The speed with which an HA coating can achieve a strong bone bond, and the fact that close approximation between bone and coating at surgery is not necessary to achieve these results, are especially striking. Although the results of this experimental study can not be fully extrapolated to the much more complex human situation, the fundamental principles involved in the concept of chemical bone bonding are of great clinical relevance. The results indicate that with HA-coated implants an implant–bone bonding of high strength can be achieved. Although this is well-known for sintered HA implants, the elimination of fatigue failure by use of HA coatings on metal substrates is a substantial improvement.

The conclusion of this plug–implant study is that HA coatings have a similar biologic response to that of sintered HA implants. Their physical strength, including fatigue strength, is much better and their biocompatibility and biostability appear the same as those of sintered HA.

## CANINE HA-COATED TOTAL
## HIP REPLACEMENT

Strong bonding properties between HA-coated plug implants and bone have been established in the previous section. A shortcoming in the plug study was that the plugs were not mechanically loaded during the time of acquiring bony fixation. According to literature reports, there can be a difference in performance of the same biomaterial under loaded or unloaded conditions (2–4). Under mechanical loading, micromotion inevitably occurs between implant and bone if there is no strong fixation between the two. The difference in the modulus of elasticity between implant material and bone, and their differences in cross-sectional geometry are important causal factors for micromotion. Micromotion at the implant–bone interface impairs the transition of capillaries across the interface and thereby the development of bony fixation (5). A fibrous tissue interface is then the end result under conditions of load-bearing, instead of solid bony encapsulation under conditions of mechanical rest. This is especially true for bioinert implant materials. The mechanical loading limits for this fibrous "pseudoarthrosis" tissue are much lower than for cortical bone. Although some authors (6) suggest that such a fibrous tissue layer can be effective in distributing interface stresses towards the surrounding bone, the mechanical loading limits for fibrous tissue are so low that it cannot be expected to bear any physiologically significant interface stresses. In addition, the thickness of fibrous tissue membranes around cementless implants appears to progress with loading and movement of the implant (7), thereby increasing (micro)motion of the implant in a vicious circle. For these reasons, "press-fit" implantation with a soft fibrous tissue interface is prone to failure.

To further investigate the mechanical and biologic characteristics of HA coatings under mechanical loading, a canine total hip replacement study was initiated. Results of HA-coated hip prostheses were compared with otherwise similar noncoated controls, both having the same initial press-fit fixation in bone. Evaluation was performed with mechanical, radiologic, scintigraphic, and histologic techniques. The objective of the study was to determine whether, under conditions of heavy joint loading, HA-coated implants provide better biologic and mechanical characteristics of implant fixation, as compared with noncoated bioinert titanium implants.

## MATERIALS AND METHODS

### Canine Total Hip Prosthesis

A canine total hip prosthesis was designed with the following required characteristics: titanium substrate; anatomic adaptation to proximal femur of dog; size adapted to dogs of initially 30–35 kg; textured surface on one side of prosthesis; HA coating on femoral stem; cement fixation of acetabular component; head diameter of 18 mm; and accurate instrumentation.

Fifteen prostheses were prepared with an HA coating, using the standard plasma-spray technique. HA coating characteristics are similar to those described in Table 1. Another 15 similar prostheses were left uncoated to serve as controls (Fig. 6). Both hips of dogs were operated on, one hip receiving an HA-coated implant, the other hip serving as a control (Fig. 7). The interval between the two surgeries was at least six weeks. Fifteen animals were operated on using standard veterinary techniques of anesthesia and surgery (8,9). Two dogs each were sacrificed at intervals of three weeks, six weeks, three months, six months, one year, and two years.

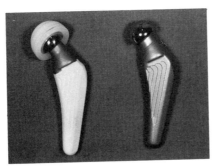

**FIG. 6.** HA-coated and noncoated canine total hip implant.

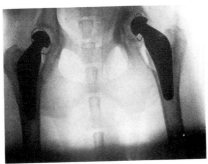

**FIG. 7.** Bilateral canine total hip implantation *in vivo*, two years.

# IMPLANTS WERE EVALUATED USING THE FOLLOWING TECHNIQUES:

## Mechanical Evaluation of Implant–Bone Interface

With implants of complex design, such as hip implants, it is very difficult to precisely quantify the mechanical characteristics of the implant–bone interface. The plug study served that purpose. Therefore, in this study we limited the mechanical evaluation of the implant fixation to clinical judgment. Moreover, forceful extractions of implants from the femur would have damaged the implant–bone interface, thereby impairing histologic evaluation. We tried to move or extract the implants from the femur by manual force. One HA-coated implant at six weeks of follow-up was extracted on the test bench with hammer and chisel to observe any unexpected events.

## Radiographic Evaluation of Implants

This included radiographic aspect of implant–bone interface, radiolucent line formation, radiodense line formation, extent of new bone formation, extent of bone resorption and general quality of bone, and adverse radiographic effects of HA coating.

## Scintigraphic Evaluation of Implants

## Histological Evaluation of Implants

Histology was reviewed with the following focus of interest: general evolution of implant–bone bonding process; character of implant–bone interface (bone/fibrous tissue); amount of new bone formation; amount of bone–resorption; density and structure of bone; potential for filling bone defects; differences in response of cortical and trabecular bone; condition of HA coating; bone marrow reactions (biocompatibility); and prosthetic neocapsule reactions (biocompatibility).

## RESULTS

## Radiographic Evaluation of Prostheses

### *Radiographic Evaluation of Noncoated Implants*

The first three to six weeks after implantation of an uncoated hip implant, radiographic appearance is indistinct from that of a coated prosthesis. The bone defects caused by the intramedullary reaming at the time of implantation were still visible. From the third week on, until longest follow-up of two years, there developed an increasing difference in bone quality between coated and noncoated prostheses. From the sixth week on, noncoated prostheses exhibited radiolucent line formation. The initial thickness of these lines was about 0.2 mm around the entire femoral stem area. With time, this line progressed somewhat and after one to two years a radiolucent line of at least 0.5 mm to 1.5 mm was visible between the implant surface and surrounding bone around the entire femoral stem area. This difference became more evident with longer follow-up and was very marked after the two-year follow-up period (Fig. 8). In some instances there was evidence of console formation, which is bone formation distally of the femoral stem tip.

### *Radiographic Evaluation of HA-coated Implants*

During the first three weeks of follow-up, the radiographic appearance of HA-coated implants was similar to that of the noncoated control implants. The bony outlines of the intramedullary reaming procedure during surgical implantation were still visible after three weeks. With six weeks of follow-up these defects had almost universally disappeared, and the implant–bone interface of HA-coated implants had a smooth radiographic appearance. Neither radiolucent nor radiodense lines were visible around the HA-coated implants. There was no visible transition zone from implant to bone.

From the sixth month on, continuing until the two-year follow-up period, there was an increasing difference in density and quality of trabecular bone in favor of the HA-coated implants. Bone density became especially high around the proximal and distal femoral stem area (Fig. 8). This increase in trabecular bone density was inversely proportional to the distance from the implant, indicating that bone density was highest at the coating/bone transition area.

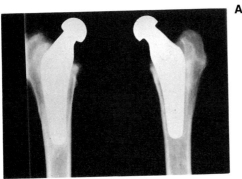
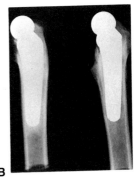

**FIG. 8.** Differences in radiolucent line formation and bone density around coated (*left*) and noncoated (*right*) canine implants at two-year follow-up. *A*: AP view explant radiograph; *B*: Lateral view of same.

## Scintigraphic Evaluation of Prostheses

### *Scintigraphic Evaluation of Noncoated Implants*

All 99m-technetium bone scans on implants with six-month to two-year follow-up showed a characteristic three-point hot spot with radionuclide accumulation. These areas with increased 99m-technetium uptake included the medial and lateral aspects of the proximal femur as well as the area around the femoral stem tip. The areas in between these hot spots did not exhibit as much uptake as the corresponding areas in their HA-coated counterparts.

### *Scintigraphic Evaluation of HA-Coated Implants*

The scintigraphic pattern of HA-coated implants after the sixth month of follow-up was characterized by a moderate uptake of 99m-technetium, with an even distribution of activity over the entire proximal femur (Fig. 9). There were no hot spots or other focal accumulations of the radionuclide, either proximally or distally in the femur.

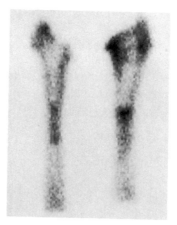

**FIG. 9.** Technetium bone scans of canine HA-coated implant (*left*) and noncoated (*right*) at two years.

## Histological Evaluation of Prostheses

### *General Comments*

With implants of complex geometry there are always areas with bone gaps and spaces. Especially around the conical distal end of the stem, slits and spaces are likely to occur despite good instrumentation and surgical technique. This was reflected in the histologic results. Early transverse sections through the proximal femur of both coated and noncoated implants, revealed that the initial mechanical stabilization of the prosthesis was achieved by three areas of point contact between implant and bone. Although both types of implants had the same initial press-fit fixation, a striking difference in histology developed between coated and noncoated prostheses.

## Histology of Noncoated Titanium Prostheses

### *General Observations*

The general evolution of the interface between uncoated titanium implants and bone was toward fibrous tissue encapsulation of the implant. There was predominant bone resorption at the implant–bone interface of noncoated implants. Although this was counteracted by the remaining bone with increased bone formation, the balance between bone formation and bone resorption remained delicate after two years.

## *Implant–bone Interface of Noncoated Implants*

Noncoated prostheses were surrounded by a fibrous tissue membrane with a thickness of between 100 and 200 μm. This fibrous tissue was visible from the third week on and became more prominent with time. In addition, there was an empty space between fibrous tissue and implant, indicating motion between the two (Fig. 10). This empty space had a thickness of up to 1.5 mm. After two years, the entire femoral stem area was encapsulated in a fibrous tissue membrane (Fig 11). The end thickness of this membrane was rather variable, between 100 and 500 μm. The bone trabeculae adjacent to the fibrous tissue membrane tended to have more parallel orientation towards the implant surface. In the microscopic sections of noncoated titanium implant–bone interfaces there were no macrophages or related cells, apart from osteoclasts, that seemed to play a role in the process of bone resorption.

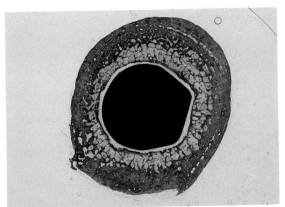

**FIG. 10.** Loose area and fibrous tissue around noncoated canine femoral component in proximal stem area. (Masson trichrome, two years, x1.)

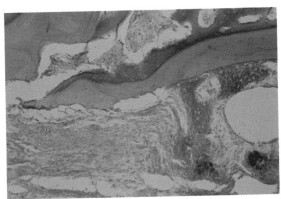

**FIG. 11.** Fibrous tissue interface with bone resorption around noncoated implant at two years (HE, x100.)

## Histology of HA-Coated Prostheses

### *General Observations*

The general evolution of the HA-coated implant–bone interface is towards complete bony coverage of implants. Within three weeks, HA-coated implants developed a close contact with the surrounding bone. Many bony defects, slits, and spaces had closed by the three-week interval, especially in the proximal stem area. At six weeks postoperatively the coated implants had a major surface covering of bone. Trabecular bone density around the implants increased with time until the bone had an almost cortical character.

### *Character of Implant–bone Interface with HA-coated Prostheses*

The characteristic interface picture of an HA-coated implant consisted of a bone plate of varying thickness against the implant. This depended on time and loading conditions. After three weeks there was clear evidence of mineralized bone condensation against the HA coating (Fig. 12). This bone plate was initially very thin, about 100 to 300 μm, but became rapidly thicker as time progressed.

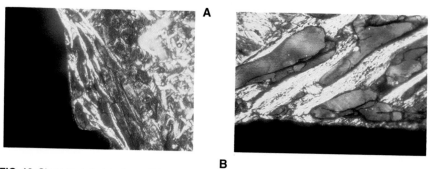

**A**

**B**

FIG. 12. Characteristic interface of HA-coated femoral stem at three weeks. *A.* Overview, area of new bone formation in implant texture area (Alcian blue, x 2); *B.* Thin bone plate on implant surface with connecting trabeculae. Older preexistent bone in upper left corner (Alcian blue, three weeks, x100.)

By the three-week interval, most bony defects, slits, and spaces had closed in the proximal stem area. At six weeks postoperatively, the coated implants were almost 100% covered with bone. The potential exists for the ultimate interface of nearly 100% mature dense bone (Fig. 13). High-magnification views (1000x) confirmed the close bonding between the HA coating and bone, without any interposition of fibrous tissue. The transition area of bone to coating showed condensation of osteoid material on the HA coating in the early follow-up period, followed later by maturation to bone and increased mineralization at the longest follow-ups of one and two years. These areas corresponded to those of increased calcium content as seen in microradiographs.

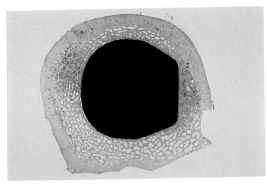

**FIG. 13.** Structure and orientation of bone trabeculae of transverse section of proximal femur. Dense bone near implant surface. (Basic fuchsin, two years, x1.)

Close approximation of HA coatings was seen not only with mature osteocytes but also with young osteoblasts. Many haversian systems exhibited direct endings on, and bonding with, the HA coating.

### Condition of HA Coating

In microscopic sections after one and two years, the HA coating was clearly discernible as such (Fig. 14). It had a smooth, dense appearance, with a sharp transition from coating to bone. There was no fragmentation of particles or delamination of coating. The thickness of the coating could be determined with the aid of a micrometer. A remaining thickness of 10 to 30 μm was regularly observed. The recorded values, however, were not very precise, because there was no guarantee that the measurements were made perpendicular to the implant surface. In addition, the initial coating thickness of the implants was somewhat variable and was not precisely known for each location. Some degradation of the HA coating was therefore present. It is known that in the first few months after implantation, during the process of bone bonding, some superficial degradation of the HA coating will occur, possibly because of increased surface porosity of the coating's outer layer. After two years of follow-up, the remaining coating thickness appears more than adequate to ensure implant fixation (Fig. 15).

The remaining coating thickness is not very critical in itself. This is because bonding to HA coatings is a surface phenomenon and is not dependent on any depth of ingrowth into the coating, which has a closed surface and a dense deep-layer structure. Longer follow-up than the current two years will be necessary to establish the long-term stability of HA coatings. After two years, polarization microscopy revealed the direction of individual bone collagen fiber systems to the implant surface. The ending angles varied between perpendicular and oblique.

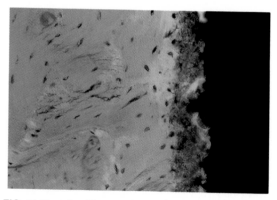

**FIG. 14.** Density of bone and structure of HA coating at two years. (Basic fuchsin, x500.)

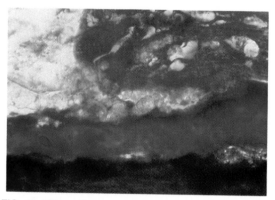

**FIG. 15.** HA coating–bone interface at two years. (Basic fuchsin, x1000.)

## DISCUSSION

These results indicate that HA-coated prostheses form very tight bonds with living bone. Despite their conical, non-retentive shape and smooth surface, extraction from the femur is not easy. Powerful extraction after three to six weeks of implantation or longer caused fissuring and fracturing. Radiology showed excellent bone quality, with condensation of endosteal bone around HA-coated implants at the implant–bone interface. Bone scintigraphy revealed an even distribution of 99m-technetium uptake over the entire coating area, without hot spots or other signs of potential instability. Histologic studies confirmed the very close bonding of the HA coating with bone. Not only did the mature osteocytes have good bonding with the HA coating, but so did the young osteoblasts. The femoral bones around the HA-coated prostheses showed hardly any evidence of early bone resorption. In addition with longer follow-up major stress-shield phenomena were not observed.

The persistent lack of adherence between the titanium surface of the noncoated implant and bone results in continuing micromotion at the interface. Persistent micromotion at the bone interface is an established cause of bone resorption (5). This bone resorption again increases (micro)motion and thereby maintains, in a vicious circle, the fibrous tissue nature of the interface. In response to this bone resorption, the bone shows an increase in osteoblasts, as evidenced by bone scintigraphy, but the net result is zero because this bone formation is just enough to compensate for the bone losses caused by the resorptive processes. Even after two years the equilibrium between these processes of bone formation and bone resorption appears delicate.

With HA-coated implants there is initially an equally large surface contact area with the surrounding bone. In the first few weeks after implantation, there is always a relative unloading of the extremity, caused by postoperative pain and discomfort. With dogs, this period is only a few weeks in duration. Even this relatively short period is long enough for rigid bony fixation to develop in the areas with primary bone contact. This process of early primary bone bonding effectively eliminates micromotion at the implant interface once joint loading commences. Afterwards, even empty areas caused by slits and spaces around the implant can ossify by secondary filling with bone. This may proceed rather fast, because filling of bony defects between bone and HA coatings proceeds from both the implant surface and the bone contact area. This is a major difference as compared with conventional implant materials, which at best can exhibit an ingrowth from bone toward the implant surface but never in the reverse direction.

In the histologic sections, ossification is well advanced within three weeks and is almost complete within six weeks, at least in the important weight-bearing areas of the implant. Only with large bony defects is more time needed for full ossification. At three months, an equilibrium is present for bone formation. Further progress of the zone of ossification is not likely after this period. Distances of up to 2 mm can fill this way from neighboring bone, as measured in the microscopic sections. There is no bone-inductive influence by the HA material itself. If no bone is present within short reach, no new bone will regenerate.

The bone bonding properties represent one major advantage of HA coatings over conventional bioinert implant materials. It could well be that a second major advantage of HA coatings on implant materials is their osteoconductive property. They provide the bone with a scaffold for ingrowth in the shortest possible time. With surgical implantation of a cementless hip implant, even accurate instrumentation cannot provide an initial bone contact area of more than 20% (10). From experimental studies (11,12), it is known that implant–bone gaps as small as 0.35–0.5 mm are never bridged by cortical bone. Instead, these gaps are filled by fibrous tissue. Other authors (13) report more favorable characteristics, especially with titanium, but even then a prolonged period of unloading of the implant is necessary to accomplish appropriate bone healing or "osseointegration." Only under conditions of complete unloading can bone grow up to bioinert titanium implant surfaces and thereby increase the initially small contact area between implant and bone. At the same time, prolonged unloading of bones is not conducive to the maintenance of good bone stock. This will lead to disuse osteoporosis of bones. In the present study, for example, the bioinert titanium control implant group consistently exhibited histologic failure of the implant–bone interface under conditions of heavy joint loading. There was a complete fibrous-tissue interface, instead of the desired "osseointegration."

HA coatings permit fast and reliable filling of bony slits and spaces that occur around cementless implants. This increases bony contact area between implant and bone from the original 20%, or lower, to near 100% in the experimental study. Even in the absence of any bone-bonding properties of HA coatings, this would decrease the relative interface stress of the implant by a factor of at least five. When the prosthesis is nearly 100% covered with dense strong bone, micromotion is largely prevented and the resultant interface stress is further reduced. In more recent studies, Stephenson et al. (14) and Søballe et al. (15) have obtained similar potentials for gap filling around HA-coated experimental implants. Especially with regard to osteoconductivity, there is a marked difference from other bioinert implant materials.

Using porous metal-coated acetabular components in the dog, some authors (11,12) could demonstrate gap areas as small as 0.35 mm not being filled by bone but instead being bridged by fibrous tissue. In a study comparing three different types of porous metal coatings—circumferential or partially-coated plasma flame-spray, sintered bead, or fiber–metal coatings—Turner et al .(16) report less ingrowth with the beaded surface at six months (25%) in comparison with the fiber–metal surface (37%). In all groups the ingrowth was incomplete, with the proximal and distal areas of the implant showing higher rates of ingrowth as compared with the midsection of the femoral stem. There was, in general, a proximal to distal gradient of loss of cortical bone at the (longest) six-months interval, a sign of bone loss by stress shielding. The magnitude of loss of cortical bone was more dependent on the extent than on the type of porous coating.

As compared with these results, HA-coated implants permit a more complete coverage with bone in a shorter period of time. Even after six weeks, HA-coated implants already have major coverage of bone around their surfaces. It is conceivable that the more complete bony integration of HA-coated implants, as compared with porous metal-coated implants, protects the implants better from stress-shielding phenomena.

Stress-shield phenomena were observed with both the noncoated and the HA-coated implants. The extent of loss of cortical thickness was related to the amount of distal fixation of the implants. Nevertheless, in Turner's study the extreme complete loss of cortical thickness with spontaneous perforation of porous and metal-coated implants into the soft tissues of the femur at six months follow-up, was not observed in the HA-coated implants of our study even at two years of follow-up. From both our study and that of Turner et al. (16), the conclusion can be drawn that it is important to confine, and indeed enforce, load transfer through implants to the proximal femur by applying coatings only to the proximal stem part of the implant.

The concept of biologic implant fixation to bone by using HA coatings on titanium substrates has proven successful under the heavy load-bearing conditions of this animal model. The original objectives of the study have been confirmed. The HA coating proves to be durable and strong without the fatigue failure problems of sintered HA. At the same time, HA coatings provide the same excellent bone bonding properties and biocompatibility characteristics of sintered HA with the added mechanical strength of metal implants. In particular, the short time interval in which an HA coating can achieve a strong bone bond and the fact that close approximation between bone and coating at surgery is not necessary to achieve good results are striking advantages over more conventional bioinert implant materials. Adverse biologic effects have not been detected, except for relatively minor proximal stress-shield phenomena that were more related to the extent of the coating on the stem than to its nature.

The general conclusion from this animal study is that the composite material consisting of an HA coating on a titanium substrate is a good material for load-bearing applications in orthopedic surgery (17). Because there were no adverse biologic effects, the chemical bone-bonding concept using HA coatings appears safe for human applications.

## REFERENCES

1. Ronningen H, Solheim LF, Langeland N. Invasion of bone into porous fiber metal implants in cats. *Acta Orthopaedica Scandinavica* 1984;55:352-8.
2. Heck DA, Nakajima I, Kelly PJ, Chao EY. The effect of load-alteration on the biological and biomechanical performance of a titanium fiber-metal segmental prosthesis. *Journal of Bone and Joint Surgery* 1986;68A:118-26.
3. Griss P, Werner E, Heimke G, Buchinger R. Vergleichende experimentelle Untersuchungen an Bioglas, Al2O3-Keramik und mit Bioglas beschichteter Keramik. *Arch Orthop Unfall-Chir* 1977;90:15-27.
4. Griss P, Werner E, Heimke G, Raute-Kreinsen U. Comparative experimental investigations with bioglass and Al2O3-ceramic coated with mod. bioglass II. *Archives of Orthopaedic Surgery* 1978;92:199-210.
5. Perren SM. The induction of bone resorption by prosthetic loosening. In: Morscher E, eds. *Cementless fixation of hip prostheses.* New York: Springer, 1983;39-41.
6. Walker PS, Onchi K, Kurosawa H, Rodger RF. Approaches to the interface problem in total joint arthroplasty. *Clinical Orthopaedics* 1984;182:99-108.
7. Hedley AK, Clarke IC, Kozinn SC, Coster I, Gruen T, Amstutz HC. Porous ingrowth fixation of the femoral component in a canine surface replacement of the hip. *Clinical Orthopaedics* 1982; 163:300-11.
8. Olmstead ML, Hohn RB, Turner TM. Technique for canine total hip replacement. *Veterinarian Surgery* 1981;10:44-50.
9. Olmstead ML, Hohn RB, Turner TM. A five-year study of 221 total hip replacements in the dog. *Journal of the American Veterinarian Association* 1983; 183:191-4.
10. Noble PC, Alexander JW, Lindahl LJ, Yew DT, Granberry WM, Tullos HS. The anatomic basis of femoral component design. *Clinical Orthopaedics* 1988; 235:148-65.
11. Carlsson L, Röstlund T, Albrektsson B, Albrektsson T. Implant fixation improved by close fit. *Acta Orthopaedica Scandinavica* 1988;59:272-5.
12. Harris WH, White RE, McCarthy JC, Walker PS, Weinberg EH. Bony ingrowth fixation of the acetabular component in canine hip joint arthroplasty. *Clinical Orthopaedics* 1983;176:7-11.
13. Albrektsson T, Albrektsson B. Osseointegration of bone implants. *Acta Orthopaedica Scandinavica* 1987;58:567-77.

14. Stephenson PK, Freeman MAR, Revell PA, Germain J, Tuke M, Pirie CJ. The effect of hydroxyapatite coating on ingrowth of bone into cavities in an implant. *Journal of Arthroplasty* 1991; 66:51-8.
15. Søballe K, Hansen ES, Brockstedt-Rasmussen H, Hjortdal VE, Johl GI, Pedersen CM, Hvid I, Bunger C. Gap healing enhanced by hydroxyapatite coatings in dogs. *Clinical Orthopaedics* 1991; 272:300-07.
16. Turner TM, Sumner DR, Urban RM, Rivero DP, Galante JO. A comparative study of porous coatings in a weight-bearing total hip arthroplasty model. *Journal of Bone and Joint Surgery* 1986;68A:1396-1409.
17. Geesink RGT, Groot K de, Klein CPAT. Chemical implant fixation using hydroxylapatite coatings. *Clinical Orthopaedics* 1987; 225:147-70.

*Hydroxylapatite Coatings in Orthopaedic Surgery,*
edited by R. G. T. Geesink and M. T. Manley.
Raven Press, Ltd., New York, © 1993.

# Hydroxylapatite-Coated Total Hip Replacement

## Five Year Clinical and Radiological Results

Rudolph G.T. Geesink, MD., Ph.D.

## CLINICAL RESULTS OF HYDROXYLAPATITE-COATED TOTAL HIP REPLACEMENT

Experimental foundations for hydroxylapatite (HA)-coated total hip replacement have been established in the last decade (1,2). They proved that HA-coated hip replacement was an attractive alternative to prevailing methods of cementless implant fixation. Consequently, the first human implantation of an HA-coated hip prostheses was performed by the author in 1986. In the following sections, clinical and radiologic details will be provided on 100 patients with 125 hip replacements and an average follow-up of five years (range 4 – 6.5 years). HA-coated total hip replacement has dramatically extended the surgeon's capabilities for treating hip joint deformities. Therefore, some introductory remarks on indications and surgical technique seem necessary. They reflect the author's opinion and may differ from those of others.

### SURGICAL ASPECTS

#### Patient Selection

The best candidates for HA-coated implants appear to be younger, active patients with good primary bone stock, younger than 65 years of age. Here, long-term results of cemented total hip replacement are less satisfactory (3–8). Typically, these patients have high bone metabolism that responds rapidly to a cementless hip implant with its altered stress pattern in the bone. In addition, posttraumatic deformities and avascular necrosis of the hip joint represent excellent indications for HA-coated total hip replacement.

Rheumatoid arthritis and metabolic bone disease, such as severe osteoporosis, represent less clear indications for HA-coated implants. Although, in the same circumstances cemented hip prostheses also have lower performance, they are probably a better choice for realizing satisfactory short-term results. This does not mean that biological fixation using HA-coated prostheses in less than ideal bone quality should be less satisfactory.

Experimental studies (9) prove that there is no difference between normal and osteoporotic bone response to HA coatings. In addition, there are literature reports on high-age human autopsy retrievals of HA-coated hip prostheses. Osborn (10), Bauer et al. (11), Furlong, and Osborn (12), Søballe et al. (13), and Hardy et al. (14) have reported on autopsy retrievals of clinically well-functioning hips. Without exception, all high age (up to 98 years!) retrievals showed excellent degrees of osseointegration, similar to those at lower ages. They prove that biologic fixation is possible in older patients. HA-coated total hip replacement in older age groups certainly poses a greater risk of perioperative cracks or fractures, caused by the generally higher degree of osteoporosis. However, many patients fall between these two categories who may have less than ideal bone quality but still have a relatively long life expectancy. The ultimate choice therefore depends on the individual characteristics of the patient, including lifestyle and general health, and on the implant selection.

For reliable biologic fixation to occur, the implant needs sufficient initial mechanical stability in a well-vascularized implant bed. To ensure sufficient load-sharing between implant and bone suggests a more or less anatomic implant design. In practice, however, there is wide variation in the size and geometry of both the proximal and the distal femur. To limit the number of available implant sizes to a practical level, it is necessary to apply proper sizing instruments to adapt the femoral bone to the prosthesis. These include intramedullary reamers and calcar rasps. After proper reaming, a slightly oversized prosthesis, in relation to the prepared intramedullary canal, is press-fit into the femoral shaft to provide a tight initial fit. This ensures good initial mechanical stability of the stem, still enhanced by the HA's high degree of surface roughness ("sandpaper surface"). Additional biologic fixation of the implant to bone by the HA coating will then be obtained within three to six weeks in areas with primary bone contact. Any remaining slits and spaces will ossify in the subsequent weeks and months, provided the space is not more than a few millimeters wide.

### Implant Characteristics

The Omnifit HA-coated hip system used (Fig. 1) has the following characteristics: titanium stems in ten sizes; macro-textured normalization surfaces; proximal 40% HA coating of femoral stem; exchangeable femoral heads; acetabular cups in 12 sizes and three designs; and separate polyethylene liners.

The characteristics of HA coating include thickness of 50 μm (range 45–65), full-density coating (porosity < 2%), content of HA after spraying >= 95%, crystalline phase of HA after spraying >= 70%, tensile bond strength >= 65 MPa, and fatigue life > $10^7$ tensile/tensile cycles at 8.3 MPa.

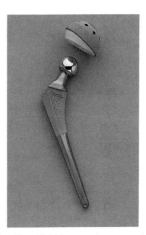

**FIG. 1.** Omnifit HA-coated stem and cup.

In the early years of HA-coated total hip replacement, there was only a screw cup available with HA coating. Later developments include the HA dual-geometry press-fit cup and the HA dual-radius press-fit cup. The press-fit cups have a macrotextured, wafer-like surface structure.

## Preoperative Planning

It is generally believed that preoperative planning adds to the accuracy of the operative procedure (15). With the aid of specific templates, the probable implant size can be determined and the optimal calcar resection level selected for best fit of the implant in the bone and preservation of correct leg length. Especially with difficult reconstructions, preoperative planning is useful.

## General Surgical Principles

Even with good implants, the surgeon in the operating room is responsible for accomplishing correct implant fit in the bone. Primary mechanical stabilization of the prosthesis in the bone is necessary to prevent early micromotion. Because biological processes are involved in the process of achieving bony union, vascularization of the implant bed is an equally important factor. This dictates, for example, that acetabular reaming should proceed until at least some bleeding is encountered in subchondral bone.

On the femoral side, reaming should not go too far. Excessive reaming can cause thermal necrosis of bone while exposing the prosthesis to low-vascularized cortical bone. Reaming should proceed until the transition area of strong cortico-spongious to cortical bone is reached. A good level of surgical skill is necessary to accomplish "primary close fit" between implant and bone. Good instruments and judicious preoperative planning can prevent many problems. Although the procedure of implanting an HA-coated prosthesis is certainly more forgiving than an otherwise similar noncoated one, too much motion at the prosthesis–bone interface, through malposition or undersizing of the implant, can adversely influence bony fixation. The exact limits of this tolerance are not yet known, although they appear to be larger than those of other cementless implant devices (16).

### Surgical Technique

After adequate surgical exposure of the diseased hip joint, the femoral head is luxated and its neck resected at the predetermined level with the aid of specific instruments (Fig 2). Intramedullary reaming is then performed with incremental sizes of reamers until adequate surgical "feel" of proper reaming is achieved. The calcar area is prepared with the corresponding calcar broach, which also serves as a trial implant. Femoral preparation is slightly undersized (0.7 mm) in comparison to the final implant to allow a mechanically tight fit between implant and bone. Acetabular preparation consists of the usual incrementally-sized spherical reamers until spherical congruency at the edges of the acetabulum (using the dual-radius press-fit cup) is achieved.

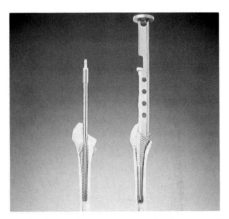

**FIG. 2.** Instruments used for femoral preparation: axial intramedullary reamers and calcar broaches.

After adequate trial reduction and positioning of the implants, the final implants are selected and inserted in the femoral canal and acetabulum. Because of the high surface microroughness of HA-coated implants, there is more frictional resistance with insertion of these implants in comparison with smoother metal implants. Further surgical technique is similar to conventional hip replacement surgery (Fig. 3).

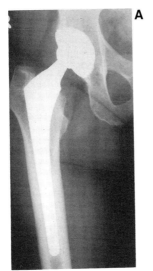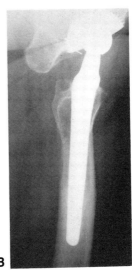

**FIG. 3.**   Typical implantation of HA-coated total hip replacement. **(A)** AP and **(B)**   lateral radiographs.

## Postoperative Management

Routine postoperative management currently includes: 24 hours of intravenous antibiotic prophylaxis (cephalosporin); peri- and postoperative anticoagulation using dicumarins for three months; indomethacin prophylaxis (75 mg daily) against ectopic bone formation for two weeks; immediate full weight-bearing is allowed after surgery if surgical conditions permit (primary surgery without "cracks"), using crutch or cane as long as comfortable. In all other circumstances  six  weeks of partial (25%) weight-bearing is allowed with crutches.

## MATERIALS AND METHODS

The first implantations of HA-coated total hip prostheses were performed by the author in 1986. Until the end of 1988, 125 primary hips of 100 patients had been operated on. Before this period, some cases were operated on using noncoated cups. Because clinical results for this specific group were somewhat less than optimal, caused by the noncoated cups (17), they are discussed separately. The current series of results has both components HA-coated. The average follow-up is five years, with a minimum of four years. Longest follow-up is well over six years. Indication for use of HA-coated implants was  below age 65 for all primary implantations. Revision surgery is discussed in a separate chapter. There were no specific exclusions for the use of HA-coated devices.

All patients were included in a prospective follow-up study with informed consent obtained. There were 100 patients with an average age of 53 years (range 21– 65 years);  31 patients were younger than 50 years. The male to female ratio in the entire group was 1:1.7. Twenty-five patients had bilateral surgery with follow-up for both hips of more than two years. The patient population is described with more detail in Table 1 for preoperative diagnosis and Tables 2 and 3 for Charnley classification and description of associated problems. Fourteen hips had a previous hip osteotomy for osteoarthritis and an additional seven various other operative procedures. Cases were operated on by the author, other staff and residents, through a posterolateral approach. Tables 4 and 5 show the Omnifit components used in this series. On the average, men needed larger components. Femoral head size is 26 mm (Table 6).

**TABLE 1**. Preoperative diagnosis of patients with HA-coated THR (% cases)

| | | |
|---|---|---|
| Osteoarthritis | | 74 |
| Dysplastic | 23 | |
| Idiopathic | 49 | |
| Post-infectious | 2 | |
| Avascular necrosis femoral head | | 15 |
| Idiopathic | 5 | |
| Alcohol abuse | 3 | |
| Steroid induced | 7 | |
| Inflammatory disease | | 5 |
| Ankylosing spondylitis | 3 | |
| Juvenile rheumatoid | 2 | |
| Posttraumatic conditions | | 5 |
| Acetabular fracture | 3 | |
| Neck fractures | 2 | |
| Tumor (chondroblastoma) | | 1 |

**TABLE 2**. Charnley classification of patients (% cases)

| | | |
|---|---|---|
| A | Unilateral, healthy | 56 |
| B | Bilateral, healthy | 25 |
| C | Uni/bilateral, medical problems | 14 |

**TABLE 3**. Associated problems of patients in Charnley category C

| Diagnosis | No. patients | No. hips |
|---|---|---|
| Ankylosing spondylitis severe | 2 | 3 |
| Juvenile rheumatoid, mult: joints | 2 | 3 |
| Bilateral osteoarthritis knee | 3 | 5 |
| Myocardial infarction | 2 | 2 |
| Pulmonary diseases | 2 | 2 |
| Neurologic diseases | 2 | 3 |
| Psychiatric disorders | 1 | 1 |
| Total | 14 | 19 |

**TABLE 4.** Femoral component size (% cases)

| Size femur | Female | Male |
|---|---|---|
| 7 | 16 | 7 |
| 8 | 34 | 10 |
| 9 | 36 | 44 |
| 10 | 10 | 29 |
| 11 | 4 | 10 |
| Average size | 8.5 | 9.3 |

**TABLE 5.** Acetabular component size (% cases)

| Size (mm) | Female | Male |
|---|---|---|
| 44 | 3 | – |
| 46 | 7 | 4 |
| 48 | 26 | 2 |
| 50 | 15 | 3 |
| 52 | 28 | 29 |
| 54 | 11 | 10 |
| 56 | 11 | 32 |
| 58 | – | 15 |
| 61 | – | 5 |
| Average (mm) | 50.6 | 54.7 |

**TABLE 6.** Head and neck size implants (%)

| | |
|---|---|
| 26-mm head | 96 |
| 32-mm head | 4 |
| 0 -mm neck | 86 |
| 5 -mm neck | 12 |
| 10- mm neck | 2 |

## Clinical Evaluation

All patients were included in a prospective follow-up study with informed consent obtained. Before surgery each patient was evaluated with the modified Harris Hip Score (HHS) (18). At follow-up intervals of three, six, and 12 months and yearly thereafter, all patients were recalled and evaluated using the same HHS system. Emphasis was placed on evaluation of pain or limp problems, especially occurrence and localization of pain, start-up pain or pain after a long walk.

Rate of obesity of patients was calculated using the Quetelet index (weight in kg divided by the squared length in meters). Normal values are around 25.

Obesity was assumed with a Quetelet index of 30 or higher; 23% of women and 9% of men were in this category. There were no patients lost to follow-up, although two patients died of non-hip-related causes (myocardial infarction and cardiac surgery).

All clinical, radiographic and laboratory data are collected in a prospective follow-up study. Many rating systems are available for evaluating hip surgery. The HHS, the modified HHS, the Mayo, the Iowa, the Hospital for Special Surgery rating system or the PMA ratings all aim at the most objective evaluation of postoperative hip performance. Some systems use only clinical parameters, whereas others also include radiographic parameters. When compared (19), most rating systems prove equally capable of separating good or excellent clinical results from moderate or poor clinical results. Because radiographic parameters and findings for this new type of HA-coated hip implant are not yet fully defined, it is more appropriate to choose a rating system based on clinical results. This seems all the more important because in the clinical use of noncemented hip implants, pain is the most obvious complaint. Although pain is a subjective phenomenon, it still should be an important criterion for evaluating hip surgery. For these reasons, clinical performance of patients in our group with HA-coated prostheses are rated according to the standard modified HHS (20) as well as the PMA ratings. These are the most widely accepted hip rating scales.

## Radiological Evaluation

During each follow-up visit an AP view of the lower pelvis was obtained together with a lateral X-ray of the involved hip. X-rays were evaluated per Gruen zone (21) of stem and cup for radiologic signs of endosteal bone formation ("spot welds"), reactive line formation around both HA-coated and noncoated parts of the femoral stem, pedestal formation around the distal stem tip, periosteal bone reactions, calcar atrophy, bone resorption, subsidence, interface deterioration and ectopic bone formation according to the Brooker classification (22). In addition, all implants were graded for their bone ongrowth characteristics according to the radiologic fixation and stability score for cementless implants of Engh et al. (23).

In interpreting the results, we must realize that the distal termination of the HA coating is half-way in femoral Gruen zones 2 and 6. For this reason, in these areas the subdivisions A (upper HA-coated part) and B (distal noncoated part) are used. In the acetabular area, the HA coating is in zones I and III, while zone II is exposed to the noncoated part of the screw-cup or the polyethylene liner. Because the HA coating has a fully dense structure and bone bonding is a surface phenomenon, the term "ingrowth" is not quite appropriate for HA coatings and we will use the term "bone ongrowth" or condensation.

## Statistical Methods

Statistical analysis was applied to the results, and influences of both clinical and radiologic variables were studied. In particular the influences on clinical results of age, sex, Charnley class, obesity, diagnosis, previous surgery, surgeon, type of acetabular component and radiological aspects of bone ongrowth were studied. Differences were calculated using *two-tailed t-test, Mann–Whitney U test,* or *logistic regression* depending on the group characteristics. Results, if significant, are specified with their respective $p$ values, assuming $p < 0.05$ as significant.

## CLINICAL RESULTS

### Complications

Complications are summarized in Table 7. One patient died 11 months after surgery of a myocardial infarction, and another died after cardiac surgery 18 months after hip replacement. Both implants had functioned without problems during their lifetime. There was one case of an unrecognized intraoperative fissure with a normal postoperative x-ray. At six weeks follow-up there was some pain, and the x-ray showed minimal displacement of a calcar fracture with 1 cm subsidence of the collarless stem. After six additional weeks of protected weight-bearing, the fracture healed and the implant appeared stable, although with 1 cm leg shortening. The clinical result remains excellent (Fig. 4).

**TABLE 7.** *Complications of HA-coated total hip replacement*

|  | (N Cases) |
| --- | --- |
| Superficial or deep joint infection | – |
| Thromboembolic complications | – |
| Dislocation of hip | 4 |
| Intraoperative fissures | 7 |
| Postoperative fracture | 1 |
| Ankylosis of hip by ectopic bone | 4 |
| Died of unrelated cause | 2 |
| Reoperations |  |
| Recurrent dislocation of hip | 1 |
| Removal of ectopic bone | 2 |
| Loosening of components | – |

### Reoperations

There were three reoperations. One case of ectopic bone formation caused complete ankylosis of the total hip joint (Brooker grade IV). One year after initial surgery the ectopic bone mass was excised and the patient regained 110 degrees of hip flexion. She is now pain free. In another case (Fig. 5) the Brooker IV ectopic bone mass was excised 18 months after surgery with full restoration of 130 degrees of hip flexion. Two more hips in one patient with

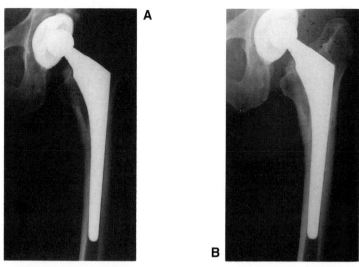

**FIG. 4.**   Postoperative fracture complication **(A)** Six- weeks postoperative x-ray showing 1cm subsidence after calcar fracture. **(B)** Five-year postoperative x-ray showing good osseointegration and stable fixation.

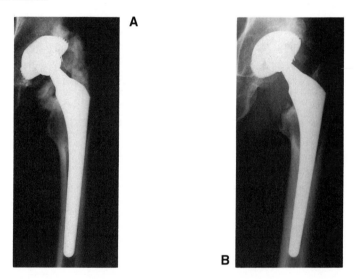

**FIG. 5.**   Complications of heterotopic bone formation. **(A)** One-year postoperative x-ray showing Brooker grade IV heterotopic bone formation. **(B)** Three-year postoperative X-ray after excision of heterotopic bone formation.

Brooker IV ectopic bone formation caused significant impairment of hip flexion, although the patient does not feel the need for reoperation because he is pain-free and his range of motion is somewhat better than before surgery (ankylosing spondylitis with complete fusion of both hips).

The third reoperation was a case of recurrent dislocation of components caused by malposition of the beveled polyethylene cup insert (Fig. 6). This was corrected by changing the position of the cup insert and a change to 32-mm head

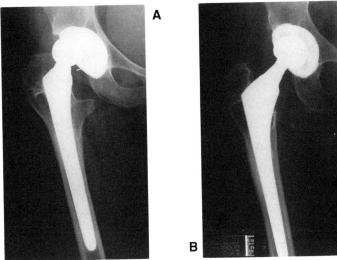

**FIG. 6.** Postoperative complication of recurrent dislocation. (*A*) Malposition of acetabular cup insert. (*B*) Revision of acetabular cup insert, 5-year postoperative x-ray.

size with a longer neck. The hip has been stable since. Bone biopsy at time of surgery revealed the presence of bone up to the implant surface for both cup and stem, although of course the interface itself could not be visualized. There were no other reoperations and, specifically, no surgery for loosening of components, nor are there cases of impending implant loosening.

### Clinical HHS

Using the HHS ratings, the clinical results are specified in Table 8 for overall HHS. Results are specified with regard to Charnley classification. In addition, the average PMA ratings with follow-up are listed in Table 9 with a more specific listing of individual classes at five-year follow-up in Table 10.

Results indicate a very low incidence of pain from early after surgery onwards. Absence of pain really means complete absence of pain under all conditions, including vigorous activities. If a patient had pain of even minimal degree after more than 1hr. of vigorous activity, he was classified in the group of occasional minimal pain. Sometimes these complaints were accompanied by a slight limp.

One year after surgery, 4% of cases had remaining complaints of clinical significance. Three of these patients had moderate pain, usually not related to level of activity, but without impairment of daily activities. The localization of pain was variable, some involving the midthigh area. One patient had more severe pain persisting after one year, even at rest. She underwent more extensive analysis. X-rays confirmed excellent bony fixation of components. Digital subtraction arthrography did not show any loosening and aspiration cultures were negative. The technetium bone scans were normal, without signs of infection. Arthroscopy of the hip did not reveal any synovial or other

**TABLE 8.** *Harris Hip score by follow-up and Charnley group*

| Group | Pre-Op | 3 m | 6 m | 1 yr | 2 yr | 3 yr | 4 yr | 5 yr |
|-------|--------|-----|-----|------|------|------|------|------|
| A | 35 | 90 | 96 | 97 | 98 | 99 | 99 | 99 |
| B | 32 | 90 | 95 | 97 | 98 | 99 | 99 | 98 |
| C | 28 | 77 | 84 | 86 | 90 | 95 | 96 | 97 |
| All | 33 | 88 | 94 | 95 | 97 | 98 | 98 | 98 |

**TABLE 9.** *PMA classification by follow-up (average)*

| Class | 3 m | 6 m | 1 yr | 2 yr | 3 yr | 4 yr | 5 yr |
|-------|-----|-----|------|------|------|------|------|
| Pain | 5.6 | 5.7 | 5.7 | 5.8 | 5.9 | 5.9 | 5.9 |
| Motion | 4.4 | 5.0 | 5.2 | 5.4 | 5.6 | 5.6 | 5.7 |
| Ability to walk | 5.6 | 5.7 | 5.8 | 5.9 | 5.9 | 5.9 | 5.9 |
| PMA sum | 15.6 | 16.4 | 16.7 | 17.1 | 17.4 | 17.4 | 17.5 |

**TABLE 10.** *PMA ratings for HA-coated hips at five years (% cases)*

| Value | Pain | Motion | Ability to walk |
|-------|------|--------|-----------------|
| 1 | – | – | – |
| 2 | – | – | – |
| 3 | – | 2 | – |
| 4 | 2 | 9 | 2 |
| 5 | 8 | 11 | 7 |
| 6 | 90 | 78 | 91 |

abnormalities around the joint space of the implant. The patient had three hip surgeries before her total hip replacement. Ultimately, a herniated disc was diagnosed and she had much relief after lumbar disc surgery. In general, all the hip complaints improved with time, and after three to five years the incidence of remaining mild pain was even lower than 4%.

## RADIOLOGICAL RESULTS

### General Remarks

In the first three months after surgery, hardly any changes in bony structure are evident. The trabecular structure of the bone is well-preserved and there is complete absence of any radiolucent line formation or any other specific interface line development. From the third month on, there is a gradual increase in density of the bone in contact with the HA coating. This increase in bone density is most pronounced over the distal medial area of the HA coating. Between six and 12 months, this process of condensation of endosteal bone around the HA-coated part of the implant becomes more pronounced. It extends both proximally and distally in area as well as showing a further increase in bone density. Radiolucent lines around coated parts of implants remain completely absent up to longest follow-up.

On the acetabular side of the prosthesis, changes in bony structure are much slower to appear. Most signs of bone condensation appear between the first and third years. Also on the acetabular side, bone quality remains good and there is complete absence of radiolucent line formation around HA-coated parts of implants.

### Endosteal Bone Apposition

The development over time of areas with endosteal bone formation ("spot welds") of more than 10 mm in length is shown in Table 11. The typical pattern is one of endosteal bone condensation against the medial distal coating area in Gruen zone 6A (Fig. 7). These spot welds in zone 6A first appear between the third and sixth month and are present in 90% of cases at the one-year interval. The same phenomena, but to a lesser degree and visible between six and 12 months, are seen at the lateral side in Gruen zone 2A. Between 12 and 24 months, the medial spot welds expand more proximally into Gruen zone 7 in approximately 75% of cases (Fig. 8). Between the first and second year these localized spot welds fuse together to form a bigger mass of endosteal "weld area" on the whole medial coating area (Fig. 9).

At the one-year interval, approximately 10% of cases do not yet show any signs of endosteal bone formation against the femoral stem. There is not a single case, however, with pedestal formation around the stem tip, detectable subsidence, or other signs of instability at the implant–bone interface. A few cases show minor signs of bone formation adjacent to the stem tip, especially when it touches one cortex of the femur. Nowhere does this bone formation extend to more than 50% of the medullary canal diameter. From two years on, all HA-coated stems show positive signs of bony ongrowth over some area of the HA coating. Up to longest follow-up, now well over six years, there is continuing expansion of the area of bone ongrowth around the implant, even extending beyond the distal termination of the HA coating (Table 11B) (Fig. 10).

### Bone-Reactive Lines

The development of bone reactive lines with a length of more than 10 mm is shown in Tables 12A and B. Bone-reactive lines are completely absent in all cases around all HA-coated parts of the femoral stem in Gruen zones 2A, 6A, and 7. In a few cases, reactive line formation is visible in the upper part of Gruen zone 1A, near the shoulder of the stem, where the HA coating begins. This line does not extend distally for more than one centimeter (Fig. 11). More often, there is a small triangle of bone densification in this area, where the HA coating starts. Reactive line formation is regularly seen around the distal noncoated part of the stem. It usually starts around the stem tip in Gruen zone 4 and becomes visible after the sixth month, a small delay (approximately three

**TABLE 11A.** *Bone formation per Gruen zone femur HA-coated femoral stems (% cases)*

| Zone | 3 m | 6 m | 1 yr | 2 yr | 3 yr | 4 yr | 5 yr |
|------|-----|-----|------|------|------|------|------|
| 1 | 4 | 23 | 37 | 64 | 83 | 92 | 93 |
| 2A | 5 | 33 | 70 | 92 | 99 | 100 | 100 |
| 2B | – | 3 | 12 | 24 | 47 | 53 | 61 |
| 3 | 1 | 1 | 2 | 18 | 33 | 42 | 56 |
| 4 | – | 1 | 1 | 1 | 2 | 2 | 2 |
| 5 | – | – | 1 | 13 | 35 | 37 | 57 |
| 6B | – | 11 | 14 | 23 | 46 | 51 | 63 |
| 6A | 10 | 56 | 89 | 96 | 100 | 100 | 100 |
| 7 | 13 | 48 | 72 | 82 | 93 | 100 | 100 |

**TABLE 11B.** *Average periimplant area of bone ongrowth, femur*

| Length Time | 3 m | 6 m | 1 yr | 2 yr | 3 yr | 4 yr | 5 yr |
|-------------|-----|-----|------|------|------|------|------|
| millimeters | 9 | 42 | 77 | 136 | 175 | 195 | 219 |

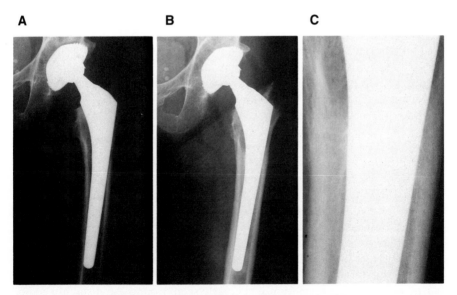

**FIG. 7.**   Development of endosteal spot welds early after operation. **(A)** Three-months postoperative, **(B)** Six-months postoperative, condensation of endosteal bone on lower medial part of HA coating, **(C)** Magnification of bone condensation area.

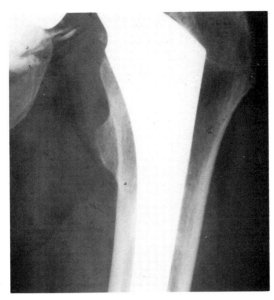

**FIG. 8.** Multiple areas of endosteal bone condensation, one year postoperative x-ray detail.

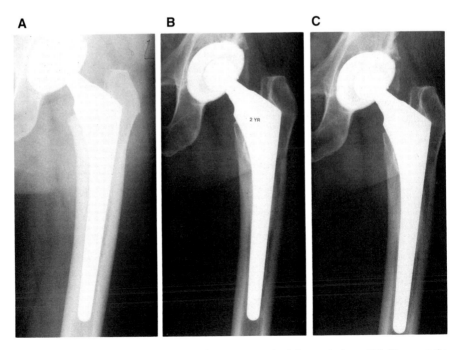

**FIG. 9.** Development of osseointegration over proximal femoral stem, **(A)** Three-weeks postoperative;. **(B)** Two- year postoperative; **(C)** Four- year postoperative. Note bone condensation below HA coating area.

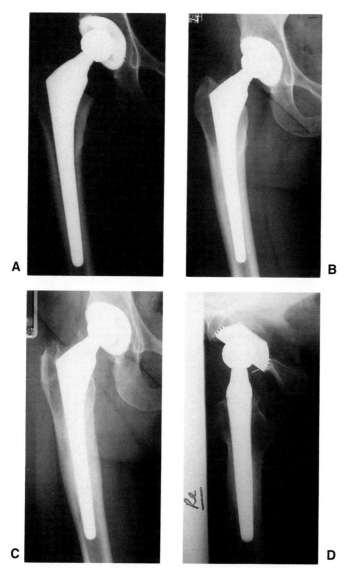

**FIG. 10.** Progressive osseointegration over distal noncoated stem area. **(A)** Early postoperative x-ray; **(B)** Two-year postoperative x-ray; **(C)** Five-year postoperative, osseointegration extending far beyond HA coating towards distal noncoated stem area; **(D)** Lateral view of same.

months) in comparison with the signs of proximal endosteal bone formation.

With time these lines extend more proximally into Gruen zones 3 and 5 and often also zones 2B and 6B. They are present in over 80% of cases at the one-year interval and are not associated with signs of local bone formation (Figs. 12 and 13). There is a strong statistical correlation ($p=0.002$) between the development of signs of endosteal bone formation in zone 6A and reactive line formation a few months later around the distal noncoated stem in zones 3, 4, and 5.

With time, especially from three years on, these reactive lines gradually diminish in length and occurrence. They fade away from proximal to distal and remain visible around the distal stem tip (Fig.14). The disappearing parts of reactive lines are being replaced by expanding areas of osseointegration of the more proximal parts of the stem.

**TABLE 12A.** *Reactive line formation per Gruen zone, HA-coated femoral stems (% cases)*

| Zone | 3 m | 6 m | 1 yr | 2 yr | 3 yr | 4 yr | 5 yr |
|------|-----|-----|------|------|------|------|------|
| 1    | –   | 1   | 4    | 4    | 3    | 3    | 2    |
| 2A   | –   | –   | –    | –    | –    | –    | –    |
| 2B   | –   | 3   | 10   | 7    | 8    | 6    | 6    |
| 3    | 3   | 13  | 41   | 46   | 47   | 47   | 28   |
| 4    | 2   | 31  | 77   | 85   | 86   | 84   | 61   |
| 5    | 2   | 16  | 36   | 34   | 35   | 37   | 36   |
| 6B   | –   | 5   | 18   | 13   | 8    | 3    | –    |
| 6A   | –   | –   | –    | –    | –    | –    | –    |
| 7    | –   | –   | –    | –    | –    | –    | –    |

**TABLE 12B.** *Average periimplant length reactive lines*

| Length | 3 m | 6 m | 1 yr | 2 yr | 3 yr | 4 yr | 5 yr |
|--------|-----|-----|------|------|------|------|------|
| Millimeters | 2 | 20 | 58 | 58 | 56 | 48 | 36 |

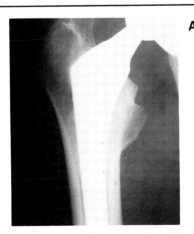
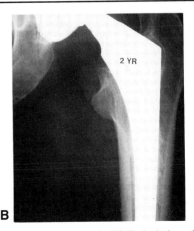

**FIG. 11.** Patterns of bone formation at shoulder area of stem in zone IA. **(A)** Typical triangular spot of bone condensation at the superior termination of the HA coating; **(B)** Less frequent line formation over shoulder of stem area extending 1 cm down the HA coating.

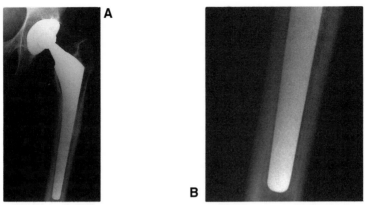

**FIG. 12.** **(A)** Reactive line formation around noncoated section of femoral component, six months postoperative. **(B)** Magnification of distal tip area.

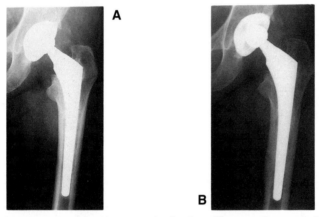

**FIG. 13.** More generalized distal bone reactive line formation around noncoated stem area. **(A)** Two year postoperative; **(B)** Five-years postoperative, disappearance of distal reactive lines and almost full osseointegration of both proximal HA-coated and distal noncoated stem areas.

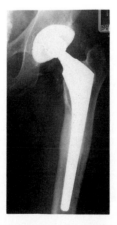

**FIG. 14.** Regression of distal bone reactive lines with time. Usual appearance at four to five years postoperative, with well-advanced bone condensation around noncoated stem section (5-year x-ray).

## Periosteal Bone Reactions

Periosteal or cortical bone remodeling reactions occur in a significant number of cases after HA-coated total hip replacement. There appear to be two distinctive patterns of bone remodeling. The first is characterized by thickening of the femoral cortex along its periphery, circumferentially in Gruen zones 2B and 6B after the first year, and extending to zones 3 and 5 between the third and fourth year. From the fourth year on this circumferential thickening of the femur gradually flattens and finally disappears. These changes always occur in combination with extensive endosteal bone formation over the HA coating in zones 2A and 6A (Fig 15). The second, asymmetric, type demonstrates very localized periosteal reactions medially or laterally on the femur near the distal stem tip. In all of these cases the distal stem was not very well-centered in the medullary canal near the stem tip but was eccentrically located and touching one inner cortex of the femur (Fig. 16). On the opposite free side of the

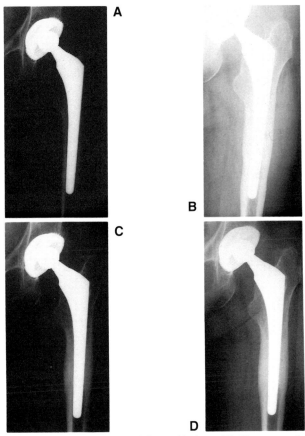

**FIG.15.** Series of typical cortical remodeling with time. **(A)** Three- months postoperative, starting point; **(B)** Two- year postoperative, early cortical thickening over zones 3 and 5, as well as medial tip. **(C)** Three-year postoperative, expansion of area of cortical thickening as well as endosteal bone condensation in zones 3 and 5; **(D)** Five-year postoperative, stabilization of remodeling reactions over distal noncoated femoral stem.

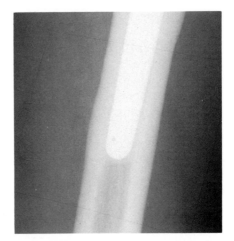

**FIG. 16.** Cortical reaction at medial distal tip of femoral component caused by slight eccentric position of tip. Reactive line on lateral side, 1 year postoperative.

noncoated stem tip, there was invariably a bone reactive line. This type of remodeling occurs earlier, sometimes only after six months, and disappears earlier, leaving a somewhat widened diameter of the femoral canal around the distal stem tip. In general, the frequency of reactive remodeling was higher in cases with a very tight fit of the stem tip in the femoral canal. The incidence of periosteal/cortical reactions is listed in Tables 13A and B.

**TABLE 13A.** *Cortical and periosteal bone reactions, femur HA-coated femoral stems (% cases)*

| Zone | 3 m | 6 m | 1 yr | 2 yr | 3 yr | 4 yr | 5 yr |
|------|-----|-----|------|------|------|------|------|
| 2 | – | 1 | 8 | 13 | 11 | 13 | 11 |
| 3 | – | 1 | 1 | 6 | 6 | 9 | 11 |
| 5 | – | 5 | 6 | 14 | 25 | 21 | 33 |
| 6 | – | – | 6 | 16 | 19 | 18 | 17 |

**TABLE 13B.** *Average periimplant length of remodeling area*

| Length   Time | 3 m | 6 m | 1 yr | 2 yr | 3 yr | 4 yr | 5 yr |
|---------------|-----|-----|------|------|------|------|------|
| Millimeters | – | 2 | 9 | 25 | 33 | 29 | 30 |

### Interface Change with Time

Once proximal bone formation and distal line formation become visible, these phenomena are progressive and occur in an increasing number of patients. At one year 97% of stems have positive signs of bone ongrowth, and at two years this is a full 100%, although the involved area of bone formation still shows further expansion until at least five years (Table 11B). There are no signs of bone formation reversal or interface deterioration with time. Figures 17 through 20 show some more samples of five-year results. At three years follow-up, there is in many cases obvious expansion of the area of osseo-integration to beyond the distal termination of the HA coating, involving not only zones 2B and 6B but also 3 and 5. Paralleling the increase of bone density in the proximal femur is a gradual disappearance of distal bone reactive lines. In many cases this is especially clear in Gruen zones 3 and 5.

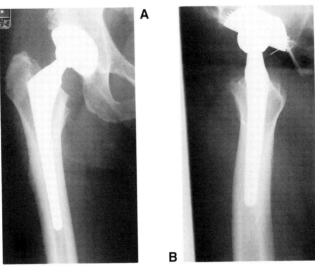

**FIG. 17.** Sample of five-year postoperative x-ray. **(A)** AP; and **(B)** Lateral radiographs.

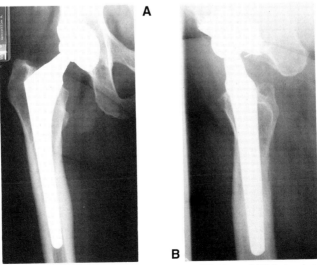

**FIG. 18.** Sample of five-year postoperative x-ray. **(A)** AP; and **(B)** Lateral radiographs.

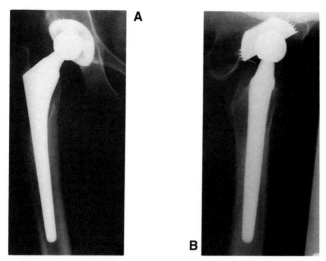

**FIG. 19.**   Sample of five-year postoperative x-ray. (*A*) AP; and (*B*) Lateral radiographs.

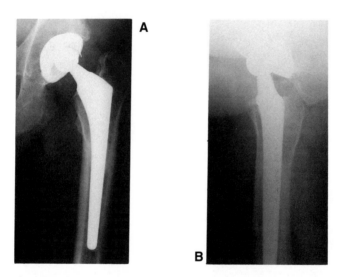

**FIG. 20.**   Sample of five-year postoperative x-ray. (*A*) AP; and (*B*) Lateral radiographs.

## Migration

There is not a single case with late subsidence of the femoral stem. Even three cases with gross undersizing or slight varus position of the femoral stem showed a stable position, with strong endosteal bone formation in zones 2A and 6A. One case showed early subsidence, caused by a postoperative femoral fracture. This stem was stable on further follow-up, as mentioned above.

## Calcar Bone Resorption

Calcar remodeling is slow to appear but is visible in some cases at one year and later. The usual appearance is one of calcar round-off and slight cortical thinning in the upper 1 cm, progressing slowly over the years. This occurs in 20% of cases at two years. Even at four to five years follow-up, however, there is not a single case with severe bone resorption at the calcar area. Many cases still have an unchanged appearance of the calcar at four to five years (Figs. 17–20). The incidence of calcar resorption is listed in Table 14.

**TABLE 14.** *Calcar bone resorption*

|          | 3 m | 6 m | 1 yr | 2 yr | 3 yr | 4 yr | 5 yr |
|----------|-----|-----|------|------|------|------|------|
| None     | 98  | 86  | 83   | 82   | 72   | 60   | 39   |
| Slight   | 2   | 14  | 17   | 16   | 21   | 32   | 44   |
| Moderate | –   | –   | –    | 2    | 7    | 8    | 17   |
| Severe   | –   | –   | –    | –    | –    | –    | –    |

## Bone Resorption

There are no signs of significant bone resorption in the femoral stem area other than moderate calcar resorption. From the second year on, a minority of cases exhibit some relative osteoporosis in zone 1B, at the level of the lateral side of the greater trochanter, rarely extending more distally into zone 2A (Fig. 21). Calcar atrophy has already been mentioned.

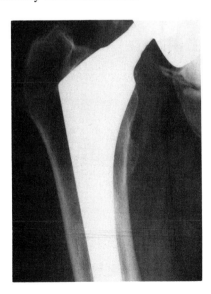

**FIG. 21.** Relative osteoporosis in greater trochanteric area 1B between areas of bone condensation (Gruen zones 1A and 2), four-years postoperative.

**TABLE 15.** *Ectopic bone formation at one and five years (% cases)*

| Brooker grade | 1 year | 5 year |
|---|---|---|
| None | 59 | 60 |
| Brooker I | 22 | 23 |
| Brooker II | 8 | 8 |
| Brooker III | 7 | 7 |
| Brooker IV | 4 | 2* |

* 2 cases reoperated

## Ectopic Bone Formation

The degree of ectopic bone formation is summarized in Table 15. Men had a moderately higher incidence of ectopic bone formation in comparison with women. Two cases of ectopic bone formation, Brooker grade IV, required excision of ectopic bone mass between the first and second years after surgery. The patients regained good range of motion. Two more cases (one patient) had significant impairment in range of motion. The lower grades (Brooker I–III) of ectopic bone formation usually had acceptable range of motion, although its speed of restoration in the hip proved to be inversely related to the degree of ectopic bone formation.

## Engh's Radiological Score

The evolution of figures for the fixation, stability and overall score are summarized in Table 16. It is apparent by virtue of their high stability and complete absence of line formation around HA-coated parts of components, that the majority of cases already have high scores early after surgery. The lowest score in the entire population is 4.5 (one case) at one year and 11.5 at two years, defining all femoral stems as having confirmed bony ongrowth at two years. Bony ongrowth confirmed is defined as a radiologic sum score of higher than plus six.

**TABLE 16.** *Average Engh's radiological score*

| | Follow-up | | | | | | |
|---|---|---|---|---|---|---|---|
| | 3 m | 6 m | 1 yr | 2 yr | 3 yr | 4 yr | 5 yr |
| Fixation score | 3.8 | 7.5 | 9.7 | 9.9 | 10.0 | 10.0 | 10.0 |
| Stability score | 8.9 | 8.1 | 5.7 | 5.6 | 5.9 | 6.6 | 10.5 |
| Total score | 12.7 | 15.6 | 15.4 | 15.5 | 15.9 | 16.60 | 20.5 |

## Acetabular Cup Ingrowth

Radiologic changes around acetabular components are much slower to appear in comparison with the femoral stem, where changes are sometimes already apparent at three months. Signs of bone formation with longer follow-up become visible in acetabular zones I and III. Approximately 65% of cases have, at one year, signs of bone densification in zone I, as opposed to 40% in zone III. Sometimes there is accompanying osteoporosis and reactive line formation in the noncoated zone II. However, radiolucent lines are absent around all HA-coated parts of acetabular components, even in zone III, which is the critical area for screw cups. Migration of cups could not be detected. The specific changes for bone ongrowth are listed in Table 17 and those for reactive line formation in Table 18. Acetabular zone II has no HA coating and is exposed to the polyethylene liner of the cup. From three years on, all HA

**TABLE 17.** *Bone formation around HA-coated cups (% cases)*

| Zone | 3 m | 6 m | 1 yr | 2 yr | 3 yr | 4 yr | 5 yr |
|---|---|---|---|---|---|---|---|
| I | 5 | 30 | 65 | 93 | 97 | 100 | 100 |
| II | – | – | – | – | 5 | 7 | 8 |
| III | 4 | 8 | 40 | 79 | 92 | 100 | 100 |

**TABLE 18.** *Reactive line formation with HA-coated cups (% cases)*

| Zone | 3 m | 6 m | 1 yr | 2 yr | 3 yr | 4 yr | 5 yr |
|---|---|---|---|---|---|---|---|
| I | – | – | 1 | 1 | 1 | 1 | 1 |
| II | – | – | – | 3 | 7 | 7 | 8 |
| III | – | – | – | – | – | – | – |

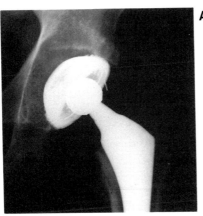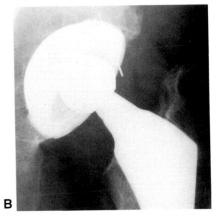

**FIG. 22.** Typical pattern of bone condensation around acetabular component. **(A)** Three-months postoperative; **(B)**: Four-years postoperative.

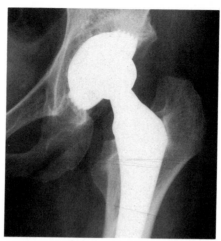

**FIG. 23.** Typical pattern of bone condensation around acetabular component in zones I and III, four-years postoperative.

screw cups have positive evidence of bone ongrowth (Figs. 22 and 23). There are no signs of secondary or impending loosening. There is one cup with questionable stability; reactive line formation in zone I, but bone condensation in zone III. There are no accompanying clinical signs.

### Polyethylene Wear

The incidence of polyethylene wear has been low until five-year follow-up. At present there is one case of a 23-year-old women with 1 mm eccentricity of the PE liner in the acetabular component. The calcar resection level does show some irregularities, caused by PE particle reactions (Fig. 24). Interface disruption, however, is not (yet) present in this case. A few more cases of young active individuals do show some irregularities at the former calcar resection line, probably caused by PE wear particle reactions. Obvious wear, however, is not (yet) visible.

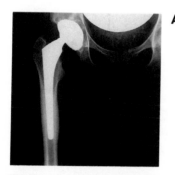
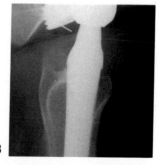

**FIG. 24.** Case with polyethylene wear five-years postoperative. **(A)** Eccentric position of femoral head in acetabular component with slight osteolytic reactions at calcar level; **(B)**Lateral view of same.

## STATISTICAL RESULTS

### Clinical Group Differences

Statistical analysis showed that there was no influence of the following variables at any time of follow-up on clinical results, as expressed in the HHS: age, sex, surgeon, or excessive weight.

The following variables showed no statistical differences in clinical results after two years, although they did so within the first year: previous osteotomy, Charnley classification, and type of acetabular component.

The early differences with patients having previous osteotomy before their total hip replacement (14 cases) were caused by both pain and a longer persisting limp after surgery. Differences in results with patients in Charnley's class C were caused primarily by limitations in such parameters as daily activities and walking distance, caused by conditions not related to the hip. The pain and limp ratings of these cases were essentially similar to those of Charnley's classes A/B. With time, their general condition improved along with their hip, and after the three-year mark, there remained virtually no differences.

The type of acetabular component used proved to have the most significant influence on clinical results. As mentioned before, some early cases had noncoated acetabular screw cups used before an HA-coated one was available. Approximately two-thirds of these patients had occasional minimal complaints of pain, usually in the groin or buttock area with activity, already suggestive of acetabular problems. Usually these pain complaints were accompanied by a limp. Although none of these pain or limp problems would seriously interfere with activities of daily living, their presence was still statistically significant at the one-year interval and before.

Even at two and five years, there was a lower performance as expressed in the HHS, although the difference was not more significant because of the small numbers involved. Table 19 describes the differences in HHS ratings for both types of acetabular components and their statistical significance. The statistical significance is $p < 0.05$ at three, six, and 12 months. At the one-year interval, patients with noncoated screw cups lose, on the average, 4 HHS points on pain rating, 3 points on limp, 2 points on support (cane), 1 point on stair climbing, and 2 points on distance walked in comparison with patients with HA-coated screw cups.

**TABLE 19.** *Harris Hip Scores and type of acetabular component*

|  | 3 m | 6 m | Follow-up 1 yr | 2 yr | 5 yr |
|---|---|---|---|---|---|
| Noncoated cup | 71 | 79 | 84 | 94 | 97 |
| HA-coated cup | 90 | 95 | 96 | 98 | 99 |
| Significance *p* | 0.01 | 0.02 | 0.03 | 0.1 | 0.4 |

Interestingly, most of these complaints improved with time and even cases with early radiolucent lines around these noncoated screw cups showed a better interface condition. However, in all cases interface quality could not match that of HA-coated cups

### Radiological Group Differences

An attempt was made at statistical correlation between radiologic parameters and clinical performance of hips as expressed in the HHS. At three, six, and 12 months follow-up, there proved to be a statistically significant correlation between signs of endosteal bone formation, especially in Gruen zone 6A, and the HHS. The results are summarized in Table 20. At six months, the average HHS was 5 points higher for the well-ongrown stems. The differences were mainly in the pain rating. After the one-year interval, there were not enough cases without endosteal bone formation to make statistical comparisons valid.

With cases of cortical bone remodeling, average HHS were somewhat higher at all follow-up intervals, however not always at a statistically significant level. They are listed in Table 21.

**TABLE 20.** *Endosteal bone formation and HHS*

|  | Follow-up | |
|---|---|---|
|  | 3 m | 6 m |
| No bone formation | 87 | 91 |
| Bone formation | 91 | 96 |
| Significance $p$ | 0.04 | 0.05 |

**TABLE 21.** *Harris Hip Score and cortical remodeling*

|  | Follow-up | | | | |
|---|---|---|---|---|---|
|  | 1 yr | 2 yr | 3 yr | 4 yr | 5 yr |
| No reactions | 96 | 96 | 98 | 98 | 98 |
| Bone reactions | 99 | 99 | 99 | 100 | 100 |
| Significance $p$ | 0.02 | 0.07 | 0.12 | 0.05 | 0.09 |

There was no statistically significant correlation between clinical parameters and radiological signs of reactive line formation around the distal noncoated stem, calcar resorption, or other radiologic signs.

### DISCUSSION

### Complications

There were no complications specifically related to the method of implant fixation using HA coatings. Intraoperative fissures and/or fracture are more related to surgical technique and can be avoided with more experience and less aggressive reaming. There were a few postoperative dislocations. One of these was caused by malposition of the cup insert and could be avoided. The amount of ectopic bone formation was comparable to figures from the literature (22–26). In theory, one might conceive that this complication could be somewhat higher with such a "bone-friendly" material as HA. There was no radiologic evidence to support this view. An occurrence of 11% of combined Brooker III + IV compares favorably with the 21% from recent studies (25, 26), although the differences are probably not significant. In addition, there were four cases in the author's series with a contralateral uncemented (non-HA) total hip and extensive ectopic bone formation. Without prophylaxis the HA-coated total hip did not form ectopic bone. Yet, with such good overall results, even relatively minor problems contribute much to the overall end results. This has lead the author to institute indomethacin prophylaxis (25 mg t.i.d. for two weeks) to decrease ectopic bone formation. This regimen is now active for over two years and seems to be successful without adversely influencing bony ingrowth to any significant clinical degree. Nevertheless, we should be aware of the theoretical possibility of indomethacin adversely influencing bony ongrowth.

## Clinical Results

In general, the results of HA-coated total hip replacement were quite satisfactory. The almost complete absence of clinically significant pain problems very early (three-month visit) after surgery was especially striking. This is quite new to cementless hip surgery. An incidence of persisting pain of 4% is comparable to references from the literature on cemented total hip replacement (27). There were no cases of loosening or even suspected radiologic loosening at the five-year interval for the young age population in this series. Remaining problems of limp or restrictions in activities of daily living were negligible at longer term follow-up.

## Radiological Changes

The radiologic pattern of bone ongrowth for HA-coated stems is one of early endosteal bone condensation over the distal half of the HA coating on the femoral stem between the third and sixth months. Somewhat later, this is followed by reactive line formation around the distal noncoated stem section. From 12 months on, slight calcar atrophy becomes evident, together with more proximal expansion of the area of endosteal bone formation at the medial side. At some level, proximally in the femur, these processes of proximal atrophy and more distal bone formation will counter-balance each other, leaving a more or less stable equilibrium, dependent on local stress patterns. Over 90% of cases show these radiologic signs of bone ongrowth at one-year and virtually all cases at two years. In this first year, a strong positive statistical correlation exists between proximal endosteal bone formation and somewhat later formation of distal reactive lines. The proximal bone formation comes first, and the distal lines follow three months later.

These distal reactive lines are probably the expression of some micro-motion between the stiff distal stem and the more elastic bone, caused by their relative differences in modulus of elasticity. This phenomenon is enhanced because of the strong proximal fixation, which causes a larger deflection of the distal stem tip (a "micro windshield-wiper sign") in comparison with a stem without proximal fixation. This phenomenon will even be enhanced because of the implant's strong fixation in the proximal femoral stem area. Under these circumstances of implant proximal fixation, the deflection of the stiffer implant against the bone by load-bearing forces will be largest near the femoral stem tip. Because the cortical bone of the femur is more elastic than the metal of the implant (even made out of titanium) some micromotion is inevitable between implant stem tip and bone. This is not necessarily accompanied by significant load-bearing in this part of the implant, as evident by the absence of console formation below the stem tip. The micromotion between implant and bone, through mismatch of modulus of elasticity between metal and bone, will cause a very localized zone of bone resorption, which appears on radiographs as a thin radiolucent line around the distal noncoated parts of the femoral stem. The development of these bone reactive lines is at its maximum between 18 and 24 months after surgery. Later, there is still a significant increase in bone density of the proximal femur (see above) with subsequent stiffening of the proximal femur. This decreases distal micromotion, and therefore it is understandable why the distal bone reactive lines go into regression after two to three years. This process is most evident from the increase in Engh's stability score after three years (Table 16).

The radiologic findings at follow-up appear similar to those of the previous experimental studies. The complete absence of radiolucent lines around the HA-coated part of the implant suggests a very close condensation of bone against the prosthesis, and the increase in bone density with condensation of endosteal bone-to-bone of almost cortical structure indeed suggests stress transfer through the coating.

This process of endosteal bone densification is limited to the coated part of the prosthesis, and is accentuated near the termination of the coating at the femoral midstem section where the coating ends. This may prove that this process is the predominant effect of the HA coating in conjunction with a good prosthetic cross-sectional geometry. It also suggests that load-carrying is lim-ited to the HA-coated part of the femoral component, at least during the first two years. With longer follow-up there is increasing expansion of the area of bone ongrowth beyond the HA-coated stem section. This is caused by the very rigid fixation over the proximal HA-coated part of the stem. With time there is an increase in bone density of the proximal femur to bone of almost cortical structure. Together with the very rigid fixation, this decreases micromotion between stem and bone in the noncoated stem section to very low levels. Then, the titanium stem is by itself capable of spontaneous secondary osseo-integration over its noncoated section. This is understandable from the results of experimental studies (28), as it is known that titanium can achieve spontaneous osseointegration provided that micromotion between bone and implant is very low. This could not be achieved without the initial fixation by the HA coating in the proximal femoral stem area (29).

In addition, there were no signs of stress shielding in the proximal femur up to current follow-up of five years. Although in theory, this can not be excluded for longer follow-up, the presence of proximal densification of trabecular bone appears reassuring in the prevention of stress shielding osteoporosis. The proximal presence only of the coating is important in this respect. The distal tip of the femoral stem does not appear to take any major load-bearing. Console formation near the stem-tip was not seen, although regular formation of a very thin radiolucent line was seen around the distal part of the noncoated femoral stem. This can be explained by the difference in modulus of elasticity between bone and the metal of the implant.

Although there is an expansion of the area of bony fixation to the more distal stem section with longer follow-up, there are currently no signs of increasing proximal bone resorption by possible stress shielding. The figures for proximal calcar atrophy, however, are slowly progressive over the years. Cases of severe proximal bone loss through stress shielding have not yet been observed, even after follow-up of six years.

### Periosteal Changes

Many cases showed periosteal or cortical bone remodeling reactions. Two patterns have evolved: a symmetric and an asymmetric type, the first one being the more common. The symmetric type is characterized by circular widening and thickening of the femoral cortex in Gruen zones 2B and 6B, in combination with intense bone densification in zones 2A and 6A. This probably reflects an adaptive remodeling response of the femur to high local stress patterns. This process appears at 12 months, and reaches its maximum at four years. Thereafter, the cortical response fades away with increasing flattening of the outer femoral cortex.

The other more asymmetric response of periosteal thickening with subsequent cortical widening usually occurs at the stem-tip level, either medially or laterally in zones 5B or 3B. In all cases the distal stem-tip was not very well-centered in the medullary canal and "touched" one inner cortex of the femur. The opposite, free side of the stem tip invariably showed a thin bone reactive line. These periosteal reactions are probably an expression of irritation of the inner cortex of the femur by the implant. This response is at its maximum around three years after surgery. Thereafter, there is increasing flattening of the outer cortex with an increase in inner femoral space around the stem tip.

In general, the frequency of this local reactive remodeling appeared higher in cases with a very tight fit of the distal stem in the femoral canal. This indicates a close coupling of interface forces from stem to bone and points to the interaction of stem design and stem fixation.

One might worry about the severity of such bone remodeling phenomena. However, on statistical analysis of these cases, the average HHS for these cases with cortical remodeling is somewhat higher as compared to those without (Table 21). Differences are not statistically significant at all follow-up intervals, but the mean value is always higher for those cases with cortical remodeling. Therefore, these cortical remodeling changes should be interpreted as signs resultant of good quality bone fixation similar to the more elementary signs of bone condensation on the HA coating.

### Engh's Radiological Score

In Engh's stability score, minus 3.5 points are given for extensive line formation around noncoated parts of implants and thus reflect a negative sign with regard to implant stability. This is certainly true for stems without signs of proximal bone ingrowth. In this case, the lines are the only signs and reflect micromotion within the bone of the stem as a whole, and thus indicate a loose stem. Distal reactive lines in combination with proximal bony ongrowth reflect a completely different mechanism of origin (well-fixed proximal stem with distal elastic modulus mismatch) and therefore should be handled differently. This method of calculation is responsible for the paradoxical lowering of the stability score up to two years (Table 16), in contrast to all other positive signs of implant stability. With longer follow-up, these reactive lines go into regression and subsequently there is a rise in the stability score. The average fixation score is, however, already at its maximum at this interval. Using this score in its current definition, at the one-year interval all but one case falls in the category of confirmed bone ongrowth (total score higher than plus six), and at two years and later all implants have confirmed bone ongrowth at the femoral side

At the acetabular side, the percentage of ongrowth phenomena for HA-coated cups is lower; 65% at one year, increasing to 97% after three years and longer. Definitions of acetabular bone ongrowth phenomena have not yet been established, because they are so rare with other methods of cementless socket fixation. In the author's material, the signs appear comparable to those of femoral bone ongrowth. They consist of bone condensation and densification against the coated parts of the cup in combination with some relative osteoporosis in the noncoated zone II. In some cups there is line formation in zone II, which could be caused by the exposure of bone to the bare polyethylene of the cup insert or to fluid pressure from within the hip joint capsule space.

### Statistical Results

In the analysis of clinical and radiologic results, there were some interesting findings. It was surprising that there was no influence of age, sex, or obesity on clinical results. Even more-or-less-experienced surgeons had similar results. When we examine the influence of clinical variables, we can distinguish between factors related to the patient, the hip or the implant itself. The first two are given; the last is under the surgeon's control.

The somewhat lower performance in the group of Charnley C patients was mainly due to differences in activities of daily living, caused by conditions not related to the hip. There was no difference in pain or limp ratings. In addition, patient satisfaction with the procedure was good.Therefore, this probably is a patient-related factor.

In previous osteotomy cases the differences are mainly in the pain and limp ratings up to two years. Osteotomy usually implies two surgeries (including plate removal), and with a varus osteotomy there is usually shortening of the leg, causing a limp. Although leg length differences are usually fully restored at the time of total hip replacement, pain and limp can still persist for more than a year. At two years, results of ex-osteotomy cases have improved and differences with "virgin hips" are only marginal and no more statistically significant. It seems probable that the surgically-induced changes in anatomy are responsible for the complaints rather than the surgical intervention as such, because similar complaints were not seen in patients with other types of previous surgeries (eg; osteosynthesis for fractures). Even restoration of leg length needs a long time of adaptation for the patient to recover good muscular control over the hip. Therefore, differences with previous osteotomy cases are probably more related to the condition of the hip, which is only partly under control of the surgeon.

In the acetabular area, the correlation between ongrowth and clinical performance is less clear. Acetabular bone takes much more time to develop endosteal bone condensation on HA-coated cups. At 12 months, 65% of cases with HA-coated cups have clear evidence of bone condensation against the coating, vs. 97% at three years. Radiolucent lines are absent around all HA-coated parts of cups, even in the critical zone III for screw cups. There is no migration of any cup, not even in some valgus-oriented cups. There is, however, another method for comparison. As mentioned earlier, some earlier cases had noncoated screw cups of identical design used in combination with an HA-coated stem, and the clinical performance in this specific group was significantly lower as compared with the group with HA-coated screw cups, even in this small group. Complaints were usually mild. Differences between the author's current series and this earlier series are listed in Table 19.

Even at two years, however, the performance was not at the same level as those of HA-coated cups, although the differences were not very significant because of the small numbers involved. In comparison to HA-coated screw cups, patients with noncoated screw-cups lose at one year, on the average, 4 HHS points on pain rating, 3 points on limp, 2 points on support (cane), 1 point on stair climbing, and 2 points on distance walked. In addition, radiographs confirm the presence of radiolucent lines in zone I or in all zones, indicative of less-optimal fixation (Fig. 25). These uniformly poorer results with noncoated screw cups are in agreement with literature findings (30). In the author's study, the addition of an HA coating to the screw cup improved clinical results and radiological ongrowth to a statistically significant degree. There are no failures or impending failures of HA-coated screw cups up to six years follow-up.

Therefore, the conclusion is also clear for acetabular components that HA coatings improve both fixation and clinical performance. Many other para-

**A**

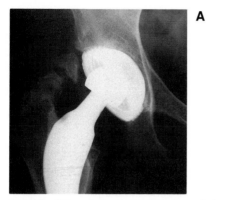

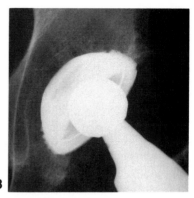

**B**

**FIG. 25.**   HA-coated and noncoated acetabular components. **(A)** Five-year postoperative x-ray of noncoated screw cup, radiolucent lines in zone I, absence of bone condensation in zone III;. **(B)**Five-year postoperative x-ray of HA-coated screw cup. Bone condensation in zones I and III.

meters were investigated, but there was no correlation between radiologic signs, other than endosteal bone condensation or cortical remodeling, and the clinical performance of HA-coated total hip components. For this reason, the main sign for positive confirmation of bony ongrowth is the presence of endosteal bone condensation and densification ("spot welds") against the coating. All other signs, including absence of reactive lines around the coating, only prove that the components are stable, and if there is no interface deterioration with time they surely do so. Nevertheless, it is a kind of "inverse proof" of bone ongrowth. Evaluation of the longer-term x-rays makes it clear that all components, if they really have any potential for bone ongrowth, do show signs of endosteal bone condensation at one time or another.

An interesting item for study is the correlation between clinical results and quality of fixation of components, in both the femur and the acetabulum. As evident from Table 20, there proves to be a statistically significant positive correlation between the degree of endosteal bone formation, especially in Gruen zone 6A, and the clinical performance of the involved hip. The average difference in HHS is 4 points at three months and 5 points at six and 12 months. The differences are mainly in the pain rating and, to a lesser degree, in limp and stair ratings.

Most of the ongrowth signs become visible within six and 12 months. Then the differences became more striking. After one year, virtually all cases show positive evidence of endosteal bone condensation, making statistical correlations impossible due to lack of numbers of noningrown implants. The conclusion of the analysis for the femoral stem is clear: adequate bony fixation does indeed improve clinical results.

In answering the question, "Do HA-coatings act only as a bone filler for empty spaces or do they really provide biological fixation?", the proof is in the x-rays when we compare them with radiologic findings after cemented hip replacement. PMMA bone cement acts as a good filler, even providing interlock with the surrounding bone when applied with modern cementing techniques. Some changes in bony architecture certainly occur after cemented implant fixation, but changes, comparable in degree and speed of development to those around HA coatings have not been described. If HA were to act only as a biological filler, the x-rays would never show such extensive remodeling with densification of bone.

Specifically, the pattern of bony changes around HA-coated implants is very similar to that described for well-ingrown porous metal-coated devices (31, 32). This concerns the pattern of endosteal bone formation ("spot welds") around the coating, proximal calcar atrophy, and reactive line formation around the distal noncoated portion of the stem, and makes Engh's radiologic fixation and stability score also applicable to HA-coated devices.

However, there are also differences. The time for development of the described bony changes is much shorter for HA-coated implants as compared with porous-coated ones. The difference in speed appears to be a factor of two. In addition, the amount of new bone formation appears to be greater for HA-coated devices. The discussed figures for bone ongrowth make HA-coated total hip replacement a reliable procedure as regards bony fixation of implants. Cementless hip surgery has always been a very critical procedure and will remain so. Very satisfying results are possible, however (32, 33), using current porous metal-coated devices applied with meticulous surgical technique. This proves that the basic principles involved are sound.

In clinical practice, however, there are often problems associated with the necessary critical maximum press-fit required at surgery. Even then, there is a high percentage of remaining complaints, especially during the first two years. The literature mentions percentages of midthigh pain up to 30% during this period (33). This proves that the clinical results do not always match the enthusiasm, based on experimental studies with the same materials (34). It could well be that the magnification and acceleration of bony ongrowth that HA coatings provide gives cementless hip surgery just the push needed beyond the critical limit of fixation and performance to let it become a procedure with reliable results. The clinical results support such a mechanism.

Human retrieval studies of well-functioning HA-coated total hip replacements also support the clinical data. Bauer et al. (11), Furlong and Osborn (12), Kroon and Freeman (35), Osborn (10), Søballe et al. (13), and Hardy et al. (14) have shown that HA-coated hip components are fully capable of achieving good-quality bony ongrowth over the majority of the HA-coated part of the implant. Dr. Bauer and I found an average surface area bone contact of 65% for primary hip replacements and still 45% for an HA-coated revision arthroplasty without bone grafting. These figures are very high, compared with those known for porous-coated hip replacements (36,37).

Some reports (38), suggest that implants without bony fixation might be able to perform properly. This includes the "press-fit" fixation theory. These reports depend only on the definition of good clinical performance. Most literature reports mention categories of good to excellent results depending on HHS ratings. "Good" means an HHS of between 81 and 90, whereas "excellent" means an HHS from 91 to 100. Analysis of data and comparison of clinical differences makes it clear that most of the reported HHS for porous-coated or press-fit, cementless implants are below 90, which is almost 10 points lower compared with what HA-coated devices allow. Certainly, we need a redefinition of " good" and "excellent" results of hip surgery. A decade ago, with the advent of porous-coated devices, 88 was certainly a good HHS for a cementless implant. Ten years later, the average HHS available with HA-coated cementless hips has risen 10 points to an average of 98. The majority of the patient population has an HHS of a full 100. Therefore, the HHS is no longer capable of expressing the real performance of HA-coated devices.

## CONCLUSIONS

Based on the current five-year results, still relatively short, the conclusion can be drawn that HA-coated total hip replacement contributes to a significantly improved postoperative result as compared with other cementless implants, the largest gain being absence of pain. This in itself allows a higher activity level to be reached in a shorter period of time. Still, long-term performance is the most important criterion. There are some prognostic factors for the life expectancy of HA-coated implants. Radiography of HA-coated prostheses shows excellent quality of bone around implants, without any radiolucent line formation around coated parts of implants. Often there is an increase in bone mass around the prosthesis, still improving five and six years after surgery with no signs of adverse bone remodeling or interface deterioration. Therefore, clinically significant problems are not to be expected in the next few years. The life expectancy of HA-coated implants theoretically should be satisfactory, clinical observation being the final answer. This study represents current knowledge on HA-coated implants and is only a starting point for further developments. Future research must focus on the consequences of the biologic bonding concept on implant design. Careful monitoring of clinical and radiologic results will certainly provide important criteria for further developments.

Refinements can be expected with regard to implant geometry as well as the area of HA-coating on the femoral stem. For example, the persisting tip activity with bone scintigraphy, in conjunction with the radiologic findings of radiolucent line formation around the distal non coated part of the femoral stem, probably proves that implant stiffness in the distal stem area is too high. Although there are no relevant accompanying clinical signs, it is certain that implant geometry can be improved. This is possible either by shortening the distal stem section or by enhancing its flexibility. Still, we must realize that if the problem of cementless implant fixation is solved, which probably is true, the next problem will be polyethylene wear. We now must determine how polyethylene wear particles will affect the HA interface and implant stability. When we want to drastically extend the lifetime of our implants, we certainly need lower-friction materials.

Nevertheless, current clinical results of HA-coated implants are excellent and are among the best available with any hip system. The most important criterion for success is still long-term performance. Although these implants may equal or even outperform cemented hip implants on short-term follow-up, we must await at least 10–15 years of clinical follow-up to make proper comparisons for survival with our present generation of hip prostheses.

## REFERENCES

1   Geesink RGT, de Groot K, Klein CPAT. Chemical implant fixation using hydroxylapatite coatings. *Clinical Orthopaedics* 1987;225:147-70.
2   Geesink RGT. Hydroxylapatite coated hip implants. *Thesis.* State University of Limburg, Maastricht, 1988.
3   Collis DK. Cemented total hip replacement in patients who are less than fifty years old. *Journal of Bone and Joint Surgery* 1984;66A:353-9.
4   Collis DK. Long-term (12-18 year) follow-up of cemented total hip replacements in patients who were less than 50 years old. *Journal of Bone and Joint Surgery* 1991;73A: 593-7.
5   Dorr L, Takei GK, Conathy JP. Total hip arthroplasties in patients less than forty-five years old. *Journal of Bone and Joint Surgery* 1983;65A:474-9.
6   Dorr LD, Luckett M, Conaty JP. Total hip arthroplasties in patients younger than 45 years. A nine to ten-year follow-up study. *Clinical Orthopaedics* 1990; 260:215-19.
7   Cornell CN, Ranawatt CS. Survivorship analysis of total hip replacements. Results in a series of active patients who were less than fifty years old. *Journal of Bone and Joint Surgery* 1986;68A:1430-34.
8   Halley DK, Wroblewski BM. Long-term results of low-friction arthroplasty in patients 30 years of age or younger. *Clinical Orthopaedics* 1986;211:43-50.
9   Søballe K, Hansen ES, Brockstedt-Rasmussen H, et al., Fixation of titanium and hydroxylapatite-coated implants in arthritic osteopenic bone. *Journal of Arthroplasty* 1991;6:307-16.
10  Osborn JF. The biological behaviour of the hydroxylapatite ceramic coating on a titanium stem of a hip prosthesis - the first histological evaluation of human autopsy material. *Biomed Technik* 1987;32:177-83.
11  Bauer TW, Geesink RGT, Zimmerman R, McMahon JT. Hydroxyapatite-coated femoral stems. *Journal of Bone and Joint Surgery* 1991;73A:1439-52.
12  Furlong RJ, Osborn JF. Fixation of hip prostheses by hydroxylapatite coatings. *Journal of Bone and Joint Surgery* 1991;73B:741-5.
13  Søballe K, Gotfredsen K, Brockstedt-Rasmussen H, Nielsen PT, Rechnagel K. Histologic analysis of a retrieved hydroxylapatite-coated femoral prosthesis. *Clinical Orthopaedics* 1991;272:255-8.
14  Hardy DCR, Frayssinet P, Guilhem A, Lafontaine MA, Delince PE. Bonding of hydroxylapatite coated femoral prostheses. *Jounral of Bone and Joint Surgery* 1991;73B:732-40.
15  Capello WN. Preoperative planning of total hip arthroplasty. *Instructional Course Lectures* 1986;35:249-57.
16  Søballe K, Brockstedt-Rasmussen H, Stender Hansen E, Bunger C. Hydroxyapatite coating modifies implant membrane formation. *Acta Orthopaedica Scandinavica* 1992;63:128-40.
17  Geesink RGT. Hydroxyapatite coated total hip replacement, two year clinical and radiological results. *Clinical Orthopaedics* 1990;261:39-58.
18  Harris WH. Traumatic arthritis of the hip after dislocation and acetabular fractures: treatment by mold arthroplasty: an end result study using a new method of result evaluation. *Journal of Bone and Joint Surgery* 1969;51A:737-55.
19  Editorial JBJS. The need for a standardized system for evaluating results of total hip surgery. *Journal of Bone and Joint Surgery* 1985;67A:511-12.
20  Ilstrup DM, Coventry MB. Factors influencing the results in 2012 total hip arthroplasties. *Clinical Orthopaedics* 1973;95:250-62.
21  Gruen TA. Modes of failure of cemented stem-type femoral components. *Clinical Orthopaedics* 1979;141:17-27.
22  Brooker AF, Bowermann JW, Robinson RA, Riley LH. Ectopic ossification following total hip replacement. *Journal of Bone and Joint Surgery* 1973;55A:1629.
23  Engh CA, Massin P, Suthers KE. Roentgenographic assessment of the biologic fixation of porous surfaced femoral components. *Clinical Orthopaedics* 1990;257:107-28.

24    Ahrengart L, Sahlin K, Lindgren U. Myositis ossificans after total hip replacement and perioperative muscle ischemia. *Journal of Arthroplasty* 1987;2:65-9.
25    Ahrengart L, Lindgren U. Functional significance of heterotopic bone formation after total hip arthroplasty. *Journal of Arthroplasty* 1989;4:125-31.
26    Ahrengart L. Periarticular heterotopic ossification after total hip arthroplasty. Risk factors and consequences. *Clinical Orthopaedics* 1991;263:49-58.
27    Charnley J. The long-term results of low-friction arthroplasty of the hip performed as a primary intervention. *Journal of Bone and Joint Surgery* 1972;54B:61-76.
28    Albrektsson T, Albrektsson B. Osseointegration of bone implants. *Acta Orthopaedica Scandinavica* 1987;58:567-77.
29    Aspenberg P, Goodman S, Toksvig-Larsen S, Ryd L, Albrektsson T. Intermittent micromotion inhibits bone ingrowth: Titanium implants in rabbits. *Acta Orthopaedica Scandinavica* 1992;63:141-5.
30    Engh CA, Griffin WL, Marx CL. Cementless acetabular components. *Journal of Bone and Joint Surgery* 1990;72B:53-9.
31    Engh CA, Bobyn JD, Glassman AH. Porous-coated hip replacement. The factors governing bone ingrowth, stress shielding and clinical results. *Journal of Bone and Joint Surgery* 1987;69B:45-55.
32    Engh CA, Massin P. Cementless total hip arthroplasty using the anatomic medullary locking stem. Results using a survivorship analysis. *Clinical Orthopaedics* 1989;249: 141-58.
33    Haddad RJ, Cook SD, Thomas KA. Current concepts review. Biological fixation of porous-coated implants. *Journal of Bone and Joint Surgery* 1987;69A:1459-66.
34    Harris WH, White RE, McCarthy JC, Walker PS, Weinberg EH. Bony ingrowth fixation of the acetabular component in canine hip joint arthroplasty. *Clinical Orthopaedics* 1983; 176:7-11.
35    Kroon PO, Freeman MAR. Hydroxyapatite coating of hip prosthesis. *Journal of Bone and Joint Surgery* 1992;74B:518-22.
36    Collier JP, Mayor MB, Chae JC, Surprenant VA, Surprenant HP, Dauphinais LA. Macro scopic and microscopic evidence of prosthetic fixation with porous-coated materials. *Clinical Orthopaedics* 1988;235: 173-80.
37    Collier JP, Bauer TW, Bloebaum RD, et al. Results of implant retrieval from postmortem specimens in patients with well- functioning, long-term total hip replacement. *Clinical Orthopaedics* 1992;274:97-112.
38    Walker PS, Onchi K, Kurosawa H, Rodger RF. Approaches to the interface problem in total joint arthroplasty. *Clinical Orthopaedics* 1984;182:99-108.

*Hydroxylapatite Coatings in Orthopaedic Surgery,*
edited by R. G. T. Geesink and M. T. Manley.
Raven Press, Ltd., New York, © 1993.

# Hydroxylapatite-Coated Hip Implants
## A Multicenter Study with Three-Year Minimum Follow-Up

James A. D'Antonio, M. D. ,
William N. Capello, M.D. and William L. Jaffe, M.D.

The arthroplasty surgeon faces many challenges in attempting to provide the patient with a durable, pain-free prosthetic replacement. Since Charnley's pioneering work in the 1960s (6), it has been recognized that one of the main challenges is providing a rigid lock between the implant and the surrounding bone. Originally it was thought that polymethylmethacrylate (PMMA) could provide such an interface. Early reports using this material were, indeed, quite encouraging (1,7,12,35). However, problems began to surface. Specifically, demarcation and fibrous interposition of the interface between the PMMA and bone were noted (8). Compounding this problem, patients began complaining of pain and, if the prosthesis was not revised, the process was frequently accompanied by massive bone loss (36, 37). This bone loss was thought to be an osteolytic reaction spawned by the particulate PMMA (29).

Alternative means of fixation were sought, and by the early 1980s there was a major shift away from the use of PMMA in implant surgery and toward cementless systems (16, 28, 32). In retrospect, this move may have been hasty. Improvements in prosthetic design, along with a better understanding of the use of PMMA and the pressurization of the material at the time of implantation, have greatly improved the results of cemented total hips (24, 34, 39). Recent reports now suggest that these constructs can provide durable and long-lasting arthroplasties even in relatively young individuals (22, 40). These clinical data gain additional support from cadaveric retrievals of long-term implants showing that there is not necessarily a fibrous membrane between the bone and the PMMA (30). In fact, microscopically the bone shows no deleterious effects when in contact with PMMA over an extended period of time (9).

Recently, another benefit of PMMA has been reported; its ability to seal the proximal femur and minimize or even prevent the ingress of polyethylene wear particles that can engender osteolytic changes in the surrounding bone (23). Although the benefits from the design improvements in cemented total hips are now recognized, many orthopaedic surgeons remain reluctant to use this mode of fixation in their younger, more active patients. This reluctance is primarily because of the significant bone loss that accompanies loosened cemented implants. Therefore, work continues on alternative means of fixing implants to bone.

Three-dimensional interlock can be achieved by bone ingrowth into a porous surface (5, 16, 33). This has been confirmed experimentally and by clinical retrievals and continues to be the basis for the use of porous implants in the young, active individual.  Unfortunately, several problems exist with porous implants, especially those which the porous coating is confined to the proximal third of the implant (38). One is the seeming unpredictability of obtaining solid bone growth into the implant. Even when bone ingrowth does occur, it appears that the percentage of the surface actually occupied by bone is alarmingly small, thus providing a surface that is fixed with scattered areas of solid bone integration (9). In addition, questions remain about the integrity of the porous coating over time. Bead defoliation and subsequent loss of fixation comprise a well-recognized mode of failure of these implants (4). Yet another problem seen with porous implants is that of stress-shielding above the level of the distal-most extend of the porous surface (15, 27). This appears to relate in part to the level of the coating but probably is as much a function of the stiffness of the implant as it is of the extent of the coating. Because most implants used in cementless fixation tend to fill the canal, the implants, of necessity, are stiff relative to the surrounding bone. Hence, stress-shielding is a natural consequence of firm fixation of the implant by bone ingrowth.

Finally, there is concern regarding the overall strength of these implants. Because of their relatively large size, strength in general is not a major issue, but the fact remains that the application of a porous coating to the implant weakens the underlying substrate, leaving areas of notched sensitivity as well as making the implant weaker than a comparably-sized, noncoated implant of the same material.

Although porous coating remains the primary means of fixing cementless implants to bone, newer means of fixation are appearing.  One example is coating part of the implant with crystalline hydroxylapatite (HA).  This material, originally used in dental applications, is plasma-sprayed onto the surface of an implant, providing a thin but well-integrated surface coating to the underlying substrate (18). Coatings of 50 to 100 μm are now commonly used with various degrees of purity of the final applied product. In 1988, Geesink et al. (19) confirmed the rapid and predictable ongrowth of bone onto this bioactive surface in a series of dog experiments. Static laboratory testing showed that the bond between this sprayed material and the substrate equaled that of a porous coating to a similar substrate. Because the material is bioactive, relating to its amorphous calcium and phosphorous component, it actually fosters bone ongrowth and initially appears to be a much more rapid and predictable means of securing implants to bone. This is a feature that neither PMMA nor porous coatings have.

Other theoretical advantages of HA coating over porous coating, as cited by Geesink (20), include the fact that there is less metallic surface area in direct contact with bone. This allays some of the fears of ion release and the potential for problems associated with long-term contact of metal against bone. The process of applying the HA to the prosthesis does not degrade the underlying substrate, and the surgeon is therefore presented with an implant of high strength.  Another theoretical advantage is that because of the rapid and predictable nature of the incorporation of these implants, proximally fixed implants should enjoy a higher success rate than similar implants with only a porous coating. The theoretical advantage of using proximally-coated implants is that the stress shielding secondary to the fixation process is minimized as compared with more extensively-coated implants.

Finally, and possibly most significant, if this floored ongrowth of bone remains, then it has the theoretical potential for sealing the proximal femur much as it is assumed that PMMA seals, hence providing a barrier to the ingress of particulate polyethylene debris and thereby minimizing the risk of massive osteolysis. The association of osteolysis with cementless implants is now becoming recognized and is resulting in the failure of certain porous-coated cementless implants.

Because of these theoretical advantages and excellent experimental data, a controlled clinical trial was begun in Europe and the United States using a proximally-coated total hip prosthesis (13, 14, 20). By December 1990, sufficient clinical and radiographic data of two years or more had been gathered, and the prosthesis had gained FDA approval. This chapter details the United States experience with one such implant that now has more than four years of both clinical and radiographic data.

## MATERIALS AND METHODS

This reported series of patients are part of a multicenter United States clinical investigational device exemption trial utilizing HA-coated implants. Between January 1988 and November 1990, 436 HA-coated femoral stems were implanted in 380 patients. The femoral prosthesis utilized had a dense, 50 μm surface treatment with HA applied circumferentially to the proximal one-third of the stem. The surface of the implant was a grit-blasted, roughened, collarless straight titanium alloy implant with normalization steps on the anterior and posterior surfaces (Fig. 1).

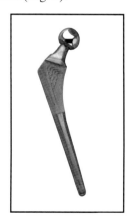

**FIG. 1.** Omnifit femoral implant: a straight titanium alloy implant with anterior and posterior normalizations and a proximal coating of 50 μm of dense HA.

The acetabular components used in conjunction with the stem included 132 porous-coated implants, 285 HA-coated, and 16 bipolar implants (Osteonics, Allendale, NJ) (Fig. 2).

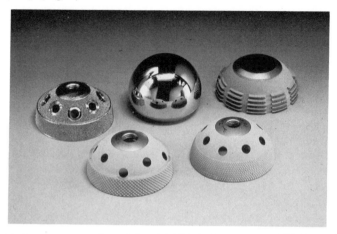

**FIG. 2.** Acetabular components; (front, left to right) HA dual geometry and HA dual radius; (rear, left to right) porous-coated dual geometry, bipolar and HA threaded socket.

This report concentrates on the 291 hips in the study that had surgery before July 1989, all of which have a minimum three-year follow-up. At three years and four years, 261 hips and 79 hips, respectively, were available for follow-up evaluation. The 30 patients excluded include eight cases that cannot be located, seven cases delayed for evaluation because of unrelated illness, change of address, or pregnancy, four deaths, and 11 revisions. Patient demographics (Table 1) reveal a majority of male patients (57%) with the young average age of 50.5 years. The most common diagnosis (Table 2) was osteoarthritis (61.2%), and 4.5% of patients received the implants in the revision setting. The acetabular components utilized with the HA-coated femoral stems in this targeted group were 125 porous-coated shells, 154 HA-coated implants, and 12 bipolar implants. The surgical technique included an attempt to achieve a maximal proximal interference press-fit using one of three surgical approaches: posterolateral (88.3%), anterolateral (10%), or lateral transtrochanteric (1.7%).

**TABLE 1.** *Patient demographics*

|  | Female | Male | Total |
|---|---|---|---|
| Hips | 124 | 1167 | 291 |
| Patients | 112 | 151 | 263 |
| Age |  |  |  |
| Mean | 50.8 | 50.3 | 50.5 |
| Range | 22/77 | 18/81 | 18/81 |
| Weight |  |  |  |
| Mean (lbs.) | 151.2 | 190.1 | 173.5 |
| Range | 79/300 | 115/305 | 79/305 |

**TABLE 2.** *Diagnosis*

| | |
|---|---|
| Osteoarthritis | 61.2 |
| Avascular necrosis | 18.2 |
| Rheumatoid arthritis | 6.2 |
| Posttraumatic arthritis | 5.2 |
| Revision arthroplasty | 4.5 |
| Congenital dysplastic hip | 3.8 |
| Other diagnosis | 1.0 |

Postoperatively, patients were instructed to use protected weight-bearing for six weeks while participating in an early, aggressive range-of-motion physical therapy program.

The study protocol required radiographs and clinical data collection preoperatively, early postoperatively (six to eight weeks), at six months, one year, and annually thereafter. Pain and functional parameters, such as stair climbing, the need for external support, mobility range, sitting ability, limp, hip range of motion, and participation in recreational activities, were evaluated at each visit and a composite Harris Hip Score (HHS) was calculated. Pain was classified as slight when it was occasional, nonspecific, and not activity-related. Mild pain was recorded when it occurred consistently and was activity-related but did not require medication or alteration of activity level. Moderate pain was recorded either when medication was required or when a decrease in activity level resulted from the symptoms.

Anteroposterior and lateral radiographs of the hip were obtained at all reactive line formations in the modified Gruen zones (21), and calcar resorption, subsidence, periosteal cortical hypertrophy, cancellous condensation, cortical erosion, and heterotopic bone formation were graded according to the Brooker classification. The modified Gruen zones 1 and 7 in the anteroposterior and zones 8 and 14 on the lateral radiograph represent the proximal HA-coated areas on the femoral implant. The appearance must have encompassed at least 50% of the zone length to be recorded. Periosteal cortical hypertrophy was recorded for an obvious and measurable increase in the outside diameter of the cortex at the point of maximal hypertrophy. Femoral cancellous condensation is defined as new bone formation occurring between the implant and the femoral cortex when compared over time to the immediate postoperative radiograph. The acetabular shells were evaluated for reactive line formation, component migration, cortical erosion, and bone condensation.

## CLINICAL RESULTS

Analysis of the clinical results demonstrates a mean HHS of 48 preoperatively, with an increase to 93 at six months, 95 at one and two years, 96 at three years, and 95 at four years (Table 3). Comparing the HHS for acetabular components over a four-year period, no statistically significant

**TABLE 3.** *Harris Hip Score*

|                    | Pre-op | 1 Yr | 3 Yr | 4 Yr |
|--------------------|--------|------|------|------|
| HHS (all hips)     | 48     | 95   | 96   | 95   |
| HHS (HA cups)      | 49     | 96   | 97   | 97   |
| HHS (porous cups)  | 47     | 94   | 96   | 94   |

**TABLE 4.** *Clinical parameters (percent)*

|                              | Pre-op | 1 Yr | 3 Yr | 4 Yr |
|------------------------------|--------|------|------|------|
| Pain-free                    | 1      | 95   | 96   | 95   |
| Thigh pain                   | 31     | 3    | 1.1  | 3.8  |
| No/mild limp                 | 27     | 97   | 97   | 95   |
| Stairs foot over foot        | 37     | 87   | 95   | 95   |
| No need for external support | 59     | 95   | 97   | 97   |
| Use of any chair             | 69     | 97   | 99   | 98   |
| Mobility range unlimited     | 10     | 81   | 88   | 86   |

difference was found for patients receiving HA-coated cups ($p = 0.125$). Pain evaluation revealed that 94% of patients were essentially pain-free at six postoperative months. At three and four years, respectively, 96% and 95% of patients were pain-free (Table 4). Thus, at four years 5% of patients complained of mild or moderate activity-related hip pain. No patients suffered marked pain or were disabled as a result of pain. When thigh pain was isolated from groin and buttock locations, activity-related thigh pain was found in 1.1% of patients at three years and 3.8% of patients at four years.

Evaluation for limp revealed that at three and four years, respectively, 97% and 95% of patients had no limp or mild limp (Table 4). The functional need for external support was present in three patients at three-year follow-up and two patients at four-year follow-up. In none of these cases was support required for the operative hip, but instead the need for support was for contralateral hip disease, contralateral girdlestone arthroplasty, femoral fracture nonunion, and contralateral hip infection. Findings for other functional measures are reported in Table 4.

## COMPLICATIONS

The orthopaedic complications in this patient population are outlined in Table 5. The two most common orthopaedic complications were intraoperative femoral cracks (7.6%) and dislocations (4.1%). A total of six femoral revisions (Table 6) were performed for the following reasons: two for infections, two for aseptic loosenings, one for postoperative periprosthetic fracture, and one for thigh pain. There have been a total of eight acetabular revisions (Table 6) for the following reasons: two for infections, four for chronic dislocations, one bipolar for pain, and one for thigh pain.

**TABLE 5.** Complications

|  | Number | Percent |
|---|---|---|
| Femoral cracks (Fx) Intra-op. | 22 | 7.6 |
| Femoral Fx post-op. | 5 | 1.7 |
| Deep joint infection | 2 | 0.7 |
| Aseptic loosening, stem | 2 | 0.7 |
| Aseptic loosening, acetabulum | 1 | 0.3 |
| Dislocation | 12 | 4.1 |

**TABLE 6.** Revisions

| Surgery date | Revision | Revision date | Reason for revision |
|---|---|---|---|
| 7/88 | Acetabular and femoral | 3/90 | Deep joint infection |
| 5/88 | Acetabular and femoral | 4/90 | Deep joint infection |
| 10/88 | Acetabular | 1/91 | Recurrent dislocation |
| 10/88 | Acetabular | 8/90 | Recurrent dislocation |
| 1/89 | Acetabular | 7/91 | Recurrent dislocation |
| 12/88 | Acetabular | 11/91 | Recurrent dislocation |
| 4/88 | Acetabular | 4/92 | Painful bipolar |
| 4/89 | Femoral | 5/89 | Post-op femoral fracture |
| 3/88 | Femoral | 1/90 | Subtrochanteric nonunion osteotomy, loose |
| 10/88 | Femoral | 10/90 | Aseptic femoral loosening |
| 3/89 | Acetabular and femoral | 2/91 | Thigh pain without loosening, revised |

Aseptic loosening occurred on the femoral side in two cases. The first revision of a femoral stem for aseptic loosening was performed two years postoperatively and was associated with a subtrochanteric nonunion resulting from an osteotomy performed at the time of the index operation for an angular deformity of the proximal femur. The second revision for femoral aseptic loosening occurred in an active farmer who at one year was pain-free and who, on returning to vigorous farm-related activities, developed progressive pain and subsidence within three months, leading to a revision two years postoperatively. Although the overall femoral revision rate is 2.1% at three to four years, the mechanical loosening rate, which includes stems that have been revised for aseptic loosening (two cases) and stems that are radiographically loose (no cases), is 0.68%.

Aseptic loosening on the acetabular side was seen in one case: an HA-coated socket showing progessive migration associated with groin pain and awaiting revision. The overall acetabular revision rate is 2.7%. The mechanical loosening rate on the acetabular side, including revised aseptically-loose sockets (no cases) and radiographically unstable acetabular components (one case), is 0.34%. The femoral and acetabular revision performed for thigh pain occurred two years postoperatively at a site out of the study group. At two years both components appeared well-fixed radiographically, and at the time of revision surgery were recorded to be solidly fixed and extremely difficult to remove.

## RADIOGRAPHIC RESULTS

Reactive line formation, as shown at four years in Figs. 3A and 3B for the anteroposterior and lateral radiographs, occurs most often around the uncoated distal tip (75%). These reactive line formations develop during the first year postoperatively and at 12 months this finding was noted in 57% of cases in zone 4 and 75% of cases in zone 11. Rarely were reactive lines noted in HA-coated zones 1 (1%), 7 (0%), 8 (3%), and 14 (1%). The incidence of reactive line formation changed little from one through four years in both HA-coated and uncoated zones.

Bone condensation at four years was found circumferentially at the transition of coated to uncoated stem in 93% of cases medially, 80% of cases laterally, and 63% of cases anterior and posterior at the transition zone (Figs. 4A and 4B). This bone condensation was detected at the one-year postoperative visit in up to 63% of cases in zone 6, and there was a progressive increase through two-, three-, and four-year follow-up periods throughout all zones around the femoral stem except for zones 1 and 11. The most dramatic increases in bone condensation from one year through four years occured in zones 3, 5, and 7 on the anteroposterior radiograph and in zones 8, 10, 12, and 14 on the lateral radiograph.

Cortical hypertrophy was noted most frequently in zone 5, occurring in 45% of the cases (Figs. 5A and 5B). A progressive increase in cortical hypertrophy was detected, particularly in zones 3 and 5 (12% at one year), on the anteroposterior radiograph from years one through four of follow-up.

Subsidence measuring 10mm and 20mm in two cases of postoperative trauma was found. In both cases the implants stabilized with protected weight-bearing and are clinically and radiographically secure at four years. These two patients, the only ones with measurable subsidence of greater than 3mm, are pain-free at both three- and four-year follow-up.

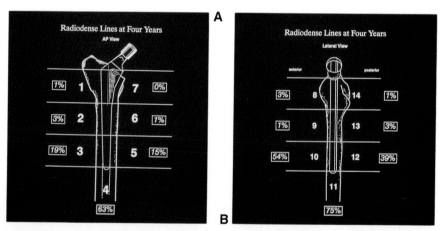

**FIG. 3A, B:**    Radiodense line formation about the femoral implant in the anteroposterior **(A)** and lateral **(B)** radiographs at four years .

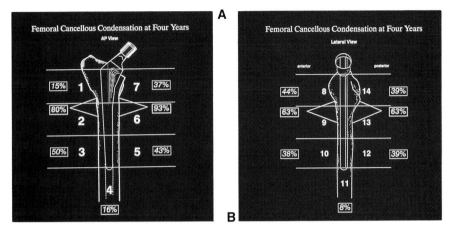

**FIG. 4A, B:** Condensation of bone between implant and cortex at four years in the anteroposterior **(A)** and lateral **(B)** x-rays.

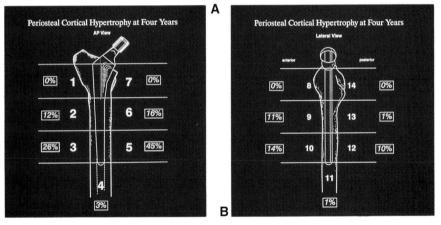

**FIG 5A, B:** Cortical hypertrophy measured as an absolute increase in width of the cortex as found in the anteroposterior **(A)** and lateral **(B)** radiographs at four years.

Scalloping at the femoral neck resection level occurred in zone 8 anteriorly (33%), zone 7 medially (24%), and zone 14 posteriorly (19%). No intramedullary osteolysis was found at the three- or four-year radiographic follow-up. In those cases with scalloping at the femoral neck resection level, although there was a tendency towards greater use of the 32 mm heads when compared with 26 and 28 mm heads, the differences were not statistically significant ($p = 0.09$).

Calcar resorption in the form of either loss of height or width was detected in 66% of cases.

Radiographic evaluation of acetabular components reveals that bone condensation begins to occur in over 40% of cases by one year with both porous- and HA-coated cups, but by four years condensation with HA cups was seen in 93% of cases in zone 1 and 57% in zone 3, compared with 65% in zone

**TABLE 7.** *Heterotopic Bone Formation (Percent)*

|  | 3 Yr | 4 Yr |
|---|---|---|
| Absent | 71.6 | 70.1 |
| Brooker I | 14.4 | 13.0 |
| Brooker II | 9.1 | 9.1 |
| Brooker III | 4.5 | 6.5 |
| Brooker IV | 0.4 | 1.3 |

1 and 44% in zone 3 with porous ingrowth cups. Reactive line formation, on the other hand, was found in only 7% of the HA-coated cups in all three zones, whereas with porous-coated cups it was seen in 9% of cases in zone 1, 11% in zone 2, and 13% in zone 3. Prosthetic migration was noted with a single porous ingrowth cup of the dual geometry design and was initially seen at the four-year follow up. The migration was superior with a radiolucency in zone 3, and the patient had an HHS of 91 and complained of no pain. Three HA-coated cup migrations have been detected, two of the dual geometry design and one of the dual radius design. Although one of these patients has radiolucencies in zones 1, 2, and 3 and complains of groin pain, the other two show no progressive migration and the patients are pain-free.

Heterotopic bone formation (Table 7) was found in 28.4% of cases at three years and 29.9% at four years. None of these patients have clinical symptoms or limitations as a result of this radiographic finding.

## DISCUSSION

The experience of the 1980s has demonstrated that bony ingrowth into an appropriate porous surface can be achieved when a well-designed implant can be rigidly implanted into bone (2,3,16). However, these experiences have taught us that the amount of bony ingrowth is limited, the amount of osteolysis about the porous noncemented implants is higher than what we had previously seen with cemented implants, and activity-related pain, particularly thigh pain, can be a problem. In addition, porous ingrowth femoral implants that are extensively coated and achieve fixation in the diaphysis of the femur can lead to unwanted and significant proximal femoral bone loss (15, 27).

HA has bioactive characteristics that permit rapid bone formation and bonding to its surface without an intervening fibrous tissue layer and without the need for a porous-coated surface (11, 18, 19). The three- and four-year clinical and radiographic results presented here compare favorably with the best cemented and cementless series reported in the literature (4, 10, 16, 24, 25, 31, 33). Second-generation cement technique as reported by Rusotti et al. (34), Harris and Maloney (24), and Maloney and Harris (31), has led to improved femoral fixation, with these groups reporting aseptic femoral loosening rates of 1.6%, 0%, and 0% of cases, respectively, with follow-up of two to seven years. Harris and Maloney (24) further noted that 5.6% of cemented femoral stems had possible radiographic loosening at 42-month average follow-up. These three cemented series also report that 94% to 99% of patients were essentially pain-free, with a zero incidence of activity-related thigh pain and composite HHS of 97, 93, and 96, respectively. The acetabular loosening rate in these series, with and without cement , was one percent or less. Collis (10), with a longer follow -up (five to 11 years) in a younger patient population, used cement on both sides of the hip joint and reported a  loosening rate of 6.7% on the femoral side and 2.2% on the acetabular side. He noted also that radiographic evidence for loosening existed in an additional 6% of femoral components. In comparison, this HA series had a composite HHS at three and four years of 96 and 95, respectively, and the incidence of aseptic femoral loosening was 0.68%, with two stems revised and no cases radiographically loose. In addition, 95% of patients were pain-free at four years. Socket migration in this series was found in 1% of the HA-coated components (three cases) and 0.34% of the porous ingrowth implants (one case). One HA-coated cup appears radiographically loose and the patient complains of groin pain.

Reports on the use of porous-coated cementless stems have shown comparable or higher revision rates to cemented stems, but thigh pain, bead shedding, and late migration are of greater concern. Initial results of 50 proximal porous-coated implants (PCA) with a minimum two-year follow-up were noted by Callaghan et al. (4) to have 16% of patients with activity-related thigh pain not requiring medication. Bead shedding was also noted, but no aseptic loosenings were found. In a report of 100 PCA hip implants followed for two to seven years, Heekin et al. (26) found late migration and loosening in 5% of femoral and 6% of acetabular components. Furthermore, the incidence of thigh pain ranged from a low of 15% at five years to a high of 23% at three years. Their radiographic analysis revealed a high incidence of reactive line formation at the proximal porous coating in zone 1 (56% lateral) and zone 8 (38% anterior). Using Engh's criteria for bone ingrowth on the femoral side, these authors rated 94% as having bony ingrowth, 1% fibrous stability, and 5% unstable at five years.  Engh et al. (17), reported on their use of a fully porous-coated stem (AML), followed for a minimum of two years, and found 84% bony growth, 13% stable fibrous, and 2% unstable. Of these AML patients, 14% reported activity-related thigh pain.  These early results improved when, with experience, they had the availability of canal-filling stems to the point where they were able to eventually achieve 94% bony ingrowth with an 8% incidence of activity-related thigh pain.  By comparison, the proximal third HA-coated implants in this study had 100% bony ingrowth at three and four years and thigh pain of 1.1% at three years and 3.8% at four years.  Furthermore, reactive line formation with the femoral HA-coated implant reported in this series at three years was 2% in zone 1 and 4% in zone 8, and at four years was 1% in zone 1 and 3% in zone 8.

The evidence for bony ingrowth in the HA-coated stems is corroborated by the low incidence of radiolucencies at the HA-coated zones and the high incidence of femoral cancellous condensation (spot welds) seen at the transition of HA-coated to uncoated stems (Figs. 6, 7, and 8). This cancellous

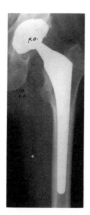 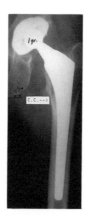 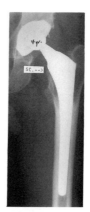

**A**   **B**   **C**

**FIG. 6.** AP radiographs in an active, 60-year-old male comparing postoperative (A), one-year (B), and four-year radiographic (C) findings in the anteroposterior view. At one year, cancellous condensation (CC) is noted at transition of coated to uncoated stem. At four years there has been progression in cancellous condensation from the transition zone through zones 3 and 5 in the mid and distal stem regions. There is no subsidence, and no proximal radiolucency, but there is a small scalloping (SC) medially at the femoral neck resection level.

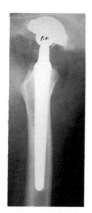 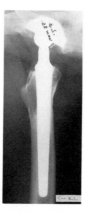 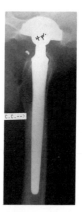

**D**   **E**   **F**

Lateral radiographs in the same patient comparing postoperative (D), two-year (E), and four-year (F) findings. At two years, there is a clear radiolucent line (RL) around the uncoated distal stem in zones 3, 4, and 5, which is similar at four years. The cancellous condensation (CC) is again noted at year two and it progresses through year four at the transition zone and distal to that zone. Again, no proximal reactive lines are noted, but there is scalloping anteriorly at the femoral neck resection level at four years.

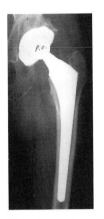 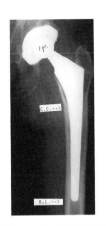 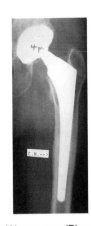

**A**       **B**    **C**

**FIG. 7.** Comparison of the anteroposterior radiographs at the postoperative (A), one-year (B), and four-year (C) periods in a 56-year-old woman with osteoarthritis and moderate osteoporosis. At one year, cancellous condensation (CC) is noted at the transition zone and a reactive line (RL) found around the uncoated distal tip. At four years, there has been progression of the condensation of bone from the transition zone distal through the mid and distal stem, progressive cortical hypertrophy (CH) throughout the same mid and distal stem regions, and the distal reactive line around the uncoated tip remains unchanged. There are no proximal reactive lines and no subsidence.

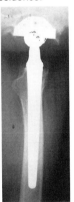 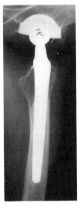 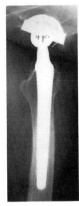

**D**       **E**    **F**

Comparison of the same patient with lateral radiographs postoperatively (D) through four years. At one year (E), a reactive line is noted around the uncoated distal tip and there is cancellous condensation noted at the transition zone. At four years (F), there has been progression of cancellous condensation at the transition zones and distal, whereas the reactive lines around the uncoated distal tip remain and no proximal reactive lines can be found.

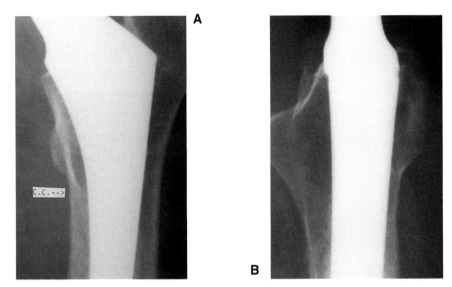

**FIG. 8.** Close-up (A) anteroposterior and (B) lateral radiographs of the HA-coated zone revealing cancellous condensation (CC) at the transition of coated to uncoated stem, with no reactive line formation and no subsidence.

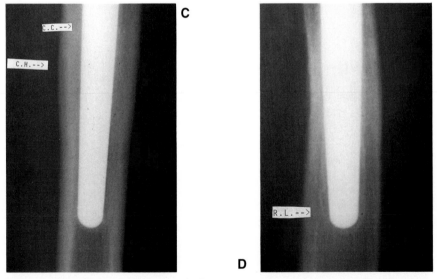

Close-up radiographs of the distal stem in the anteroposterior (C) and lateral (D) radiographs, revealing the presence of cancellous condensation (CC) of bone throughout the mid and distal stem on the anteroposterior and lateral views; a reactive line (RL) around the uncoated distal tip is most noticeable on the lateral x-ray, where the implant has not engaged cortical bone; and on the anteroposterior view, cortical hypertrophy (CH) is found.

condensation occurs within the first postoperative year and continues to increase through the second, third, and fourth years to an incidence of 80% of cases in zone 2 and 93% in zone 6 at four years. By Engh's criteria, 100% of cases at three to four years had radiographic evidence for bony stability.

Reactive line formation is an indication of relative motion between the implant and bone and characteristically occurred about the uncoated, unfixed distal stem but not at the proximal HA-coated zones or in regions where the prosthesis contacts endosteal cortical bone (Fig. 8). Although reactive lines occurred around the distal tip in up to 75% of cases within the first postoperative year, this did not increase over the four-year period and, in fact, showed a slight decrease as the incidence of cancellous condensation progressed distally along the femoral stem. Along with the increase in cancellous condensation was seen an increasing incidence of cortical hypertrophy (Fig. 7) along the mid-and distal-stem regions (zones 3 and 5). We believe that this combination of radiographic findings represents adaptive remodeling of the femur about a proximally well-fixed stiff femoral implant.

The mechanical loosening rate in this reported series for HA-coated femoral stems is 0.68% at three and four years of follow-up. Two stems have been revised for aseptic loosening and no stems are radiographically loose. One aseptically loose stem occurred in a patient who had a subtrochanteric osteotomy performed for an angular deformity and that osteotomy went on to nonunion. The second loose stem occurred in a patient who returned to heavy farming activities one-year postoperatively and within three months developed increasing pain and subsidence of the femoral components. Although there have been no revisions of either a porous ingrowth or HA-coated acetabular component for aseptic loosening, one HA socket appears radiographically loose, is associated with symptoms (groin pain), and awaits revision.

We hypothesize that distal stress transmission occurs through the stiffer stem that is well-fixed proximally, reflecting the new bone formation distally. The distal radiolucencies, we believe, are an indication of motion at an unfixed portion of the stem, which is predictable and occurs because of the mismatch in modulus of elasticity between the stiffer femoral stem and the surrounding bone where the stem remains proximally secure. It is interesting to note that as the incidence of cancellous condensation in the distal stem increases, the findings of reactive line formation show a decline, thus providing further evidence of osseous integration of the mid-distal stem. These findings of reactive line formation and cancellous condensation are described with proximally porous-coated implants. However, the onset is much slower, taking years to develop, and the consistency of findings and the magnitude of remodeling change are much less than that described with these HA-coated stems.

It is important to note that although an active assessment of bone density was not performed on a prospective basis, a visual inspection of serial radiographs from the postoperative through four-year follow-up period suggests a variable degree of stress shielding, with some loss of bone density occurring proximal to the areas of femoral cancellous condensation at the transition of coated to uncoated femoral stem. Further evidence of proximal stress relief is the finding of calcar atrophy in the form of either round-off or loss of height, which was noted in up to 66% of cases at four years. We believe that these findings are predictable as a direct result of rigid intramedullary fixation and loading with an implant that is stiffer than bone.

The results of this multicenter clinical trial using HA-coated femoral implants, in conjunction with porous-coated, HA-coated, and bipolar acetabular shells, are very encouraging. The clinical and radiologic findings have been remarkably consistent in this young and active patient population. Clinically, the patients manifest early pain relief between six weeks and six months and have three- and four-year clinical HHS comparable to the best cemented and cementless series reported in the literature. Although 5% of patients at four years complain of activity-related hip pain, only 1.1% at three years and 3.8% at four years complain of activity-related thigh pain, an incidence more comparable to the reported cemented femoral stems than cementless femoral implants. The characteristic radiographic findings about the HA-coated femoral stems are supportive of excellent early proximal fixation and predictable distal stress transmission. Comparing the use of HA- and porous-coated acetabular sockets with the same HA-coated stems, the clinical and radiographic results over three-to-four years appear similar. Continued follow-up of this patient population is desirable to establish the durability of these excellent three- to four-year results.

## ACKNOWLEDGMENT

The authors acknowledge the following investigators who contributed to the case study:

Benjamin Bierbaum, M.D. - Boston, MA
John Cardea, M.D. - Richmond, VA
Michael Christie, M.D. - Nashville, TN
Omar Crothers, M.D. - Portland, ME
Joseph Dimon, III, M.D. - Atlanta, GA
Vincent Eilers, M.D. - St. Paul, MN
Randall Lewis, M.D. - Washington, D.C.
James Lindberg, M.D. - Denver, CO

David Mattingly, M.D. - Boston, MA
Paul Pellicci, M.D. - New York, NY
Eduardo Salvati, M.D. - New York, NY
William Stillwell, M.D. - Smithtown, NY
James Turner, M.D. - Cedar Rapids, IA
Anthony Unger, M.D. - Washington, DC
Richard Zimmerman, M.D. - Portland, OR

The authors also acknowledge the efforts of Judy Feinberg, Ph.D., of Indianapolis, IN, and Alexis Ferderbar, of Sewickley, PA.

## REFERENCES

1. Amstutz HC. Trapezoidal-28 total hip replacement. *Clinical Orthopaedics* 1973, 95:158.
2. Bobyn JD, Mortimer ES, Glassman AH, Engh CA. Producing and avoiding stress shielding: Laboratory and observations of non-cemented total hip arthroplasty. *Clinical Orthopaedics J* 1992, 274:79.
3. Bobyn JD. Pilliar RM, Cameron HU, Weatherly GC. The optimum pore size for the fixation of porous-surfaced metal implants by the ingrowth of bone. *Clinical Orthopaedics* 1980, 150:263.
4. Callaghan JJ, Dysart SH, Savory CG. The uncemented porous-coated anatomic total hip prosthesis. Two-year results of a prospective consecutive series. *Journal Bone and Joint Surgery* M 1988, 70-A:337.

5.  Cameron HU, Pilliar RM, MacNab I. The rate of bone growth into porous metal. *Journal of Biomedical Materials Research* 1976, 10:295.
6.  Charnley J. Arthroplasty of the hip - A new operation. *Lancet* 1961, 1:1129
7.  Charnley J. The long-term results of low-friction arthroplasty of the hip as a primary intervention. *Journal Bone and Joint Surgery.* 1972, 54B:61.
8.  Charnley J. *Low-friction arthroplasty of the hip.* New York: Springer-Verlag, 1979.
9.  Collier JP, Mayor MB, Chae JC, Suprenant VA, Suprenant HP, Dauphinais LA. Macroscopic and microscopic evidence of prosthetic fixation with porous-coated materials. *Clinical Orthopaedics* O, 1988, 235:173.
10. Collis DK. Cemented total hip replacements in patients who are less than fifty years old. *Journal Bone and Joint Surgery.* M 1984, 66-A: 353.
11. Cook SD, Thomas KA, Kay JF, Jarcho M. Hydroxylapatite-coated titanium for orthopaedic implant applications. *Clinical Orthopaedics* 1988, 232:225.
12. Coventry MB, Beckenbaugh RD, Nolan D. Experience with two thousand Charnley total hip arthroplasties. *Journal Bone and Joint Surgery* 1972, 54A:1357.
13. D'Antonio JA, Capello WN, Crothers OD, et al. Early clinical experience with hydroxyapatite-coated femoral implants. *Journal Bone and Joint Surgery* A 1992, 74A:995.
14. D'Antonio JA, Capello WN, Jaffe WL. Hydrosylapatite-coated hip implants multicenter three-year clinical and roentgenogrpahic results. *Clinical Orthopaedics* D 1992, 285:102
15. Engh CA, Bobyn JD, The influence of stem size and extend of porous coating on femoral bone resorption after primary cementless hip arthroplasty. *Clinical Orthopaedics* 1988, 231:7.
16. Engh CA, Bobyn JD. Glassman AH. Porous coated hip replacement: The factors governing bone ingrowth, stress shielding, and clinical results. *Journal Bone and Joint Surgery* J 1987, 69B:45.
17. Engh CA, Massin P. Cementless total hip arthroplasty using the anatomic medullary locking system: Results using a survivorship analysis. *Clinical Orthopaedics.* D 1989, 249:141.
18. Geesink RGT, DeGroot K, Klein CPAT. Chemical implant fixation using hydroxylapatite coatings. *Clinical Orthopaedics* 1987, 225:147.
19. Geesink RGT, DeGroot K, Klein CPAT, Serekian P. Bone bonding to apatite coated implants. *Journal Bone and Joint Surgery* 1988, 70B:28.
20. Geesink RGT. Hydroxylapatite coated total hip prosthesis: Two year clinical and roentgenographic results of 100 cases. *Clinical Orthopaedics* 1990, 261:39.
21. Gruen TA, McNeice GM, Amstutz HC. Modes of failure of cemented stem type femoral components: A radiographic analysis of loosening. *Clinical Orthopaedics* 1979, 141:17.
22. Halley DK, Wroblewski BM. Long term results of low- friction arthroplasty in patients 30 years of age or younger. *Clinical Orthopaedics* 1986, 211:43.
23. Harris W. The role of cement in preventing femoral osteolysis. *Presented to closed meeting of the Hip Society*, Indianapolis, IN, September, 1992.
24. Harris WH, Maloney WJ. Hybrid total hip arthroplasty. *Clinical Orthopaedics* D 1989, 249:21.
25. Hedley AK, Gruen TAW, Borden LS, Hungerford DS, Haberman E, Kenna RV. Two-year follow-up of the PCA noncemented total hip replacement. In the hip: Proceedings of the fourteenth open scientific meeting, *The Hip Society*, C.V. Mosby, St. Louis, 1987:225-50.
26. Heekin RD, Callaghan JJ, Hopkinson WJ, Savory CG, Xenos JS. The uncemented porous coated anatomic total hip prosthesis: 5-7 year results of a prospective consecutive series. *Journal Bone and Joint Surgery* Accepted for Publication, 1992.
27. Huiskes R. The various stress patterns of press-fit, ingrown, and cemented femoral stems. *Clinical Orthopaedics* 1990, 261:27.
28. Judet R, Siguier M, Brumpt B, Judet T. A noncemented total hip prosthesis. *Clinical Orthopaedics* 1978, 137-76.
29. Linder A, Lindberg L, Carlsson A. Aseptic loosening of the hip prosthesis. A histologic and enzyme histochemical study. *Clinical Orthopaedics* 1983, 175:93.
30. Malcolm A. Retrieval analysis of asymptomatic Charnley total hip arthroplasty. *Presented to closed meeting of the Hip Society*, Montreal, Canada, September 1988.
31. Mahoney WJ, Harris WH. Comparison of a hybrid rough and uncemented total hip replacement. *Journal Bone and Joint Surgery* O 1990, 72-A:15.
32. Pilliar RM, Cameron HU, MacNab I. Porous surface layered prosthetic devices. *Biomedical Engineering* 1975, 10:126.
33. Pilliar RM, Cameron HU, Binnington AG, Szivek J, MacNab I. Bone ingrowth and stress shielding with a porous surface coated fracture fixation plate. *Journal of Biomedical Materials Research* .1979,13:799.
34. Russotti GM, Coventry MD, Stauffer RN. Cemented total hip arthroplasty with contemporary techniques: A five-year minimum follow up study. *Clinical Orthopaedics* 1988, 235:141.

35. Smith RE, Turner RJ. Total hip replacement using methylmethacrylate cement. An analysis of data from 3,482 cases. *Clinical Orthopaedics* 1973, 95:231.
36. Stauffer RN. Ten year follow-up study of total hip replacement. *Journal Bone and Joint Surgery* 1982, 64A:983.
37. Sutherland CJ, Wilde AH, Borden LS, Marks KE. A ten year follow-up of one hundred consecutive Miller curved-stem total hip replacement arthroplasties. *Journal Bone and Joint Surgery* 1982, 64A:970.
38. Tanzer M, Maloney WJ, Jasty M, Harris WH. The progression of femoral cortical osteolysis in association with total hip arthroplasty without cement. *Journal Bone and Joint Surgery* 1982, 74A:404.
39. Weinstein AM, Bingham DN, Sauer BW, Lunceford EM. The effect of high pressure insertion and antibiotic inclusions upon the mechanical properties of polymethylmethacrylate. *Clinical Orthopaedics* 1976, 121:67.
40. White SH. The fate of cemented total hip arthroplasty in young patients. *Clinical Orthopaedics* 1988, 231:29.

*Hydroxylapatite Coatings in Orthopaedic Surgery,*
edited by R. G. T. Geesink and M. T. Manley.
Raven Press, Ltd., New York, © 1993.

# Hydroxylapatite-Coated Implants for Total Hip Replacement: Clinical Experience in France

Jean-Alain Epinette, M.D.

For many years, non-cemented hip replacement has suffered from having to justify its existence while proving its superiority to cement. Without rejecting bone cement outright, the immediate and potential problems of cement, the doubts and questions about its future, and the increasing youth of patients led us very early to seek a cementless solution. To date, we have implanted more than 2000 noncemented stems of various designs.

In practice, "geometry" and "interface" are inseparable factors in attaining longlasting results. With respect to geometry, we sought the biomechanical elements best suited to promoting primary load transfer to the load-bearing bone. Regarding the interface, the work of Rudolph Geesink (3, 4) led us to view hydroxylapatite (HA) as the most appropriate solution for a durable, stable "bioactive" link between bone and implant.

Our first HA Omnifit stems and HA Arc 2f acetabular cups were implanted in May 1987. Since then, 945 HA components of these designs have been implanted. Our ratio of noncemented implants to cemented implants in 1987 was 1:10 for the femoral components and 8:10 for the acetabular components. Today, after five years of positive clinical experience, HA-coated stems represent over 90% of femoral implants, whereas the HA Arc 2f cup covers nearly 100% of our indications, for both primary and revision arthroplasties.

## MATERIALS AND METHODS

### Materials

We studied two HA-coated titanium (Ti) femoral hip stems: the HA Omnifit (827 cases) and the HA Omniflex (118 cases). The two models differ only in the distal geometry: The former has a long and solid stem whereas the latter is narrower in the distal two-thirds, with a polished cobalt chromium modular distal tip. The decision to use these designs was dictated by the need for the best possible solution as far as geometry and interface were concerned (7). Both give good immediate metaphyseal fixation, optimal filling of the metaphysis, and satisfactory distal contact. The Omnifit and Omniflex stems are coated only in the proximal stem third, with a 50 μm monolayer of HA deposited by a plasma-spray process onto a textured Ti substrate (Fig. 1).

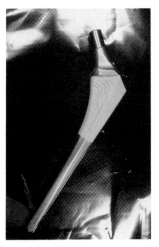

**FIG. 1.** HA Omnifit stem: Proximally-coated with hydroxylapatite.

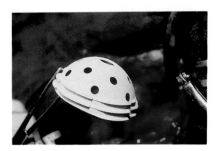
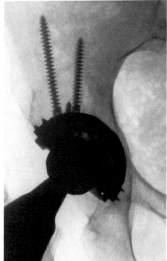

**Fig 2.** HA Arc2f Cup.

In virtually all cases in our series, both primary and revision, the acetabular component was the HA Arc 2f Acetabular Cup (93.40%) (Fig. 2). The Arc 2f cup is an HA-coated spherical cup with a thread around the equator. Initial stabilization is achieved by screwing the cup into the acetabulum. Secondary fixation is enhanced by bone screws.

## Methods

We chose both the Postel and Merle d'Aubigné clinical rating scale (PMA) and the Harris Hip Score (HHS) to evaluate our clinical results. The PMA provides an independent assessment of pain (P), range of motion (M) and functional stability (F) by ranking each clinical parameter on a scale of 0 to 6, with 6 being the best (8). The HHS, on the other hand, provides a clinical assessment by presenting a single number from 0 to 100, with 100 being the best. The HHS score incorporates the following clinical parameters and their associated scores: pain (44 points), functional ability (47 points) and range of motion (ROM)/lack of deformity (9 points) (6).

We chose the Engh and Massin (2) approach to radiographic analysis which lists the essential modifications according to the different zones, especially for the femoral component. These authors proposed combining radiographic elements as two cumulative scores (0 - 27 points): fixation and bone rehabilitation. This combination enabled a diagnosis of confirmed or suspected bone rehabilitation, fibrous encapsulation, or component loosening. To this we should add the importance of angle measurements and linear distances between reference points, well-defined by the work of Maurice Müller (9).

Our series, from 1987 through 1992, represents a total of 945 cases and 807 patients. All the implantations were performed by the same surgeon under identical operating room conditions using the same operative and postoperative protocol. The series presented is nonselective, i.e, all patients meeting the surgical criteria of good primary stability and satisfactory bone stability were fitted with HA-coated implants without discrimination as to age, etiology, or whether they took part in a randomized study.

The clinical follow-up was carried out as part of the work of the Centre d'Etude des Prothèses Articulaires (CDPA) under the aegis of the Apatite Group for Orthopaedic Research on Arthroplasties (AGORA group). The results were collated with use of a computer program (O.Soft2) and underwent statistical processing (Statis). Roentgenographic films were digitized by scanner and stored in a computer for subsequent radiographic analysis.

All the prostheses implanted were included in the overall statistical data on epidemiology, operating criteria, and immediate or secondary complications. We used only dossiers containing full clinical and radiographic data dating back at least two years for determining the overall clinical results. The rate of subsequent clinical observation of the patients involved in this study was over 94%.

The first HA implants were reserved for our youngest patients and in cases where bone cement was contraindicated. As initial observations proved favorable, we gradually expanded our indications for HA. A breakdown of the method of fixation according to year shows a gradual increase from 1987 to 1992 resulting today in a ratio of 9:1 HA stems to cemented stems in primary surgery (Table 1). Press-fit stems, (noncemented and non-HA-coated), were definitively abandoned in 1989.

**TABLE 1.** *Breakdown of HA vs. cement vs. press fit stems according to year*

|           | 87    | 88    | 89    | 90    | 91    | 92    |
|-----------|-------|-------|-------|-------|-------|-------|
| HA        | 31    | 104   | 168   | 180   | 231   | 200   |
| Press fit | 28    | 23    | –     | –     | –     | –     |
| Cement    | 108   | 38    | 22    | 14    | 8     | 5     |
| %HA/total | 18.6% | 63.0% | 88.4% | 92.8% | 96.7% | 97.6% |

## CLINICAL RESULTS

For the 945 cases using HA-coated stems in the present series, the mean follow-up period was 23.04 months. Of these 945 cases, women represented 61.15% and men 38.84%. In nearly 75% of the patients, activity was recorded before the operation as "not very active" or "inactive." The mean weight and height were 73 kg (160.94 lb) and 1.66 m (65 inches), respectively. Fourteen percent of patients weighed over 90 kg (198.4 lb) at the time of the operation. In our series, only 35% of subjects were considered of normal weight, 43% were overweight, 17% obese, and 5% severely obese. The age ranged between 19 (aseptic posttraumatic total osteonecrosis of the femoral head) and 95 years with a mean of 65.36 years. Seventy-three patients (8%) were younger than 50 and 331 (35%) were older than 70 (Table 2).

**TABLE 2.** *Distribution of patients among different age ranges*

| Age/yrs | ≤20 | No. of cases (%) of patients in indicated age range (y) | | | | | | | |
|---------|-----|------|------|------|-------|-------|------|------|------|
|         |     | ≤30  | ≤40  | ≤50  | ≤60   | ≤70   | ≤80  | ≤90  | ≥90  |
| No. cases | 1 | 7    | 24   | 41   | 163   | 330   | 247  | 80   | 4    |
| %       | 0.1% | 0.8% | 2.6% | 4.5% | 17.8% | 36.1% | 27%  | 8.8% | 0.4% |

Osteoarthritis was the most common etiology, representing over 80% of cases (Table 3). Revision cases numbered only 40 (4.45%). There was a fairly low percentage, 3.79%, of posttraumatic cases following fresh fracture of the femoral neck. These fractures were generally treated with cemented stems, at least at the beginning of the series.

The HA Omnifit stem was used in 827 cases and the HA Omniflex in 118 recent cases. The acetabular component was an Arc 2f cup in 93.4% of cases. (The remainder were HA pressfit, Harris, cemented and bipolars.) The most common stem size was size 9 (23%). Early head diameters were 32 mm. The head diameter used today is 28 mm. The mean cup size was 52 mm, used in 29.03% cases (Table 5). We never used sizes 44 or 46 mm, even for dysplasia or the sequela of congenital dislocation of the hip (CDH). Generally, three screws were often used for ancillary fixation (63% of cases). The mean duration of the operation, whether for primary or revision surgery, was 77 minutes.

**TABLE 3.** *Breakdown of etiology among 914 cases.*

| Etiology | No. | % |
|---|---|---|
| Osteoarthritis-arthritis | 736 | 81.69% |
| Avascular necrosis | 81 | 8.99% |
| Rheumatoid | 19 | 2.11% |
| Femoral neck fracture | 34 | 3.77% |
| Tumoral | 2 | 0.22% |
| Neurometabolic | 2 | 0.22% |
| Revision | 40 | 4.44% |

## Operative Complications

We must stress the absence of operative complications over the five years we used the HA Omnifit prosthesis and Arc 2f acetabular component. Neither vascular wounds nor nerve trauma occurred, especially of the sciatic nerve. This is an important point, considering the potential risk feared by those who view acetabular screws unfavorably. With more than 3,000 screws implanted, there has never been any complication.

Unlike our experience with other designs, we have not had one diaphyseal fracture among the more than 900 arthroplasties using the HA Omnifit or Omniflex prostheses. This is certainly the result of meticulous "line to line" preparation with the associated reaming and rasping beforehand. Twelve cracks occurred at the proximal section of the calcar during the operation. Cracks occurred six times with the Omnifit (approx. 1%), and six times with the Omniflex (approx. 5%).

## Early Complications

The general complications were the same as in any hip surgery (Table 4). We recorded 32 cases of thrombophlebitis (3.38%), including five of pulmonary embolism, one of which resulted in early death. There were two postoperative deaths. One resulted from a thromboembolism, the other from massive intestinal ischemic syndrome with extensive necrosis. A transient paresis of the external popliteal sciatic nerve did occur on postoperative day 3 with no other satisfactory etiological explanation other than a hypothesized compressed hematoma as explanation for the delayed appearance of neurological disorders in one patient. This resolved within three months. Postoperative hematoma were recorded in 17 cases (1.7%), six of which were evacuated by puncture or debridement. Six cases of cutaneous disunion occurred, three of which were dealt with by use of secondary sutures. Five cases of superficial wound infection following a hematoma or cutaneous disunion required local revision for washing and irrigating, while the prosthesis remained in place; no extension to deeper layers occurred. Four cases of deep infection occurred, including one in an iterative revision surgery and three after primary arthroplasty of the hip.

The infection rate with HA-coated prostheses found in this study is similar to that reported in other series. The absence of cement allows for direct contact of antibiotics transported by the vascularized tissue in direct contact with the prosthetic implants. This would explain the favorable results during the time the prosthesis was still in place for all our cases of infectious complications.

## Late Complications and Adverse Effects

Dislocations occurred in 23 cases (2.4%). The dislocations were first recorded between weeks 4 and 10 in 20 of 23 cases, at a time when return to functional activity was good, pain was absent with satisfactory functional abilities and cicatrization of the posterior periarticular region was still not entirely complete. Only one case of secondary, nontraumatic subsidence was observed in the whole series. One sudden case of subsidence at two years occurred in a patient whose course had been excellent. Revision was carried out with an Omnifit HA stem one size larger, and the findings on clinical follow-up one year later were excellent (Table 4).

## Complications: Failures and Prosthetic Revisions

We reoperated on 14 stems in our series as follows: four tenoarthrolyses with the components remaining in place; five periprosthetic fractures with replacement of the prosthetic stem; three deep infections (one involving revision surgery), the other components remaining in place; one subsidence of the stem and replacement of the femoral component (HA Omnifit); and one prosthesis painful at the end of a year, with no radiographic or scintigraphic explanation (HA Omniflex prosthesis in a young and obese patient).

In the seven cases where the femoral component was replaced, only two were due to failures of the HA stem, i.e., 0.2% of our series. As to the Arc 2f cup, no revision and replacement of the acetabular component was required.

## Summary of Two-Year Clinical Results

A total of 483 HA Omnifit stems were available for two-year followup, of which 448 were nontraumatic primary arthroplasties. Among this total, 372 cases were observed in a regular manner, consistent with the parameters of the study; 12 deaths occurred, from causes not related to the prosthesis; 18 patients were not included because of concurrent problems rendering any functional assessment impossible (polyarticular disorders, major cardiac problems, nonmatched contralateral amputation, blindness, myelopathy or serious neurological problem, etc.); and 15 patients were lost to follow-up.

The result obtained for pain was convincing because this was the main reason for the arthroplasty: before the operation, > 70% of the patients felt great pain, whereas afterwards, > 98% felt either none at all or merely slight pain (Table 5).

Lack of mobility is not the classic reason for consulting a doctor; indeed fewer than 25% suffered from severe stiffness before the surgery. Afterwards, the results were nevertheless an improvement, because 93% of the hips were completely mobile (Table 6).

**TABLE 4.** *Complications and adverse effects*

*n=945*

• **Operative:**

| | | | |
|---|---|---|---|
| Vascular wound | 0 | 0% | |
| Nerve trauma | 0 | 0% | |
| Calcar cracks | 12 | 1.3% | 6 Omnifit / 6 Omniflex = 4 secondary fractures |
| Diaphyseal fracture | 0 | 0% | |

• **Early:**

| | | | |
|---|---|---|---|
| DVT | 32 | 3.4% | |
| Pulmonary embolism | 5 | 0.5% | 1 Death |
| Transient paresis | 1 | 0.1% | External popliteal sciatic nerve |
| Hematoma | 17 | 1.8% | 6 Evacuated |
| Cutaneous disunion | 6 | 0.6% | 3 Secondary sutures |
| Superficial infection | 5 | 0.5% | Local irrigating/no extension |
| Deep infection | 4 | 0.4% | 1 Iterative revision surgery/ 3 primary |
| Death | 2 | 0.2% | 1 Pulmonary embolism/ 1 intestinal necrosis |

• **Late:**

| | | | |
|---|---|---|---|
| Dislocation | 23 | 2.4% | Between weeks 4 and 10 in 20 cases |
| Tendonitis | 14 | 1.5% | 9 Calcifying periarthritis cases = 4 tenoarthrolysis |
| Nontraumatic subsidence | 1 | 0.1% | At 2-year follow-up |
| Secondary fracture | 7 | 0.7% | 5 Re-operated on |
| Pain | 1 | 0.1% | HA Omniflex: no explanation |
| Loosening | 0 | 0% | |

• **Revision:**

| | | | |
|---|---|---|---|
| Overall | 14 | 1.5% | 7 Stems retrieved/ zero cup retrieved |
| Stem retrieval | 7 | 0.7% | 5 Secondary fractures/ 2 failures |
| Stem failure | 2 | 0.2% | 1 Subsidence (Omnifit)/ 1 painful hip (Omniflex) |
| Cup failure | 0 | 0% | |

**TABLE 5.** *PMA scores for pain (n=372)*

| | Percentage of patients with indicated PMA score | | | | | |
|---|---|---|---|---|---|---|
| | 1 | 2 | 3 | 4 | 5 | 6 |
| Preop | 0 | 71 | 0 | 25.7 | 2.1 | 1.2 |
| Postop | 0 | 0.3 | 0 | 1.2 | 11.3 | 87.1 |

**TABLE 6.** *PMA scores for range of motion (n=372)*

| | Percentages of patients with indicated PMA score | | | | | |
|---|---|---|---|---|---|---|
| | 1 | 2 | 3 | 4 | 5 | 6 |
| Preop | 1.8 | 2.5 | 4.9 | 15.3 | 41.9 | 33.6 |
| Postop | 0 | 0.3 | 0.6 | 1.2 | 4.6 | 93.3 |

Before the operation, the functional aspects are generally in a state of deterioration, but this may also depend on other general or polyarticular factors. Before surgery, more than 95% of subjects could not leave home, climb stairs normally, or walk without limp. Nearly 60% of cases resulted in total recuperation of function, as compared with < 3% confined to the home (Tables 7 and 8).

**TABLE 7.** *PMA scores for function (n=372)*

| | Percentages of patients with indicated PMA score | | | | | |
|---|---|---|---|---|---|---|
| | 1 | 2 | 3 | 4 | 5 | 6 |
| Preop | 39.8 | 55.7 | 1.8 | 2.5 | 0.3 | 0 |
| Postop | 0.6 | 1.8 | 7.3 | 23.6 | 9.5 | 57.2 |

**TABLE 8.** *Total PMA scores (n=372)*

| | Percentages of patients with indicated PMA score | | | | | |
|---|---|---|---|---|---|---|
| | ≤8 | ≤10 | ≤12 | ≤14 | ≤16 | ≤18 |
| Preop | 37 | 38.8 | 20.5 | 2.5 | 1.2 | 0 |
| Postop | 0.3 | 0 | 1.5 | 4 | 30 | 64.2 |

The overall clinical results for the population was determined as follows: "excellent" for the PMA score for hips described as "forgotten," i.e., having the best result (6) for each scoring parameter, and with an HHS score of ≥98 points; "Good" for a total PMA of ≥15 and between 80 and 97 for the HHS; "Fair" for a total PMA between 14 and 12, and between 60 and 79 for HHS; and "Poor," if the PMA score was ≤ 11 and ≤ 59 for HHS. As assessed by PMA, we obtained over 95% excellent or good results with only one graded as poor. The HHS was very similar with 96% good or excellent with only one patient having a score of less than 60 points. Overall scores are given in Table 9.

**TABLE 9.** *Overall rating by Postel and Merle D'Aubigné (PMA) and Harris Hip Score (HSS) (n=372)*

| | Preop | | Postop | |
|---|---|---|---|---|
| in % | PMA | HHS | PMA | HHS |
| Poor | 84.71 | 91.44 | 0.31 | 0.61 |
| Fair | 14.98 | 6.42 | 3.99 | 3.06 |
| Good | 0.31 | 1.83 | 43.87 | 38.23 |
| Excellent | 0 | 0.31 | 51.84 | 58.1 |

The percentage of painful hips was particularly low. All hips had either zero or "slight" pain, except for five cases, only one of which one was really painful. All painful hips were found in patients of 74 to 80 years of age exhibiting invalidating degenerative joint disease of the spine and, for two of them, a past history of neurological problems. The pain was never isolated and always occurred in association with lumbosacralgia or lumbocruralgia.

Six patients had stiff hips. In the first group, there were preoperative factors hinting at immobility, such as a past history of infectious coxitis, ankylosis accompanied by severe osteophytosis, or a long history of bilateral disorders of flexion contracture and hyperlordosis. In these cases, limitations to flexion were often pain-free, and the patients rarely required tenoarthrolysis.The second group presented normal preoperative mobility whereas major calcification and painful stiffness of the hip occurred after the operation. In this case, stiffness was most frequently due to inflammatory capsulitis.

Finally in this analysis of two-year data, we defined three patient age-groups: those aged less than 55; those between 55 and 70; and those over 70 (Table 10).

**TABLE 10.** *Clinical results by patient age*

| Categories | No. | Results PMA Score | | | | Mean Harris |
|---|---|---|---|---|---|---|
| | | EXCELLENT | GOOD | FAIR | POOR | |
| <55 yrs | 78 | 68% | 28% | 4% | 0% | 97.83 |
| 55-70 yrs | 196 | 61% | 38% | 1% | 0% | 97.26 |
| >70 yrs | 91 | 23% | 65% | 11% | 1% | 91.91 |

The first two groups, all below 70 years old, were relatively homogeneous in terms of results, with an HHS above 97 points. By comparison, the results were distinctly and significantly less positive for the oldest subjects with a total HHS of only 91.91 points and only 23.18% with a PMA of excellent.

This decline in the results with increased age, observed clinically with no radiological correlation, does not seem to cast doubt on the quality of prosthetic fixation. It is mainly the functional handicaps which increase with age. This analysis suggests that younger subjects are associated with better clinical results because of generally superior function.

### Summary of Five-Year Clinical Results

The detailed examination of 28 patients operated during 1987 is very important since these were our first cases, and the follow-up period for these patients now exceeds five years. This five-year period is the first "hurdle" for arthroplasties, and, for a good number of our earlier series of non-cemented and non-HA press-fit stems, the percentage of failure and retrieval of the prosthesis at five years was already unacceptable at approximately 15-20%.

Thirty-one HA Omnifit stems were implanted in 28 patients in 1987, 29 primaries and two revisions. Out of this total, 30 were re-examined and the dossier completed with full clinical and radiographic details. Only one primary case was lost to follow-up. The results of initial check-ups were positive but we have been unable to trace her for further examination.

These 30 prostheses are still in place and no surgical reoperation has been required. The two revisions have been dealt with in a separate section. The 28 re-examined cases with primary arthroplasty in which the follow-up exceeds five years have been studied in detail and systematically compared with the overall two-year series (Table 11).

**TABLE 11.** *Comparison of two-year and five-year followup*

**Mean Results/>2 Year Followup**

| PMA | P:Pain / 6 | M:Motion / 6 | F:Function / 6 | Total / 18 |
|---|---|---|---|---|
| Preop | 2.62 | 4.93 | 1.56 | 9.12 |
| 2 years | 5.85 | 5.89 | 5.11 | 16.85 |
| % over postop | 53.8% | 16% | 59.2% | 43% |

**Mean Results / >5-year follow-up (n=28)**

| PMA | P:Pain / 6 | M::Motion / 6 | F:Function / 6 | Total / 18 |
|---|---|---|---|---|
| Preop | 1.64 | 4.89 | 1.71 | 8.21 |
| 5 years | 5.82 | 5.86 | 5.46 | 17.14 |
| % over postop | 69.7% | 16.2% | 62.5% | 49.6% |

A comparison of the results using the PMA criteria showed no significant difference between the two- and five-year groups. Although the five-year numbers are small, there appears to be no deterioration of results with time. The percentage of "excellent" hips is almost the same for the three PMA criteria.

In summary, those patients operated on in 1987 showed no prosthetic failure after five years; no ablation of the prosthesis, no negative score and no deterioration of results with time. The scores compared during the postoperative followup years (one to five) appear to remain stable from the first to fifth year.

## RADIOGRAPHIC RESULTS

### Reactive Lines / Lucencies

Reactive lines are to be differentiated from lucencies. We consider a lucency to be a light border next to the stem and to signify a space of variable size at the metal-bone interface. This space, filled with connective tissue, always means a break of contact between bone and stem. It is always a warning sign.

A reactive line, on the other hand, is defined as a thin, dense border, separate from the metal and the prosthesis by about 1 mm, with identical bone density on either side of the line. What it signifies may vary according to location, but it always corresponds to a necessary adaptation between the stem's stiffness and the bone's elasticity with no direct bone-prosthesis transfer of stress. The location of a reactive line is crucial to its significance. Finding a reactive line in contact with a surface supposedly providing bony ingrowth is always a negative sign, because it expresses the lack of cohesion between the implant and the adjacent bone. However, it is normal to find lines in contact with the smooth distal parts of the prosthesis. The presence or absence of lines in these areas depends essentially on the shape of the medullary canal, the fit of the stem, and the elasticity of the bone shaft.

Reactive lines may be systematically recorded according to the zones developed by Gruen (5). With the stems used in the study, the HA coating descends to the middle of zones 2, 6, 9, and 13. We did not wish to complicate matters by re-dividing the zones into even more parts. We therefore define the entire surface of the HA coating on the HA Omnifit stem as zones 1, 7, 8, and 14.

## Cancellous Condensation

This radiographic phenomenon of cancellous condensation can be described as bony bridges and spot welds. Their significance is open to question; however, one may presume they are due to a local adaptive effect of the bone to point contact with the implant surface, creating rigid endosteal bone instead of soft spongy tissue.

We regularly observed this phenomenon immediately below the HA-coated zone, at the beginning of the smooth part. It had a tendency to spread, or flow, distally and stiffen the bony segment. Only rarely did these spots occur at the lowest part of the HA coating and never at the upper part. This cancellous condensation was also occasionally encountered at the tip of the stem and, in terms of disease classification, are borderline with the pedestal sign.

## Pedestal

Pedestals are an extremely important radiographic sign, for they express the femoral response to the stem at the crucial transition point of distal "bone-prosthesis" to "free bone." Pedestals are medullary bone with a distinct, inverted "egg-cup base"-shaped border. The pedestal is called "stable" if this osseous condensation is in direct contact with the metal distal stem part and "unstable" if separated from the stem by a lucency.

A pedestal indicates end loading of bone by the implant. We found them in virtually all of our noncemented, non-HA coated stems and considered them as a sign of proximal stabilization having failed. Often the pedestal was associated with a reactive line running at least along the proximal (if not the whole) part of the implant.

## Cortical Thickening

Many interpretations have been offered concerning long-term diaphyseal thickening. Thickening of the cortex may occur without periostitis or reaction of the adjacent soft tissues. True cortical thickening is easily recognizable. Often during the second year postoperative, a regular lump-shaped arch appears, interrupting the femur's overall continuity of curvature. For some time, distal cortical thickening was considered harmful. It was thought to be an irritant response to the bone being in contact with the metal tip of the prosthesis. Over the years, our experience has led us to propose a different interpretation based on a changed state of stress on the bone. This, however, will require further corroboration and longer-term statistical analysis.

### Calcar Remodeling

The calcar is a special surgical zone since it is at the superointernal tip of the osseous femur at the point where the bony structure is continuous with the internal part of the prosthetic neck. Structural modifications of the osseous framework here have given rise to great controversy as to their meaning. In fact, for the intact femur, the calcar transmits stress to the proximal femur from the acetabular zone. Substituting a prosthetic stem neck will induce major modifications in how these stresses are distributed in accordance with Wolff's law.

Special mention must be made of radiographic scalloping of the calcar (Fig. 3). This usually occurs at the junction where the stem's medial zone meets the superointernal tip of the calcar. We generally encounter this after some three or four years in porous stems and believe it is due to polyethylene wear debris.

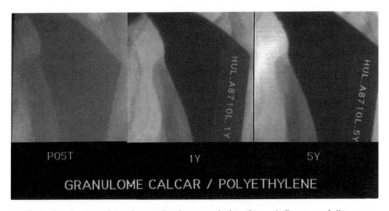

**FIG. 3.** Scalloping of the femoral calcar: evolution through five-year follow-up.

### Position of the Stem (AP - Lateral View)

The position of the HA Omnifit stem has been examined from both AP and lateral views for correlating bone reactions with the stem position and bone-metal contact points (Fig. 4). We have defined five frontal positions:

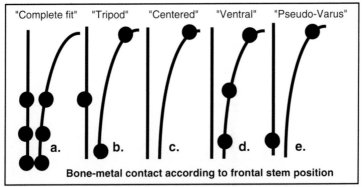

**FIG. 4.** Patterns of implant-bone contact.

(a) "**Complete fit.**" Complete contact of the stem throughout the mediodiaphyseal and distal part, occurring along more than half the femoral component. This type of fit is most commonly found in the "blunderbuss" femurs, or "champagne-flute," femurs. Primary support is most likely mediodiaphyseal with direct, but optional, contact at the calcar.

(b) "**Tripod.**" Support is provided at three points: the calcar, the medioexternal and distal internal parts. Tripod fixation is most commonly found with cylindrical femurs or in cases of coxa valga.

(c) "**Centered.**" Bone-metal contact occurs only at the calcar. The stem is not undersized if shown to be of correct size on the profile roentgenogram.

(d) "**Ventral.**" Contact is obtained all along the internal part of the cortex from the calcar to the distal stem with no contact along the external cortex. This often occurs in broad femurs with a standard cervicocephalic angle.

(e) "**Pseudo-varus.**" Distal contact occurs at the external cortex with the stem appearing to rest on the calcar. If the profile appears to fit correctly, the stem is in this position because of abnormal curvature of the diaphyseal shaft. It is neither in varus nor malposition and the term "pseudo-varus" has no pejorative connotation.

### Additional Acetabular Parameters

Radiographic evaluation of the acetabulum traditionally divides the implant into three zones: superoexternal, central, and inferointernal. To these we added zone 4, corresponding to the site of additional bone screws. Zone 4 is of capital importance because the appearance of lucencies or mobilization areas expresses without a doubt instability of the prosthesis and incipient subsidence, as does a secondary rupture of the screw. Demonstrating the reactive lines or lucencies is often difficult because cup orientation and poor quality roentgenograms can be very misleading. With this in mind, a detailed radiographic analysis from AP and lateral views is often possible, particularly if the roentgenograms are not consecutive.

### Heterotopic Calcifications

We used Brooker's scale of 1 through 4 for grading heterotopic calcifications, where 1 corresponds to a small amount of periprosthetic calcification and 4 corresponds to the greatest.

### Radiographic Analysis

The radiographic analysis involved 223 full dossiers. For purposes of comparison, we were able to use all the radiological dossiers on the prostheses implanted in 1987 and thus have follow-up data through five years. Our previous experience with 500 noncemented, non-HA stems added to our first series of cemented stems helped us understand how the osseous changes related to implant type. We never encountered reactive lines in contact with the HA-coated zones during primary surgery (Table 12). Thus, the enchondral condensation spots (Table 13) were found immediately below the HA / smooth zone junction. Only rarely did the condensation increase by 1 or 2 cm and "infringe" upon the HA zone.

**TABLE 12.** *Reactive lines: femur*

|  | R.L. in % (n=223) |
| --- | --- |
| None | 34.08 |
| HA zone | 0 |
| <50% smooth | 34.53 |
| >50% smooth | 14.35 |
| Zone 4 only | 16.59 |

## Enchondral Ossification (Subcortical Cancellous Bone Formation)

**TABLE 13.** *Enchondral ossification: femur*

|  | in % (n=223) |
| --- | --- |
| Yes | 42.41 |
| Moderate | 9.82 |
| None | 47.77 |

## Pedestal

We found a very low incidence of pedestal formation (2.57%) (Table 14). Pedestal formation used to be a classic phenomenon in noncemented, non-HA stems, indicative of distal fixation.

**TABLE 14.** *Presence or absence of pedestals*

|  | in % (n=223) |
| --- | --- |
| **None** | **97.44** |
| Incipient | 2.05 |
| Stable | 0.26 |
| **"Unstable"** | **0.26** |

Nearly 30% of cases exhibited cortical thickening (Table 15). The most common were found either in zone 5, or in zones 3, 10, 12, and 5, corresponding to a container-contents adaptation of elastic gradient. In these cases, not once did thigh pain occur. According to our experience, these changes occurred between the second and third year and remained stable with time.

**TABLE 15.** *Cortical thickening*

|  | in % (n=223) |
| --- | --- |
| **None** | **70.40** |
| Zone 5 | 15.35 |
| **Zone 3** | **0.45** |
| Distal "Ferrule" | 13.90 |
| Overall | 4.48 |

No modification of the calcar was demonstrated in > 50% of cases (Table 16). Slight resorption occurred in one-fourth of the cases, moderate resorption in 10% and severe resorption in 6% but without any associated anomalies such as signs of stem loosening. Hypertrophy was never encountered in this entire series of primary hip arthroplasty.

**TABLE 16.** *Calcar changes*

| Calcar Resorption | in % (n=223) |
| --- | --- |
| **No modification** | **55.51** |
| Slight Resorption | 24.67 |
| Moderate Resorption | 10.13 |
| Severe Resorption | 5.73 |
| Calcar Scalloping | 3.96 |
| **Hypertrophy** | **0** |

Special attention must be paid to the "droplet" osteolysis (4% of cases), signifying, in our opinion, the presence of polyethylene debris. It always occurred after the second year and, at five years, has been nonprogressive. Its presence has never been associated with a non-neighboring cyst or granuloma.

### Other Radiographic Signs

Other than a traumatic occurrence, stem subsidence was observed once in the entire series, representing < 0.15% of cases. In successive checkup visits, no evidence of incipient subsidence or stem destabilization has been observed. Osseous osteolysis and stress shielding of the greater trochanter were never evaluated.

### Position of the Stem Frontal / Profile

Stems were analyzed with use of both AP and lateral roentgenograms. A crossed study on 194 observations confirmed the statistically large number of "complete fit" adaptations found in nearly half of the frontal roentgenograms, and 36% of cases for both frontal and profile. The "centered" position was rarer for frontal, occurring in less than one-fourth of cases, of which only 10% were found for both frontal and profile. The "varus position," found in 5% of cases, occurred in only two "centered" profile observations. These two cases could thus represent, in the absence of abnormal femur curvature, malposition

(1.03% of cases). On the other hand, of five cases that qualified as "undersized" on frontal roentgenograms, they were in fact found in only two cases.

## ACETABULUM

### Reactive Lines

Since we started using the HA-coated Arc 2f acetabular cup, we have never observed a reactive line in zone III (Table 17). However, with the Ti plasma-coated Arc 2f acetabular cup, reactive lines were commonly observed in zone III and in zone II. This reveals the positive effect HA has on a geometrically identical acetabular component with the same additional screws implanted by the same surgeon.

**TABLE 17.** *Arc 2F: Reactive lines: plasma vs. HA*

| Reactive line | Plasma Ti | HA |
|---|---|---|
| Zone I | 0% | 0% |
| Zone II | 26% | 0% |
| Zone III | 52% | 0% |
| Zone IV | 0% | 0% |

### Migration

With five years follow-up and over 1,150 Arc 2f acetabular components in our series, we never encountered a case of acetabular protrusion or ascending migration. This finding compares favorably to a prior series of first-generation smooth screwed rings, the mean rate of acetabular movement was 5 - 10% after three years.

### Loss of Screw Fixation

We should also mention the importance we ascribe to the nonoccurrence of secondary rupture of the screw. Because of their divergent and nonparallel positions, a "hasp" effect occurs that locks the acetabulum in place. Movement can occur only if one or more screws are ruptured. This has never happened in any of the 3,200 Arc 2f acetabular cups implanted to date.

### Heterotopic Calcifications

Secondary periarticular calcifications were studied according to Brooker's classification (Table 18). The number of cases lacking significant calcification

**TABLE 18.** *Calcifications: percent and effect on flexion*

| | No. | Percent | Mean Flex |
|---|---|---|---|
| None(St.. 0) | 115 | 71.3 | 126° |
| Slight (St. 1) | 25 | 15.9 | 122° |
| Average (St. 2) | 12 | 7.6 | 124° |
| Severe (St. 3) | 6 | 3.2 | 88° |
| Bridge (St. 4) | 4 | 2 | 41° |

is high (over 70%). Evaluation, however, is in fact both difficult and controversial. It would seem wiser to note the percentage of grades 2, 3, and 4 (which add up to less than 12%, 2% of which are bridges corresponding to Stage 4).

A crossed-study on the mobility of the hip in flexion according to the degree of calcification was carried out with 157 cases. We calculated the flexion means using Brooker's calcification grade and found an identical flexion mean of greater than 120° for Brooker Stages 0, 1 and 2. Mean flexion is distinctly decreased (< 90°) for Stage 3 and too low for Stage 4 and constantly required revisions for tenoarthrolysis.

## Comparative Study of Two-Year and Five -Year Data

The detailed examination of the radiographic dossiers on the 31 patients currently at five years is of especial interest because of their homogeneity. Comparisons were made with the results of the entire two-year series (Table 19).

**TABLE 19.** *Comparison of reactive lines at five-year and 2-year followup*

| Reactive Line | Five-year Group (n=28) | Two-year Group (n=223) |
|---|---|---|
| None | 37.50% | 34.08% |
| HA Zone | 0% | 0% |
| <50% Smooth Z. | 29.17% | 34.53% |
| >50% Smooth Z. | 16.67% | 14.35% |
| Zone 4 Only | 16.67% | 16.59% |

Comparing the results of reactive lines at five years with the overall results of the two-year series demonstrates the absence of distortion among the different groups. Within each category, the results are virtually identical. This finding supports our opinion that if stem fixation and stability remain perfect, the reactive lines in the smooth zones are derived from an adaptation between the femoral shaft and the metal stem. Persistent fixation at five years is confirmed by the lack of reactive lines.

Cortical remodeling proves particularly interesting at five-year follow-up (Table 20). The percentage of cases without cortical remodeling is 48% compared with 70% for the overall two-year series. This may be explained by the late occurrence of these changes, often at two or three years. In our experience, the modifications that do occur—and this has no pejorative conno-

**TABLE 20.** *Comparison of cortical thickening at five-year and two-year followup*

| Cortical Thickening | Five-year Group (n=28) | Two-year Group (n=223) |
|---|---|---|
| None | 48.00% | 70.40% |
| Zone 5 | 40.00% | 15.35% |
| Zone 3 | 0.00% | 0.45% |
| Distal Ferrule | 4.00% | 13.90% |
| Overall | 8.00% | 4.48% |

tation except for the reactions in zone 3—do not change noticeably over annual follow-up visits. Not one of these 13 patients exhibiting a cortical reaction felt thigh pain. In the last analysis, this crossed-comparison confirms that this type of reaction is definitely not the consequence of metal-cortex contact.

At five years, remodeling of the calcar reached nearly 85% compared with 45% for the overall two-year series (Table 21). Given the increase in modifications with time this finding is normal. We tried to find a relation with other parameters for the three cases exhibiting severe resorption (Figs. 5-8). These three cases correspond to the three situations of stems "centered" in both the frontal and profile planes. The "severe" resorption is thus the result of atrophy due to "nonsupport" in this zone and has no apparent clinical consequence. In these three cases, we found one case of "overall" cortical remodeling and none for the other two. Thus, this type of atrophy does not correspond to incipient varus capping. It is worth recording the absence of hypertrophy of the calcar, even after this time frame, providing evidence that the stress is suitably and lastingly dealt with by the metaphyseal fixation.

**TABLE 21.** *Comparison of calcar resorption at five-year and two-year followup*

| Calcar Resorption | Five-year Group (n=28) | Two-year Group (n=223) |
|---|---|---|
| No modification | 16.00% | 55.51% |
| Slight resorption | 44.00% | 24.67% |
| Moderate resorption | 24.00% | 10.13% |
| Severe resorption | 12.00% | 5.73% |
| "Droplet" osteolysis | 4.00% | 3.96% |
| Hypertrophy | 0.00% | 0.00% |

## Case Studies

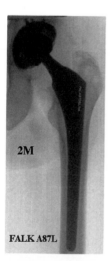
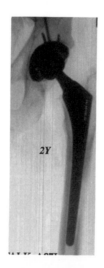
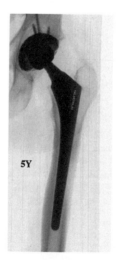

**FIG. 5.**   FALK, male 58y, 85 kg, OA. Heavy work 2 weeks after the hip replacement. Excellent result at 5y FU. X-ray: 2 mos / 2 yrs / 5 yrs = cortical thickening 5 zone - no thigh pain.

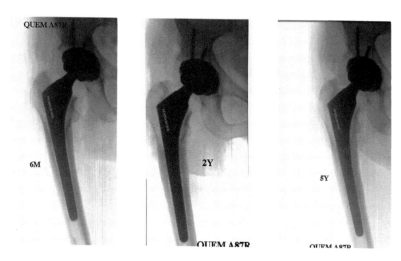

**FIG. 6.** QUEM, female 70y, OA. Excellent result at 5 year FU. X-Ray: 6 mos / 2 yrs /5 yrs = no significant change at 5 years.

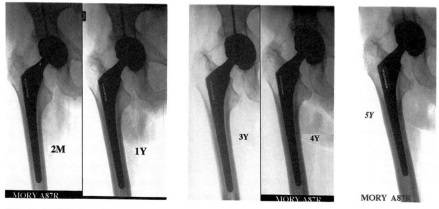

**FIG. 7.** MORY, female 69. Excellent result at 5y FU. X-ray: 2 mos / 1 yr / 3 yrs / 4 yrs / 5 yrs = No significant change.

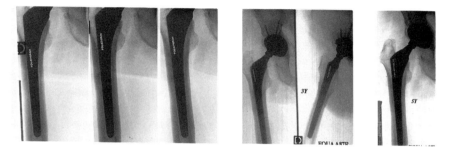

**FIG. 8.** FOUA, male 64, OA. Excellent result at 5-year FU. X-Ray: 6 mos/1 yr/ 2 yrs/3 yrs/5 yrs = cortical thickening at 1-year (circular remodeling so called "ferrule": 3-6-10-12 Gruen zone), no change at 5-year examination.

## Assessment According to the Engh Score

Although we recognize the merit of Engh and Massin (2) in having been the first to describe a semiology of radiological signs for noncemented stems, we did encounter some difficulties with Engh's score as a numerical means of assessment. Certain parameters, such as deterioration of the interface or elimination of particles, do not correspond to the character of the HA coating.

For purposes of clarity, the means were expressed according to three scores: fixation, stability and overall. Despite the random nature of some of the parameters, these results confirmed bone rehabilitation and excellent fixation in all cases ("bone ingrowth confirmed"); this diagnosis of bone rehabilitation, proposed by Engh for a score of +6 points, was obtained in 100% of our cases (Table 22).

**TABLE 22.** *Engh score: comparison of means at two and five years*

| Mean / Pts | Stability / 10 | Fixation / 17 | Overall / 27 |
|---|---|---|---|
| >2 Year Group | 6.33 | 11.37 | 17.71 |
| >5-Year Group | 9.69 | 14.96 | 24.65 |

## DISCUSSION

Experimental work has demonstrated the excellent biointegration of HA by neighboring bone tissue. The work of Geesink shows that the metal-HA link can be considered reliable. Our clinical observations support this, and we have not been disappointed with the coating's fixation and resistance with respect to the prosthetic metal.

For the acetabulum, we initially chose the Arc 2f cup designed in 1985 as an adaptation of the two models of acetabular implants used at the time. With the HA Arc 2f Acetabular Cup, primary fixation is achieved by a thread around the cup equator, and secondary "biological" fixation seems ensured by the HA. Screws provide ancillary fixation when located in the axes of stress lines. We believe that this cup is a satisfactory solution to the concept of primary fixation and that it provides the best conditions for long-term stability.

With regard to the femoral stem, we believe that the HA coating should be limited to the proximal stem third only. The metaphysis should be filled as best as possible without compromising the proximal cancellous bone. The proximal geometry should prevent rotational instability and ensure excellent frontal fit. The distal part of the stem is solid and elongated, preventing varus instability problems.

The complications were minimal with regard to the stem, with less than 0.5% of failed cases. The statistics for general complications in the series are similar to those of cemented prostheses, but there was a degree of security unequaled by previous cementless models. There were no complications with the HA Arc 2f Acetabular Cup: no pelvis fractures, no material problems, and no neurovascular lesions due to additional screws.

The results were distinctly better than those of our previous cementless series and were comparable with the short- and mid-term results found with cemented prostheses. Obviously, for a nonselective series involving elderly subjects often suffering from a polyarticular handicap not related to the arthroplasty itself, the scores of the overall assessment or results of the "function" parameter are likely to be lower. The various studies of subgroups and the crossed studies nevertheless gave excellent results in terms of pain and mobility, in particular with the complete disappearance of "thigh pain," which used to be so typical in this type of arthroplasty.

For the radiographic data, we took advantage of the lessons learned from Engh regarding femoral components implanted without cement. It is true to say that cementless femoral implants have completely altered bone-prosthesis relations and, hence, the visible signs on roentgenograms. Although each parameter has its importance in terms of bone biomechanics, the appearance of new models for HA must also be taken into consideration in drawing up score diagnoses.

The problem with radiographic interpretation is the necessity of analyzing a multitude of parameters from only two planes (AP and lateral). Among the parameters are femoral curvature, endomedullary morphology, bone elasticity, etiological components, and patient activity. These factors inevitably lead to modulation of the bone's response to the prosthetic implant.

For a number of years, we followed a set of empirical rules. The first was that the distal stem should not come in contact with the diaphysis because this could cause thigh pain or adverse cortical remodeling. We also believed that the stem should be as short as possible to prevent conflicts of elasticity and subsequently, problems of thigh pain. Finally, we believed that stem flexibility was a major factor in enabling pain arising in the mid- or long-term to disappear. And yet, the HA Omnifit stem is long, solid, and supported within the diaphysis for optimum primary fixation.

Our experience thus allows us to put forth certain different opinions:
(a) The bone-metal contact points in our series have never caused pain, "irritant" reactions, or, especially, adverse cortical remodeling or thickening. In fact, we found cortical thickening to be a response of the load-bearing bone shaft to the endomedullary component, and hence a compromise of elasticity between the container and the contents without causing any pain or change of prosthetic fixation. (b) The presence of a rigid implant such as the HA Omnifit has shown us that the bone can adapt without causing prosthetic failure.

## CONCLUSION

In summary, our five years of clinical follow-up regarding HA is distinctly positive and encouraging. A further understanding of bone reactions and improving upon articular implants will provide for even greater implant longevity. The ideal hip prosthesis will probably never exist. Nevertheless, in terms of geometry and interface, the HA Omnifit Hip Stem and the Arc 2f Acetabular Cup combination seems to be an extremely promising choice, even if adaptations can be envisaged for improving the already satisfactory results.

HA-coated stems must be distinguished once and for all from press-fit stems. The poor long-term fixation of the latter results in a high proportion of failures and hence brings the "noncemented" arthroplasties into disrepute. HA-coated prostheses provide a "bioactive" interface and have been reported as being effective by a wide variety of authors. These implants maintain bone contact in the HA zones and perform more effectively than the all-metal press-fit designs.

## REFERENCES

1. D'Antonio JA, Capello WN, Jaffe WL; Hydroxylapatite-coated hip implants: Multicenter three-year clinical and roentgenographic results. *Clinical Orthopaedics,* 1992, 285:102.
2. Engh CA, Massin P; Cementless total hip arthroplasty using the anatomic medullary system: Results using a survivorship analysis. *Clinical Orthopaedics,* 1989, 249:141.
3. Geesink RGT; *Hydroxyapatite-coated implants.* Maastricht, the Nederlands: Rijkuniversiteit Limberg te Maastricht; 1988, Thesis.
4. Geesink RGT, deGroot K, Klein CPAT; Chemical implant fixation using hydroxyl-apatite coatings. *Clinical Orthopaedics,* 1987, 225:147.
5. Gruen TA, McNeice GM, Amstutz HC; "Modes of failure" of cemented stem-type femoral components: A radiographic analysis of loosening. *Clinical Orthopaedics,* 1979, 141:17.
6. Harris WH; Traumatic arthritis of the hip after dislocation and acetabular fractures: Treatment by mold arthroplasty. An end result study using a new method of result evaluation. *Journal of Bone and Joint Surgery,* 1969, A51:737.
7. Manley MT, Kay JF, Uratsuji M, Stern LS, Stulberg BN; Hydroxylapatite coatings applied to implants subjected to functional loads. *13th Annual Meeting Society for Biomaterials,* 1987, New York, NY:210
8. Postel M, Kerboul M, Evrard J, et Courpied JP; Arthroplastie totale de hanche, *Springer-Verlag Edition,* 1985 (to come)
9. Müller ME; Total hip replacement: planning, technique and complications. In: Cruess RL, Mitchell NS: *Surgical management of degenerative arthritis of the lower limb,* Lea & Febiger, 1975, Philadelphia, PA 10:91-113.

Hydroxylapatite Coatings in Orthopaedic Surgery,
edited by R. G. T. Geesink and M. T. Manley.
Raven Press, Ltd., New York, © 1993.

# The APR-I Experience
# with Hydroxylapatite

Edward J. McPherson, M.D.,
Richard J. Friedman, M.D. FRCS (C), and
Lawrence D. Dorr, M.D.

The advances conceived by Charnley in cemented total hip technology were indeed a revolution in the fundamental ways of treating advanced coxarthrosis. The initial goals of relieving pain and restoring function to elderly patients with advanced degenerative arthritis have been realized. Long-term studies of Charnley low-friction arthroplasties (LFA) in the elderly population with follow-up between 16 and 26 years reveal that first-generation LFAs are doing remarkably well, with overall survival rates between 89 and 95% (34,36). With the advent of second-and third-generation cement techniques, survival rates of up to 97% have been reported at 11-year follow-up by Harris et al. (27).

The initial success with cemented total hip arthroplasties (THA) led to more liberal applications of this technique, with indications for cemented THA expanded to younger and more functionally active patients suffering from advanced coxarthrosis. Unfortunately, long-term studies with this group of patients have proven disappointing (7,18,19,26,30). In Dorr's study of 81 cemented THAs in patients younger than 45 years reviewed at 9- to 10- year follow-up, there were 58% clinically satisfactory results with a revision rate of 33%. This group continues to be followed, and at approximately 15-year follow-up, nearly 67% of this group has been revised (17). These results are supported by Chandler, who reported 57% incidence of loosening in patients 30 years or younger at 5-year follow-up (7).

The development and clinical use of porous-coated joint implants is a direct outcome of the poor results obtained with cemented THAs in young, active patients. It is believed that a noncemented hip implant can achieve biologic stabilization via bony ingrowth into a porous-coated implant surface provided that (a) the material is inert, (b) there is no movement at the bone implant site during healing, and (c) the porous structure has optimal pore size and pore morphology (4,6,8,12,14,25). The authors believe that the porous coating of the femoral stem must be limited to only the femoral metaphysis to minimize proximal stress shielding, as reported with fully coated stems, and promote proximal load transfer similar to the normal hip (9,20,21).

The orthopaedic literature abounds with short-term and intermediate-term clinical results of porous-coated implants. First-generation porous-coated THAs including the AML, APR-I, Harris Galante, LSF, Omnifit, and PCA, have demonstrated encouraging results ranging from 2 to 6 years (5). However, the early experience with bony ingrowth systems reveals major concerns regarding the consistency of achieving bony ingrowth into porous implants. Because of the variations of age, genetic makeup, and concurrent medical illnesses, the rate as well as quantity of bony ingrowth represents a metabolic spectrum and may be unpredictable in individual patients. Furthermore, micromotion of the implant greater than 50–150 microns ($\mu$m) at the implant/bone interface immediately after implantation might prevent appositional bone ingrowth and, in particular, prevent ingrowth of osteoid with subsequent bone formation within the pores (22).

Cook et al. (11) reported on 22 porous-coated femoral components and 14 acetabular components found to be well fixed at revision surgery. The components were of several first generation designs with varying porous surface geometries. The incidence of bone ingrowth was 82% of femoral components and 43% of acetabular components. However, only 23% of femoral components and 7% of acetabular components had more than 5% of the interface surface occupied by bone ingrowth (11 ). Collier et al. (10) studied 104 porous femoral components and 58 acetabular components of various designs retrieved for a variety of reasons including loosening. In this series, 27% of the femoral components and 16% of the acetabular components demonstrated bone ingrowth. Galante, reported more encouraging results in reviewing 14 retrieved Harris-Galante porous femoral stems removed for reasons other than loosening and infection. All components demonstrated some degree of bony ingrowth. Of the 10 primary femoral stems retrieved from femurs of normal geometry, the mean interface surface occupied by bone was 17% (23).

In an effort to improve the rate and quantity of biologic fixation of uncemented total hip systems, orthopaedic researchers have turned to their dental and oral–maxillofacial counterparts to help solve their problem. The result has been the introduction of hydroxlapatite (HA) to the orthopaedic field.

Calcium phosphate ceramics have been shown in laboratory and animal studies to be biocompatible, nontoxic, and capable of direct intimate bonding with bone because of the chemical similarity to components of natural bone mineral. The synthetic HA form of calcium phosphate closely resembles the apatite bone mineral component of vertebrate hard tissue (12). HA plays an integral part in the mineralization of bone, serving as an osteoconductive medium for the deposition of newly formed osteoid. Central to the rationale for the use of HA with total hip implantation is the concept that this substance represents a "friendly" environment for bone ingrowth into the porous coating (33).

HA has shown good ability to provide bone ingrowth fixation to implants in both animals and clinical dental use (13,15,24,28,32,35). These experiments confirmed the use of HA as an osteoconductive medium that enhanced the rate of bone formation. The mechanism of action is to allow osteoid to form on the implant. As a result, maturation of osteoid results not only in bone growing from host toward the implant, but also in bone growing from implant/HA toward the host bone. The result is a more rapid closure of gaps between implant and host bone. Secondly, growth of bone occurs around the entire implant/HA surface, which maximizes the amount of bone attached to the implant. Once bone has formed on the HA surfaces, the bond between synthetic HA and host bone is strong. Synthetically prepared HA has been shown to chemically bond with bone when implanted in a hard tissue site (30). This chemical bond results in a normal healing process and proceeds on and around the dense HA-coated implant. The bond is so strong that once bone has become attached to the surface of HA and samples are stressed to failure, the fracture occurs in the bone some distance away from the actual bone/ceramic interface (15,29).

The following discussion reviews our work with HA coatings employing the APR-I total hip implant system. This discussion will focus on our experience with HA-coated porous implants and HA-coated nonporous implants in comparison with their non-HA-coated implant counterparts.

## FEMORAL STEM FIXATION USING THE APR-I TOTAL HIP SYSTEM: COMPARISON OF HA-POROUS VERSUS POROUS

The purpose of this study was to evaluate the results of the APR-I primary total hip replacement comparing stems that achieved femoral fixation by proximal bony ingrowth into porous patches vs.proximal bony ingrowth into HA-coated porous patches. This study was performed exclusively at the Kerlan-Jobe Orthopaedic Clinic.

The APR-I primary hip (Intermedics Orthopaedics, Austin, TX) was made of titanium alloy and had "cancellous structured" patched coating, proximally placed on the anterior, posterior, and medial surfaces. There was a porous-coated collar and an anatomic posterior bow (Fig. 1). All original APR-I femoral heads were made of titanium. The pore size was 450 μm. The pore size was increased to 750 μm on the HA-coated implants to accommodate the partial closure of pores that occurs when HA is sprayed onto the coating. The thickness of the HA coating was 50 μm. The application was by a plasma- spray method developed by Calcitek, Inc. (Carlsbad, CA).

Eighty-four cementless APR-I total hip replacements were performed by the same surgeon (LDD) and followed for a minimum of three years. Forty-two hips were implanted with HA coating on the proximal porous patches. A control group of 42 hips was matched for age, sex, weight, diagnosis, Charnley class, bone quality type as described by Dorr, and surgical technique. In the surgical technique, assurance was made that each matched pair had equivalent distal femoral stem filling of the canal, which assured initial stabilization of the implant during the healing phase.

The pairs were matched for bone type as described by Dorr (Fig. 2). Type

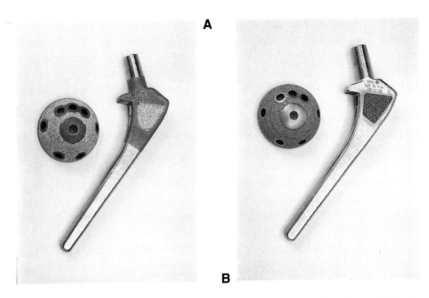

**FIG. 1.** Porous-coated APR-I primary hip stem and acetabular cup (**A**) with and (**B**) without hydroxylapatite coating.

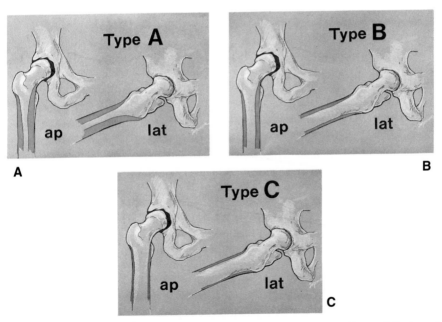

**FIG.2.(A,B,C)** Diagrams of Type A, B, and C bone. Note progressive loss of femoral diaphyseal cortex which becomes nearly indistinct in Type C bone. Also note progressive loss of posterior cortical fin. Type C femurs often have a diaphyseal diameter mismatch, with the lateral endosteal diameter measuring up to 4–5 mm larger than the AP endosteal diameter.

A bone has thick femoral diaphyseal cortices with prominent medial and posterior cortical fins. Type B bone has diminished cortical thickness. The medial and posterior cortical fins are attenuated, but the posterior fin is still distinct. Type C bone is characterized by attenuated, nearly indistinct cortices with absent medial and posterior cortical fins. Type C bone is flexible and yields a reduced strength for attachment due to its weakened architecture.

The demographics of the two groups are listed in (Table 1). Important to note is that the study groups are relatively young, and bone quality in the groups is predominantly Type A and Type B.

**TABLE 1.** *Comparison of HA porous vs. porous demographics of match pair groups*

|  | HA Porous | Porous |
| --- | --- | --- |
| Age | 55 ± 11 | 56.5 ± 11 |
| Sex | 18 Male<br>24 Female | 18 Male<br>24 Female |
| Bone Type | 11 A<br>29 B<br>2 C | 11 A<br>29 B<br>2 C |
| Diagnosis | 30 OAP<br>7 ON<br>2 OAT<br>3 DDH | 30 OAP<br>7 ON<br>2 OAT<br>3 DDH |

OAP = Osteoarthritis primary, ON = osteonecrosis, OAT=osteoarthritis posttraumatic, DDH = developmental dysplasia hip.

Clinical results were based on Harris hip scores (HHS). Patients were seen every three months for the first year and yearly thereafter. Radiographs were evaluated for fixation, bone remodeling, and osteolysis by a zonal interface analysis as developed by Gruen. A modified Engh scale for use in proximal ingrowth devices was used to grade radiographic fixation in each patient (Table 2).

**TABLE 2.** *Modified ENGH skeletal fixation score for femur*

| Fixation Grade |  | Radiolucency | |
| --- | --- | --- | --- |
|  |  | Porous<br>surface | Smooth surface |
| Bone ingrowth, stable | IA | None | None, one or two zones |
| Bone ingrowth, stable | IB | None | Three to five zones |
| Bone ingrowth, stable | IC | None | All six zones |
| Fibrous ingrowth, stable | II | Zone 7 | All six zones |
| Fibrous ingrowth, *unstable* | III | Zone 1&7 | Variable |

## RESULTS

The HHS for three-year follow-up are presented in Fig. 3. Clinical results

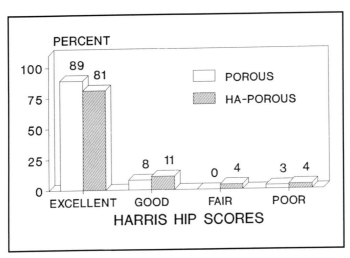

**FIG. 3.** Comparison of clinical results at three- year follow-up between HA porous vs. porous APR-I primary total hip replacements

revealed average HHS scores were not statistically different between the groups at all follow-up intervals (six months and yearly thereafter). At three-year follow-up, both groups had over 90% good or excellent results. When the pain scores were analyzed separately, there was no statistical difference in the pain scores between the two groups. Only one hip required revision surgery. This was in the HA porous group and was performed for osteolysis. Overall mechanical failure rate, defined as revision or radiographic type 3 fixation, was 2 in the porous group and 2 in the HA-porous group.

Figure 4 displays the femoral fixation scores for both groups. Bone fixation scores demonstrated similar results at six months, one year, and two years. At three years, the HA-porous group had overall higher fixation scores, but did not reach statistical significance. At three year follow-up, stable bony fixation (defined as radiographic IA, IB, or IC fixation) was achieved in 93% of the HA-porous stems and 84% of the porous stems.

One advantage found in this study was that the HA coating accelerated bone remodeling, characterized by proximal cancellous hypertrophy (Fig. 5). Table 3 compares the incidence of proximal bone remodeling detected on serial radiographic examinations. The HA porous group showed earlier evidence of proximal bone remodeling, and the percentage of femoral stems exhibiting cancellous hypertrophy was significantly greater at all follow-up intervals.

The HA coating did not alter the rate of osteolysis when comparing the two groups (Table 4). Because there was no circumferential coating proximally, wear debris was able to tract distally. The HA coating was not helpful in preventing distal osteolysis, but the rate was not increased with the HA coating.

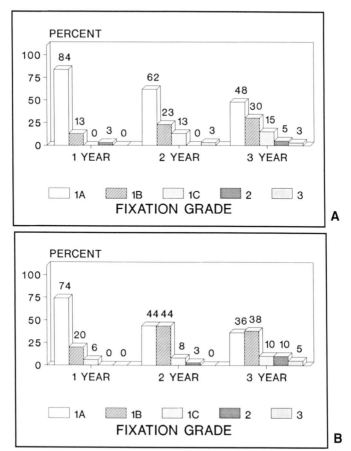

**FIG. 4.** Comparison of modified Engh bone fixation scores between HA porous group (**A**) and porous control group (**B**). Note inferior fixation scores in the porous group compared with the HA-porous group at the three-year follow-up interval.

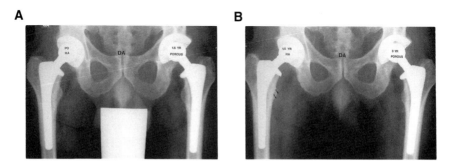

**FIG. 5.** Example of cancellous hypertrophy around proximal femoral stem in a patient who received an HA-porous APR-I THR on the right and a porous APR-I THR on the left. (**A**) Post-operative radiograph of HA-porous THR on right and 1.5-year follow-up of porous THR on left. (**B**) Radiograph of patient 1.5 years later. Compared to the left hip, the proximal cancellous bone around the right hip is more dense and is aligned along the lines of weight bearing stress (arrows). This in effect creates medial and lateral buttresses, called the *buttress sign.*

**TABLE 3.** *Proximal Bone Remodeling Cumulative Percent*

|  | Porous | HA-Porous |
|---|---|---|
| 6 Months | 3 | 15 |
| 1 Year | 9 | 44 |
| 2 Years | 41 | 68 |
| 3 Years | 47 | 79 |

**TABLE 4.** *Osteolysis Number of Cases*

|  | Proximal | Distal |
|---|---|---|
| Porous | 2 | 2 |
| HA Porous | 3 | 1 |

## FEMORAL STEM FIXATION USING THE
## APR-I TOTAL HIP SYSTEM:
## COMPARISON OF HA NONPOROUS VERSUS NON-POROUS

This study reviews the use of a press-fit version of the APR-I primary total hip in two forms: one with HA coating and one without coating. Implantation was performed under a multicenter clinical protocol that began in June 1987. Thirteen clinical investigators participated in the study.

The press-fit version of the APR-I primary hip (Intermedics Orthopaedics, Austin, TX) was manufactured in the same anatomic configuration as its porous-coated counterpart. On the femoral component of the press-fit version, grooves were placed on the proximal third of the body that added a three-dimensional geometric feature to increase the overall strength of the bony attachment. The acetabular component was of hemispherical shape and contained the same grooved features found on the femoral stem. The HA coating was placed circumferentially around the proximal third of the femoral stem and on the outside spherical surface of the acetabular component (Fig 6). The central dome of the acetabular component was not coated. The thickness of the HA coating was 50 μm, and was applied by a plasma -spray technique developed by Calcitek, Inc. (Carlsbad, CA). The HA coating was fully dense, containing more than 95% apatite after spraying. Static tensile and shear bond strengths after application were 7,051 psi and 5,920 psi, respectively.

Two hundred sixty-nine press-fit APR I total hip replacements were performed by the 13 participating surgeons and were followed for a minimum of 2-1/2 years (range 2-1/2 - 4 years). Two hundred twenty-one patients received press-fit APR-I components that were HA-coated, and 48 patients received the same press-fit components without HA. A random selection method was used to determine those patients whose implants were coated with HA and those whose implants were not coated. The ratio of HA-coated hips

**A**

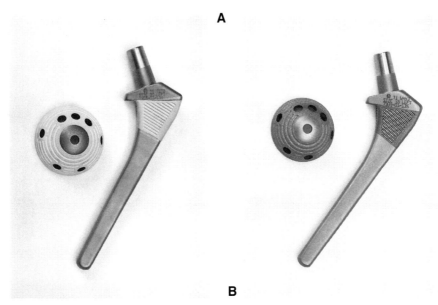

**B**

**FIG. 6.** Press-fit APR-I primary stem and acetabular cup with (**A**) and without (**B**) HA coating.

noncoated hips was 5:1 and was designed so that the patient numbers were sufficient for statistical evaluation. The demographics of the study group are presented in Table 5.

Clinical results were based on HHS scores. Patients were seen every three months for the first year and then yearly thereafter. Radiographs were evaluated for fixation and radiolucent lines by a zonal interface analysis as developed by Gruen.

**TABLE 5.** *Comparison of HA nonporous vs nonporous demographics*

| | |
|---|---|
| Average age | 58 (Range 22-88) |
| Sex | 138 Male |
| | 131 Female |
| Diagnosis | 239 Osteoarthritis |
| | 30 Inflammatory arthritis |

## RESULTS

Preoperative HHS scores were not statistically different between the two groups, with a mean of 40 points. Statistically significant improvements in the HHS of the HA group compared to the control group were evident by three months, and continued throughout the study. At 2-1/2 to 4 years of follow-up, the mean HHS was 91 points in the HA group, compared to 87 points in the control group ($p < 0.05$). When the pain scores were analyzed separately, the pain scores of the HA group were significantly better than the control group, with 91% of the HA patients having no significant pain. Two patients in the HA group (0.9%) and six patients in the control group (12%) were revised for mechanical failure. The reasons for revision are listed in Table 6.

Radiographic evaluation demonstrated significantly fewer radiolucent lines around the HA coating of the femoral component. Radiolucent lines were observed in 4% of the HA-coated stems in the coated zones (Gruen zones 1 and 7) vs. 40% in the noncoated stems ($p < 0.01$).

**TABLE 6.** *Description of revised components APR-I press-fit study*

| Component Description | Time to Revision | Reason for Revision |
| --- | --- | --- |
| 1. HA-coated stem | 2 weeks | Undersized stem |
| 2. HA-coated stem | 28 months | Loosening |
| 3. Uncoated stem | 7 months | Loosening |
| 4. Uncoated stem & shell | 14 months | Thigh & groin pain |
| 5. Uncoated stem | 17 months | Loosening |
| 6. Uncoated stem | 9 months | Loosening |
| 7. Uncoated stem & shell | 24 months | Osteolysis, loosening |
| 8. Uncoated stem & shell | 33 months | Loosening |

## DISCUSSION

In the multicenter press-fit study, the clinical and radiographic results demonstrated the beneficial effects of HA when applied to a nonporous stem. The patients with HA-coated stems had significantly better Harris Hip Scores and had less pain. Radiographic analysis of the HA-coated zones confirms that bone apposition without a radiolucent zone does occur in a consistent fashion. This study supports the concept that HA provides a new means of biologic fixation for uncemented THA that is superior to press-fit fixation alone. The FDA has declared that HA is safe and effective on press-fit nonporous surfaces subsequent to the IDE investigations done by Osteonics and Intermedics. However, the authors would caution the reader to be judicious in the use of HA on press-fit textured surfaces. Although the results obtained in the use of HA on press-fit stems has instilled enthusiasm for this coating, retrieval data from HA-coated stems creates some concern. Bloebaum has examined 14 retrieved HA-coated hip implants of various designs. He has unequivocally demonstrated the presence of HA particles embedded within the polyethylene inserts, and also within periprosthetic soft tissue surrounding the implants. Additionally, he has observed areas where HA has separated from the implant in nonporous-coated stems. The postulated loss of HA from these retrieved implants is either due to mechanical abrasion or resorption (2,3). Most likely, it is due to abrasion secondary to mechanical loosening, thereby explaining HA particles within periprosthetic soft tissue and polyethylene inserts. Although Bauer, in his retrieval study of HA-coated hip implants, proposes resorption of HA, Bloebaum, in review of over several thousand histologic sections, has

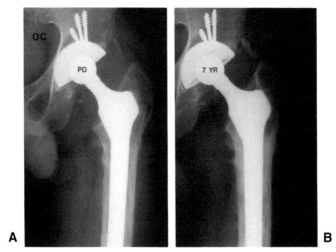

**FIG. 7.** Radiographs of a second total hip revision at seven- year follow-up in a patient who received a textured (nonporous) HA-coated APR collarless revision stem. (**A**) Immediate postoperative radiograph. (**B**) Radiograph at seven-year follow-up. Notice solid fixation about proximal femoral stem.

rarely identified osteoclastic resorption of HA (1,2,3).

It must be stressed that the bonding of HA to an implant surface represents a mechanical bond or "microscopic interlock," as opposed to a chemical bond. The question must then be raised whether this mechanical bond will ultimately fail and affect durability of fixation.

We do have HA-coated textured revision stems still well fixed without evidence of deterioration that were implanted in 1984 and 1985 (Fig. 7). This suggests satisfactory durability of HA fixation. Furthermore, we must emphasize that HA does not substitute for poor technique (i.e., a small, undersized prosthesis), nor can it be expected to be efficacious with a poorly designed prosthesis.

In the matched, controlled porous study, HA-coated stems performed well clinically, with 92% good or excellent results in Harris Hip Scores. Radiographic analysis determined stable bony fixation in 93% of femoral stems at three- year follow-up. HA coating did not alter the rate of osteolysis, but the HA coating did not increase the rate as some opponents had feared. A definite advantage of the HA coating was that bone remodeling was accelerated and enhanced. Whether this will translate into increased survival of the femoral stems is unclear, but we would predict increased survival because superior bone remodeling translates into superior long-term stability. Studies with the APR-II stem, which obtains a proximal cortical fit and eliminates patched porous coating, have achieved better results than the APR-I. HA-coated APR-II stems have a two- to three-year survival rate of 99.6% for both revision and osteolysis. The buttress bone remodeling pattern is seen by one year rather than two years with the APR-I. This confirms that stem geometry is the most critical factor for success. The accelerated bone remodeling with HA demonstrates that HA, as a surface finish, can enhance fixation and stability.

In conclusion, the authors believe that HA serves as an osteoconductive medium that provides more rapid attachment of the prosthesis to host bone, and that the bone remodeling around the prosthesis is enhanced and more complete. We believe that proximally loaded bone ingrowth stems should be the avenue taken for noncemented fixation, and that this technique will be afforded longevity equal to or better than that of cemented stems if the problem of osteolysis can be minimized. We view HA as an adjunctive agent for porous-coated surfaces that accelerates the incorporation and stabilization of the implant within the surrounding host bone. HA cannot substitute for poor surgical technique (i.e., an undersized prosthesis), and it cannot be expected to improve the results of a poorly designed implant. Based on our IDE studies we anticipate that the FDA will soon approve the use of HA on porous-coated surfaces. When approved, we intend to use HA routinely on our porous-coated APR-II implants.

## REFERENCES

1.  Bauer TW, Geesink RGT, Zimmerman R, et al. Hydroxyapatite-coated stems, histological analysis of components retrieved at autopsy. *Journal of Bone and Joint Surgery,* 1991,73A:1439.
2.  Bloebaum RD, Beeks D, Dorr LD, et al. Complications with Hydroxyapatite particulate separation in total hip replacement. *Clinical Orthopaedics.* (in press).
3.  Bloebaum RD, Dupont JA. Osteolysis from a press-fit Hydroxyapatite-coated implant: A case study. *Journal of Arthroplasty,* 1993, 8:195-202.
4.  Bobyn JD, Pilliar RM, Cameron HU. The optimal pore size for the fixation of porous-surfaced metal implants by the ingrowth of bone. *Clinical Orthopaedics,* 1980, 150:263.
5.  Callaghan JJ. Total hip arthroplasty, clinical perspective. *Clinical Orthopaedics,* 1992, 276:33.
6.  Cameron HU, Pilliar RM, Macnab I. The effect of movement on the bonding of porous metal to bone. *Journal of Biomedical Materials Research,* 1981, 15:301
7.  Chandler HP, Reineck FT, Wixon RL, et al. Total hip replacement in patients younger than 30 years old. A five year follow-up study. *Journal of Bone and Joint Surgery,* 1981, 63A:1462.
8.  Clemow AJT, Weinstein AM, Klawitter JJ, et al. Interface mechanics of porous titanium implants. *Journal of Biomedical Materials Research,* 1981, 15:73.
9.  Cohen JL, Bindelglass DF, Dorr LD. Total hip replacement using the APR-II system. *Techniques in Orthopaedics,* 1991, 6(3):40.
10. Collier JP, Mayor MB, Chae JC, et al. Macroscopic and microscopic evidence of prosthetic fixation with porous-coated materials. *Clinical Orthopaedics,* 1978, 235:173.
11. Cook SD, Barack RL, Thomas KA, et al. Quantitative analysis of tissue growth into human porous total hip components. *Journal of Arthroplasty,* 1988, 3:249.
12. Cook SD, Thomas KA, Dalton JE, et al. Enhanced bone ingrowth and fixation strength with hydroxyapatite-coated porous implants. *Seminars in Arthroplasty,* 1991, 2:268.
13. Cook SD, Thomas KA, Kay JF, et al. Hydroxyapatite-coated titanium for orthopedic implant applications. *Clinical Orthopaedics,* 1988, 232:225.
14. Cook SD, Walsh KA, Haddad RJ. Interface mechanics and bone growth into porous coated Co-Cr-Mo alloy implants. *Clinical Orthopaedics,* 1985, 193:271.
15. Denissen HW, deGroot K. Immediate dental root implants from synthetic dense calcium hydroxyapatite, *Journal of Prosthetic Dentistry,* 1979, 42:551.
16. Dorr LD. Clinical total hip replacement with hydroxyapatite from 1984 to 1991. *Seminars in Arthroplasty,* 1991, 2:289.
17. Dorr LD. *Personal communication.* September 1992.
18. Dorr LD, Luckett M, Conaty JP. Total hip arthroplasties in patients younger than 45 years. *Clinical Orthopaedics,* 1990, 260:215.
19. Dorr LD, Takei GK, Conaty JP. Total hip arthroplasties in patients less than forty-five years old. *Journal of Bone and Joint Surgery,* 1983, 65A:474.
20. Engh CA, Bobyn JD, Glassman AH. Porous coated hip replacment: The factors covering bone ingrowth, stress shielding, and clinical results. *Journal of Bone and Joint Surgery,* 1987, 69B:45.

21. Engh CA, Massin P. Cementless total hip arthroplasty using the anatomic medullary locking stem: results using a survivorship analysis. *Clinical Orthopaedics*, 1989, 249:141.
22. Freeman MAR, Tennant R. The scientific basis of cement versus cementless fixation. *Clinical Orthopaedics* , 1992, 276:19.
23. Galante JO, Jacobs J. Clinical performance of ingrowth surfaces. *Clinical Orthopaedics*, 1992, 276:41.
24. Geesink RGT, De Groot K, Klein CP. Chemical implant fixation using hydroxyapatite coating: the development of a human total hip prosthesis for chemical fixation to bone using hydroxyapatite coatings on titanium substrates. *Clinical Orthopaedics* , 1987, 225:147.
25. Haddad RJ, Cook SD, Thomas KA. Current concepts review: biological fixation of porous-coated implants. *Journal of Bone and Joint Surgery* , 1987, 69A:1459.
26. Halley DK, Wroblewski BM. Long-term results of low-friction arthroplasty in patients 30 years of age or younger. *Clinical Orthopaedics* , 1986, 211:43.
27. Harris WH, Maloney WJ, Barrack RJ, et al. Cement versus cementless for the femoral component. Modern cement wins. Presented at: *9th Combined Meeting of the Orthopaedic Associations of the English Speaking World.* Toronto, Canada. June 22, 1992.
28. Jarcho M. Biomaterial aspects of calcium phosphates. *Dental Clinics of North America* , 1986, 30:25.
29. Jarcho MJ, Kay F, Gumaer KI, et al. Tissue, cellular, and subcellular events at a bone-ceramic hydroxyapatite interface. *Journal of Bioengineering*, 1977, 1:79.
30. Joshi A, Porter M, Trail I. Total hip arthroplasty in patients of 40 years of age or younger: a survival analysis, clinical appraisal and radiologic study. Presented at: *9th Combined Meeting of the Orthopaedic Associations of the English Speaking World.* Toronto, Canada. June 24, 1992.
31. Kay JF. A new concept for noncement fixation of orthopaedic devices. *Techniques in Orthopaedics* , 1987, 2(1):1.
32. Kay JF, Manley MT, Stern LS, et al. The effect of hydroxyapatite coating on fixation of loaded metallic devices-a preliminary study.*Proceedings of the Annual Meeting of the European Society of Biomaterials,* Bologna, Italy, September 14-17, 1986.
33. Kirschenbaum IH. Basic principles of hydroxyapatite in joint replacement surgery. *Seminars in Arthroplasty* , 1991, 2:252.
34. Older J, Butorac R. Charnley low friction arthroplasty (LFA). A 17-21 year follow-up study. Presented at: *9th Combined Meeting of the Orthopaedic Associations of the English-Speaking World.* Toronto, Canada. June 22, 1922.
35. Thomas KA, Cook SD, Kay JF, et al. Attachment strength and histology of hydroxyapatite coated implants. *Biomaterial Medical Devices and Artificial Organs* 1986, 14:73.
36. Wroblewski PD, Siney PD, Raut VV, et al. Charnley low friction arthroplasty- 19-26 year results. *Poster Presentation at 9th Combined Meeting of the Orthopaedic Associations of the English Speaking World.* Toronto, Canada. June 21-26, 1992.

*Hydroxylapatite Coatings in Orthopaedic Surgery,*
edited by R. G. T. Geesink and M. T. Manley.
Raven Press, Ltd., New York, © 1993.

# A Comparison of Press-Fit, Cemented and Hydroxylapatite-Coated Femoral Components

## The Early Outcome as Judged by the Measurement of Migration

Gareth Scott, F.R.C.S., and
Michael A.R. Freeman, M.D., F.R.C.S.

The major problem concerning any total hip arthroplasty has been how to stabilize the prosthesis in the skeleton reliably and reproducibly. Various factors influence this aim: surgical factors, surgical approach; and operator skill; patient factors, bone anatomy and biology, and levels of activity; and implant factors, the biomechanical appropriateness of the materials and design. Aside from these considerations is the matter of fixation. Currently, four approaches to fixation are used: polymethylmethacrylate (PMMA) cement, uncemented press-fit (PF), porous coating, and latterly hydroxylapatite (HA) coating. Porous coating will not be considered further in this chapter.

## MATERIAL AND METHODS

At the Royal London Hospital we have been able to study the outcome of these three methods of fixation prospectively, both recording clinical outcome and by measured micromovement using a digitizer and standard radiographs. It is appropriate first to describe the implant, because it has unique features that the authors believe contribute to its stability.

Following from work with double cup arthroplasty the senior author developed a proximal femoral implant that preserved the femoral neck completely. The logic for conserving the femoral neck has been explained elsewhere (1).

Incorporated in the design and its method of introduction were features that enabled digitized measurements of distal migration to be made. These features were a straight lateral border to the intramedullary portion of the stem that lay within the greater trochanter and terminated as a point. The method of insertion used determined that the point described above lay in the same radiographic plane as the apex of the greater trochanter itself. The implant was made of TiA1V alloy and has been fully described elsewhere (2).

To maintain a clear radiographic view of the greater trochanter, myositis was inhibited by the routine use of indomethacin (3).

Regardless of the chosen method of fixation, the implant was introduced by the same operative technique. A modified anterolateral approach was used (4) and the femur prepared with milling tools, which resulted in a precise fit in the femur for the implant.

The distal portion of the stem was polished and tapered such that it did not contact the cortical bone distally but permitted the femoral diaphysis to flex around it, thereby reducing proximal stress shielding. This feature is of principal relevance in the uncemented forms.

The decision whether or not to cement the femoral component was based on the patients' age. Generally PMMA was used in those older than 60 years and uncemented stems were used in patients younger than 60 years.

The uncemented and cemented versions differed from each other in three respects. The cemented version possessed pits on the anterior and posterior surfaces of its neck where it rested within the femoral neck to enhance cement interlock with the component. The uncemented versions were provided with longitudinal ridges 1 mm high in the proximal part extending distally to the polished level. The purpose of the ridges was to cut into the proximal cancellous bone on insertion to enhance rotational stability. This requirement had been demonstrated in a cadaveric study (5). Finally, in the uncemented form, fine stipples 1 mm high were present on the anterior and posterior surfaces of the neck for bone ingrowth. Again, these stipples made the implant slightly oversized in rotation to the milled channel so that they cut into the bone on insertion. The placement of these stipples corresponds to the site of the pits on the cemented version.

In 1989, HA became available for use with the uncemented version. *In vivo* experimental work in a canine cancellous bone model at this hospital had demonstrated bone conduction to a depth of 3 mm in grooved TiA1V plates that had been coated with HA (6). These findings mirrored those reported from Denmark (7).

The proximal 3.5 cm of the femoral implant was plasma sprayed with HA to a thickness of 80–120 µm. Analysis of the coating has been undertaken by the Department of Applied Science (Division of Physics), Staffordshire Polytechnic, England. Purity was in excess of 98%, crystallinity greater than 75% and sheer strength 20–40 MPa.

Cemented components were introduced in a manner similar to the uncemented varieties, except that loose cancellous bone was curetted away before the bone trabecular spaces were opened by washing and brushing for increased cement interlock. A distal centralizing cement restrictor was used and then cement was introduced by gun. On introduction, by virtue of its shape, the prosthesis pressurized the PMMA provided the femoral neck was occluded by the operator's finger until the neck portion of the prosthesis engaged the bone.

Each patient was x-rayed immediately postoperatively and thereafter at six, 12, and 24 months. The radiographic requirements were for the thigh to be flat on the film cassette, the source-to-plate distance to be constant at 1 meter, the exposure to be centered on the palpable greater trochanter, and the patella to be pointed vertically (8). The film included the full length of the femoral component.

Measurements were made on each radiograph using an Orthographics Inc. digitizing table. Measurements were recorded and processed by a Dell computer with a dedicated program.

Prior to any measurements of migration, the coordinates of the femoral head size were entered to correct for magnification, and apparent prosthetic length was measured to ensure the suitability of the positioning. The digitizer could then be used to record distal prosthetic migration.

A vertical proximal line was extended from the straight lateral border of the prosthesis. From this line two perpendiculars were dropped: one passed through the tip of the prosthesis' lateral border and the other intersected the most proximal part of the greater trochanter at a tangent. The vertical distance between these two levels was recorded (8,9). These two points lay in the same radiographic plane. All measurements were made by a single observer not involved in the provision of clinical care to the patients.

The digitized measurements have been estimated as being accurate to 1 mm ($\pm$ 0.5 mm) (8). The technique is similar to the method of matched indicators for radiographic assessment, which has been validated against roentgen stereophotogrammetric analysis as accurate to $\pm$ 0.5 mm. (10).

Additionally, the radiographs were inspected for the emergence of radiolucent lines (RLL) as described by Gruen et al. (11). The nature of the cement restrictor engaging the stem in the PMMA group may well have reduced the apparent number of RLLs encountered in zone 4.

Clinical data were also recorded for the three groups. The patients were questioned regarding their maximum continuous walking times and their pain levels. A simple pain scale of 1 to 4 was applied: grade 1, no pain; grade 2, mild pain requiring no analgesia; Grade 3, moderate pain controlled by simple analgesia; grade 4, any pain more severe than grade 3. The patients were asked to grade pain at three different activity levels: walking, sitting at rest and lying at rest. The worst score was used for this analysis. Grades 1 and 2 were considered satisfactory in outcome and grades 3 and 4 unsatisfactory.

Because of the manner in which this prosthesis has been developed, three groups of patients receiving primary total hip replacement have become available for prospective study. The cemented group was created from patients receiving primary total hip replacements between the latter part of 1986 (when the current version of the cemented implant became available) and the end of 1989. The press-fit group consisted of patients receiving the uncemented version during the same period as the PMMA group. The HA group consisted of those patients from 1989 onwards who received the HA-coated version that superseded the PF in clinical practice. In each group, patients were included for analysis only if *all* the necessary data had been recorded in a prospective manner and the radiographs had been of sufficient quality for measurement. No case had been withdrawn because of revision surgery up to the time of the report. It is accepted that the groups are not randomized, as PMMA had been considered inappropriate in the younger patients. The two uncemented varieties (PF and HA) have been used in the same population pool, and this is reflected in the demographic data (see Tables 1 and 2). The results presented here, therefore, consist of clinical parameters and measured micromovement data at two years for three different methods of fixation.

The validity of early reporting (i.e., at two years) is acceptable only because micromovement results are presented, it having been shown that early micromovement reflects the late clinical outcome (14).

## RESULTS

The walking abilities of each group are shown in Table 3. Higher levels of activity were present in both uncemented groups.

The analgesic requirements of each group are shown in Table 4.

Radiolucent lines (RLLs) were found in at least one zone in 23 (49%) of PMMA hips, 24 (58%) of PF hips-and 15 (50%) of HA hips. RLLs represented as percentages of the proportion of each stem type that had any RLL are shown in Figs. 1 A- C. Because of the probable under-recording of zone 4 RLLs in the PMMA group, no firm conclusion can be drawn from the zone pattern for PMMA.

RLLs were absent proximally around the stem in the HA group (Fig. 1C): Presumably, the osteoconductive properties of HA led to complete bone apposition against the implant proximally. In this context we include a

**TABLE 1.** *Age and sex distribution for the three stem types*

|  | PMMA | PF | HA |
|---|---|---|---|
| Number | 47 | 41 | 30 |
| Mean age (yrs) | 70 (59-83) | 50.5 (27-72) | 50 (27-63) |
| M:F | 15:32 | 12:29 | 18:12 |

**TABLE 2.** *Diagnostic distribution for the three stem types.*

|  | Fixation Type | | |
|---|---|---|---|
| Diagnosis | PMMA | PF | HA |
| OA | 44 | 35 | 28 |
| RA | 1 | 4 | 1 |
| Other | 2 | 1 | 1 |

**TABLE 3.** *Percentage of patients able to walk uninterruptedly for 30 or more minutes*

| PMMA | PF | HA |
|---|---|---|
| 68% | 78% | 80% |
| (37/47) | (32/41) | (24/30) |

**TABLE 4.** *Percentage of patients requiring no analgesia*

| PMMA | PF | HA |
|---|---|---|
| 89% | 95% | 93% |
| (42/47) | (39/41) | (28/30) |

photographic example of an HA coated stem that was retrieved (not from our series of patients) at eight weeks showing bone densely adherent to the HA-coating of the implant (Figs. 2A-C). We believe that the distal RLLs in this group represent flexing of the diaphysis around the implant.

The assessment of each method of fixation was not based primarily on the clinical results, but rather on the measured micromovements. In this respect the greatest stability was seen in the HA-coated stem. These results are presented in Table 5. The ranking order of stability by micromovement mirrored that of the clinical results.

Statistical analysis of the migration was undertaken using the paired *t*-test with Satterthwaite's approximation for unequal variance. The results are presented in Table 6.

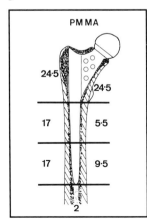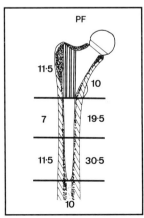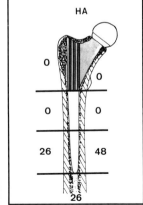

**FIG. 1. A-C.** The distribution of RLLs represented as percentages of that proportion of each stem type which demonstrated any RLL.

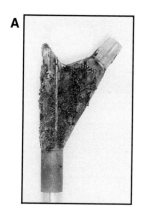
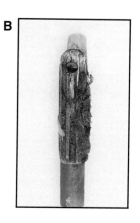
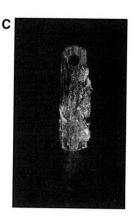

**FIG. 2. A-C.** Densely adherent bone in the proximity of the HA coating. **(A)** View of the anterior surface of the implant. **(B)** Lateral view of the same implant. **(C)** Lateral view of same implant under ultraviolet lighting to demonstrate the bone as white.

**TABLE 5.** *Mean migration of the three types of fixation at 2 years*

|  | PMMA | PF | HA |
|---|---|---|---|
| Mean mm | 0.78 | 1.7 | 0.3 |
| Range mm | -0.5 to +3.6 | -0.6 to +10.4 | -0.6 to +1.8 |
| SD | 0.86 | 1.91 | 0.61 |

**TABLE 6.** *Levels of significance for comparison of stability afforded by the different methods of fixation*

| PMMA - PF | $p = 0.0063$ |
|---|---|
| HA - PMMA | $p = 0.0055$ |
| HA - PF | $p = 0.0001$ |

## DISCUSSION

It can be seen from these results (Table 4) that the most stable fixation was achieved with HA, the least stable with a press-fit and PMMA intermediate between the two. This finding is particularly striking when one considers that the mean age for the HA group was 20 years younger than that for PMMA. This was reflected in an increased walking duration for the HA when compared to the PMMA group.

A question remains with regard to the outcome of HA. It has been reported that HA is removed by osteoclasts around the implant (13). The problem then arises: If all the HA is resorbed, will a "perfect" press-fit remain or will the loss of HA lead to rapid loosening? Hopefully, if the HA-coated implant had been textured to enable trabecular interlock by bone ingrowth (the HA acting as a "drug" to induce bone rather than as an adhesive on a smooth surface), then long-term stable fixation may continue after the HA is lost. Furthermore, assuming comparable loosening rates it would seem preferable to revise a young person's hip in the absence of cement than undertake a revision procedure in its presence.

Finally, the question arises as to whether the chosen age limit for the use of HA in this study is appropriate in clinical practice when better stability appears to be achieved with its use than either with PMMA or with press-fit. Experimental data have shown that an HA coating produces an enhanced trabecular bone anchorage even in osteopenic bone (14). It might be appropriate, therefore, to extend the use of HA to a higher upper age limit in view of the increasing life expectancy and greater activity of today's older people.

## REFERENCES

1. Freeman M A R. Why resect the neck? *Journal of Bone and Joint Surgery* 1986 68B:346.
2. Albrektsson B E J, Freeman M A R, Carlsson L V, et al. Retention of the femoral neck: a method to enhance prosthetic fixation. *Journal of Orthopaedic Surgical Techniques*, 1987, 3(2): 99.
3. Levack B, Freeman M A R. The value of indomethacin in the prophylaxis of myositis ossificans after hip replacement surgery. *Communication to the Royal Society of Medicine.* London, February 1986.
4. Stephenson P K and Freeman M A R. Exposure of the hip using a modified anterolateral approach. *Journal of Arthroplasty* 1991, 6(2): 137.
5. Nunn D, Freeman M A R, Tanner K E, Bonfield W. The torsional stability of a femoral total hip replacement component in response to an anteriorly applied load. *Journal of Bone and Joint Surgery* 1989, 71B: 452.
6. Stephenson P K, Freeman, M A R, Revell P A, et al. The effect of hydroxylapatite coating on ingrowth of bone into cavities in an implant. *Journal of Arthroplasty* 1991, 6(1): 51.
7. Søballe K, Hansen E S, Brockstedt-Rasmussen H, et al. Hydroxyapatite coating enhances fixation of porous coated implants. *Acta Orthopaedica Scandinavica* 1990, 61(4): 229.
8. Braud P, Freeman M A R. The effect of retention of the femoral neck and of cement upon the stability of a proximal femoral prosthesis. *Journal of Arthroplasty* 1990, 5:55.
9. Scott G, Kroon P O, Freeman M A R. Immediate measurements of proximal femoral stability after addition of an hydroxylapatite coating. *Proceedings of Micromovement in Orthopaedics,* Oxford Orthopaedic Engineering Centre, April, 1992.
10. Carlsson L V, Albrektsson B E J, Freeman M A R, et al. A new radiographic method for detection of tibial migration in total knee arthroplasty. *Journal of Arthroplasty.* In Press.
11. Gruen T A, McNeill G M, Amstutz H E. Models of failure of cemented stem-type femoral components. *Clinical Orthopaedics,* 1979, 141:17.
12. Grewal R, Rimmer M G, Freeman M A R. Early migration of prostheses related to long-term survivorship. *Journal of Bone and Joint Surgery* 1992, 74-B: 239.
13. Bauer T W, Geesink R G T, Zimmerman R, McMahon J T. Hydroxyapatite-coated femoral stems. *Journal of Bone and Joint Surgery* 1991, 73-A: 1439.
14. Søballe K, Hansen E S, Brockstedt-Rasmussen H, et al. Fixation of titanium and hydroxylapatite coated implants in osteopenia. *Journal of Arthroplasty* 1991, 6(4): 307.

Hydroxylapatite Coatings in Orthopaedic Surgery,
edited by R. G. T. Geesink and M. T. Manley.
Raven Press, Ltd., New York, © 1993.

# Revision Arthroplasty with Hydroxylapatite-Coated Implants

Rudolph G.T. Geesink, M.D., Ph.D.

The excellent clinical results of implant fixation using hydroxylapatite (HA) coatings have been discussed in previous chapters. They are based on the good osteoconductive properties of HA, resulting in well-fixed implants. Application in revision surgery might be even more challenging. Often there are significant bone deficiencies, and under these circumstances HA can be pushed to its limits of clinical application.

## MATERIALS AND METHODS

Clinical and radiologic results of 50 consecutive revision cases performed between 1987 and 1989 will be discussed. This was a relatively young group of patients, with an average age of 55 years. The male:female ratio was 1:1, which is higher in comparison with the primary group (1:1.7). Of the cases, 29 were first-time revisions and 21 were multirevisions, ranging between second- and fifth-time revision. Revision was performed for both loose cemented hips and loose cementless hips of various types, including some revisions of well-fixed implants for nonloosening-related problems. The numbers and implants involved are listed in Table I. Ten cases were infected arthroplasties for which a two-stage exchange procedure was performed using gentamicin beads after implant removal. Reimplantation was usually done two weeks later.

Current follow-up was an average of four years and up to five years for the oldest patients. All patients were in a prospective follow-up protocol with follow-up visits at three, six, and 12 months and yearly thereafter. No patient was lost to follow-up. One patient died of non-hip-related causes. His hip was available for histologic analysis and will be discussed below.

To evaluate the stability of implants more objectively, x-rays were digitized, comparing early postoperative and two-year x-rays for subsidence.

Standard treatment after revision surgery included intravenous antibiotic prophylaxis for 24 hrs, usually with cephalosporin, anticoagulation with

TABLE 1. *Specification of revision implants*

| Number and type of revision | Total no. | Multirevision | Infected |
|---|---|---|---|
| Cemented THR | | | |
| Muller curved/straight | 24 | 13 | 5 |
| Others | 3 | 1 | |
| | | | |
| Cementless THR | | | |
| Mittelmaier | 4 | 1 | |
| Thomas | 5 | 3 | 3 |
| Judet | 2 | | |
| CLS | 6 | 2 | 1 |
| Others | 2 | | 1 |
| | | | |
| Double cups | 4 | 1 | |
| | | | |
| Total numbers | 50 | 21 | 10 |

TABLE 2. Average Omnifit component size in hip revision arthroplasty

| | Primary THR | First revision | Multirevision |
|---|---|---|---|
| Acetabular cup | 52 | 56 | 61 |
| Femoral stem | 8.4 | 9.3 | 10.5 |

dicumarin for three months, and ectopic bone prophylaxis with indomethacin (25mg daily) for two weeks. The usual operative approach was posterolateral, although some of the more difficult cases required a transtrochanteric or transfemoral approach. Patients were mobilized after surgery as early as surgical stability permitted. In contrast to primary surgery, where immediate full weight-bearing is the rule, in revision surgery protected weight-bearing is recommended for at least six weeks and, after difficult reconstructions, up to three months.

In virtually all cases, the standard Osteonics Omnifit-HA prosthesis was used. Although this stem is not specifically designed for revision surgery, it can still be used regularly because it is longer than most of the older cemented or cementless stems. Second, the HA coating is long enough to permit direct bone contact in the metaphyseal part of the femur, just distal to the usual area of proximal bone loss. One case necessitated the manufacturing of a custom long stem with longer HA coating. Even without the use of custom implants, we should to be aware of the occasional need for very large components, i.e. acetabular size of 72 mm or even larger, as well as large stem sizes. Average component size is listed in Table 2 for comparison with the author's primary group.

If bone deficiencies are present in the more distal stem area, bone grafting is necessary with protected weight-bearing for several months. The author believes that even in the case of proximal bone loss, the aim should be to reconstitute as good proximal bone stock as possible. The application of bone grafts with HA hips is probably different from other cementless components. The theory is to let the smaller defects fill in spontaneously, which means gaps of up to 2 mm. These are probably more easily filled in by direct osteoconduction through HA (1, 2, 3), in comparison with the process of transformation and revascularization of dead bone auto- or allograft. Bone deficiencies larger than 2 mm are grafted if they are located in important weight-bearing areas. In the author's series, 10% of cases had bone grafting on the femoral side, in comparison with 35% on the acetabular side. If available, autologous bone from the iliac crest is preferred, otherwise bone bank allograft is used.

## RESULTS

Results are best detailed by some clinical examples, which will illustrate how HA can influence clinical judgment.

### Case #1

The very first revision case was a 72-year-old woman who needed removal of a well-fixed cemented stem with excessive amount of bone cement, high varus position with excessive leg length, periarticular calcification, and sciatic nerve impairment (Fig. 1). Attempts at removal of bone cement resulted in splitting and fracturing of the femur, creating seven or eight pieces of femoral bone. Cementing these pieces together would have impaired fracture healing, so all fragments were adapted around an HA-coated stem with only marginal initial stability. Fracture healing could be expected but not surgical stability of the implant, and the plan was to change the stem for a bigger one after three months or so. Interestingly, however, the fractures healed and the implant became stabilized, showing nice osseointegration with good bone fixation. The patient was pain-free very early, with only a limp caused by a trochanteric nonunion. This was repaired after two years. The last x-ray at five years shows a good implant/bone interface with healthy bone condensation against the implant coating and no radiolucent line formation.

### Case #2

A similar case concerned revision of a loose, recurrently dislocating cementless cup in a 59-year-old woman. Placing a smaller cup slightly eccentric in the existing larger cup area made cup revision easy. The removal of a rigidly fixed distal part of the cementless stem (Judet type) with severe metallosis necessitated complete longitudinal splitting of the femoral shaft (Fig. 2). In this

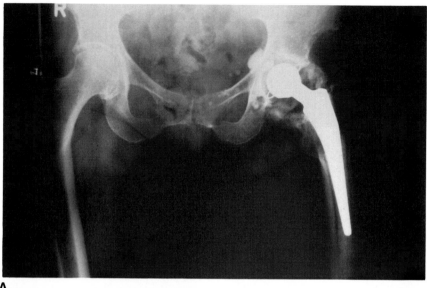

**FIG. 1.** Femoral fracture healing and stem osseointegration. **A**: preoperative condition; **B**: two months postoperative; **C**: five years postoperative after repair of trochanteric nonunion. Note good quality bone in contact with proximal medial side of femoral component.

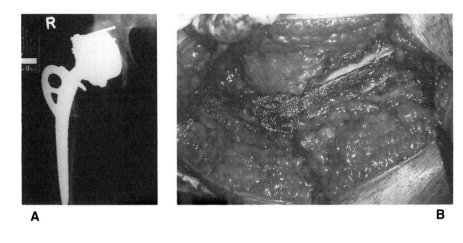

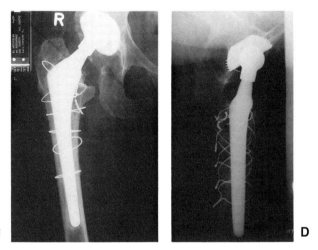

**FIG. 2.** Transfemoral approach for removal of well-ingrown porous-coated stem. **A**: preoperative condition; **B**: operative view with transfemoral approach to stem; **C**: 5-year postoperative; **D**: lateral view of same.

case, internal fixation was also done with multiple cerclage wires, without bone grafting, showing good clinical and radiologic results. There were several more cases like this, and the principles of a transfemoral approach always proved reliable.

### Case #3

This case was not specifically difficult, but it underscores the bone-reconstituting properties of HA based on its osteoconductivity. It was a case of a loose Mittelmaier stem and cup in a 52-year-old man (Fig. 3). Of interest is the fact that the lucent lines of the previous loose stem are still visible on the early postoperative x-ray. Over the HA-coated part of the stem, these lines gradually disappear and fade away in newly formed bone condensation around the proximal stem. The ultimate implant/bone interface, now at five years, shows

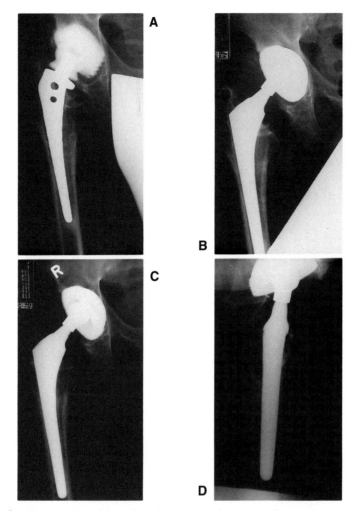

**FIG. 3.** Spontaneous osseointegration after previous loosening of cementless components. **A**: preoperative condition; **B**: three weeks postoperative; note still present lines around proximal interface; **C**: five years postoperative with good bone condensation around proximal interface and disappearance of lucent lines; **D**: lateral view of same.

excellent bone quality and stability, with complete absence of lucent lines around the coating area of the stem.

### Case #4

A more difficult case was this multirevision, infected after cemented hip replacement, in a 62-year-old woman (Fig. 4). There was extensive bone loss, with splitting and fracturing of the femur. In addition, the cup had to be completely reconstructed. After reconstructing both stem and cup with grafting, the patient recovered very satisfactorily. After two years there is an almost primary-case bone stock, with full regeneration of bone in the proximal femur and healing of bone deficiencies. Only the fixation wires of the bone grafts are reminiscent of the previous problems. Bone stock is improving yearly.

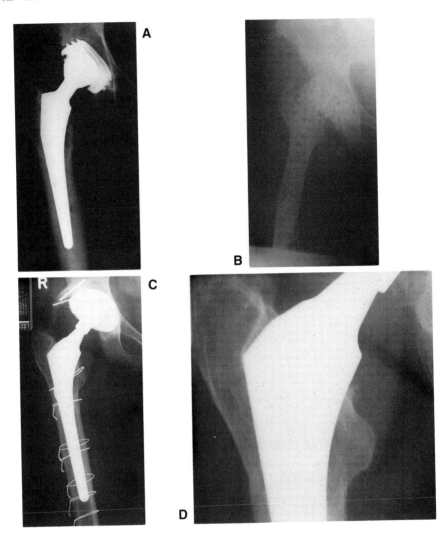

**FIG 4.** Infected multirevision. **(A)**: preoperative condition with infectious loosening of cemented femoral stem and cementless acetabular component; **(B)**: postoperative condition after removal of components and implantation of gentamycin beads; note fractures and bone loss. **(C)**: two years postoperative condition with good restoration of bone stock; **(D)**: detail of femoral HA/bone interface at four years after removal of wires.

## COMPLICATIONS

Surgical complications were somewhat more frequent in revision surgery, especially dislocation and intraoperative cracks. No complications were related to the method of implant fixation using HA coatings. One patient died from a non-hip-related cause six months after surgery. This case will be detailed below. Complications are listed in Table 3 and reoperations in Table 4.

TABLE 3. *Complications in revision arthroplasty (50 cases)*

| | |
|---|---|
| Dislocation | 5 |
| Deep joint infection | – |
| Recurrent infection | 3 |
| Cracks or fractures | 5 |
| Died of unrelated cause | 1 |

TABLE 4. *Reoperations in revision arthroplasty (50 cases)*

| | |
|---|---|
| Implant removal sepsis | 2 |
| Joint debridement sepsis | 1 |
| Mechanical loosening | 1 |
| Trochanteric nonunion | 1 |
| Removal osteosynthesis | 2 |

## REOPERATIONS

There was one case with secondary loosening of the femoral component. The history follows.

### Case #5

A 62-year-old woman underwent fourth time revision arthroplasty for loosening of a cemented femoral component. The femoral cortical wall was not unlike an eggshell in mechanical strength and there were multiple perforations of the shaft on the lateral side (Fig. 5). On revision arthroplasty, bony defects were autografted on the lateral side, but not on the medial side. The patient received an HA-coated femoral stem and cup and early postoperative recovery was uneventful. There was apparent bone regeneration and the grafted areas improved in appearance. Two-and-one-half years postoperatively the hip became symptomatic after the patient fell. The hip was painful, and x-rays showed 1cm subsidence of the stem. Because symptoms persisted, reoperation was performed and the femoral component was found to be loose. Still, overall bone quality was already better in comparison with the previous revision. The next larger size of HA stem was implanted, in combination with more extensive bone grafting of slits and spaces around the stem. Follow-up at one year is satisfactory and the patient is pain-free.

More specifically, recurrent infection was the single most important cause of failure in this series. Of ten previously infected cases, three failed by recurrent, early deep wound sepsis. In two cases, implants were removed after two and three weeks, leaving a Girdlestone resection condition. In one more case the implant was saved two weeks after surgery by early debridement,

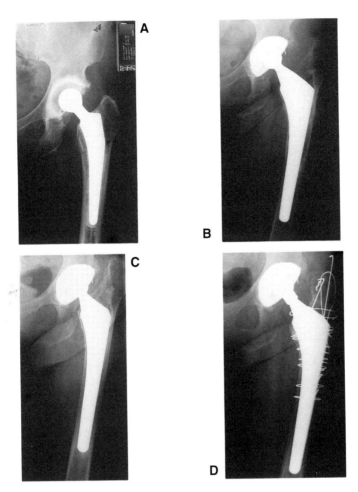

**FIG 5.** Mechanical failure of HA-coated revision for cemented multirevision. **(A)**: preoperative condition; note very thin bone loss and big cement mass; **(B:)** two years after third revision, stable position of HA-coated stem; **(C)**: two years postoperative with subsidence of stem; **(D)**: one-year after fourth femoral revision, new HA-coated femoral stem.

temporary implantation of gentamicin beads, and antibiotic suppression for six months. The patient is now free of complaints four years after surgery (Fig. 6). ESR, x-rays and bone scans are all normal.

Ectopic bone formation was recorded using the Brooker classification. There were only grades one and two, but no cases with clinically significant impairment of function by ectopic bone. Indomethacin prophylaxis was used for two weeks and appears to be an effective regimen, without adverse effects on bone ingrowth.

## CLINICAL RESULTS

Although the postoperative course after revision arthroplasty is usually more prolonged, the ultimate clinical results are very encouraging. Harris Hip

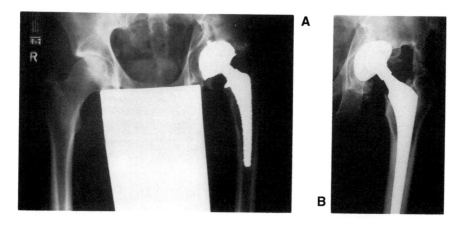

**FIG 6.** Revision of infected cementless components. **(A)**: preoperative condition; **(B)**: five years postoperative condition; note good overall bone quality of stem and lack of osteolytic reactions after early implant-retaining treatment for postoperative infected hematoma.

Score ratings (HHS) are listed in Table 5.

Two years after surgery the average HHS is 91 and continues to show improvement. At some of the shorter follow-up intervals, first-time revisions appear to do somewhat better overall. However, there is little difference in results between first-time and multirevisions. After two years the HHS for

**TABLE 5.** *Harris Hip Scores in revision arthroplasty (50 cases)*

| | Pre-op. | 3 m | 6 m | 1 yr | 2 yr | 3 yr | 4 yr | 5 yr |
|---|---|---|---|---|---|---|---|---|
| | 32 | 81 | 85 | 86 | 91 | 94 | 96 | 96 |

multirevisions is 89, indicating a good clinical result. Points are lost in these cases, not by pain, but by residual limp or impairment of range of motion.

PMA ratings, listed in Table 6, show similar results. Most patients are completely pain-free, including early "midthigh" pain. Average pain rating is 5.7 from two years onward. Some patients have some residual limp, causing a lower but still acceptable walking rate (5.5). Similarly, function scores are

**TABLE 6.** *PMA classification of revision arthroplasty (average)*

| Follow-up | 3 m | 6 m | 1 yr | 2 yr | 3 yr | 4 yr | 5 yr |
|---|---|---|---|---|---|---|---|
| Pain | 5.3 | 5.6 | 5.6 | 5.6 | 5.7 | 5.7 | 5.7 |
| Motion | 4.2 | 4.6 | 5.0 | 5.2 | 5.3 | 5.5 | 5.5 |
| Ability to walk | 4.8 | 4.9 | 5.2 | 5.2 | 5.4 | 5.5 | 5.6 |
| PMA sum | 14.3 | 15.1 | 15.8 | 16.0 | 16.4 | 16.7 | 16.8 |

somewhat less than optimal (5.6) because some cases exhibited restrictions in range of motion. Overall, patients say that there is a major improvement over their preoperative condition.

## RADIOLOGIC RESULTS

Measurements of radiologically detectable migration of clinically satisfactory cases (thus excluding the case with mechanical loosening) show some scatter around the zero line, but the average subsidence is only 0.8 mm, signifying zero significance in a statistical *t*-test comparison. This means that HA-coated stems are stable and do not migrate because they are well-fixed to the bone.

Radiologic signs of bone ongrowth are visible on femoral stems from the third month on, analogous to primary stems. These "spotwelds," or better "weld areas," are somewhat more irregular in shape in comparison with primary arthroplasties, but ultimately almost the entire proximal HA-coated part of the stem becomes osseointegrated (Fig 7). Fine lucent lines are regularly found around the distal noncoated part of the stem. These are the result of some micromotion between the more rigid metal of the titanium stem versus the more elastic femoral bone. No clinical signs are associated with this phenomenon, which also occurs in primary arthroplasty and is extensively described in that section.

In general, the process of bone ongrowth is very similar to that described for primary arthroplasty. Only the speed of bone formation, as measured by areas of bone condensation, is somewhat lower during the first two years. At two years and later, many revision arthroplasties have recovered almost primary hip bone stock. Engh's radiologic scores for implants are listed in Table 7. At the two-year interval all femoral stems have confirmed bone ongrowth.

On the acetabular side, the situation is less clear. Many cups do indeed show clear signs of bone condensation. There were, however, several cups with extensive bone allografts. Some of these were also fixed with screws or other devices. Many of them did not show clear signs of bony fixation, although the great majority remained in a stable position. Two cups with massive allograft did show changes in position within six months after surgery ("settling"), after which these cups were able to retain their position. Both patients are free of complaints and are able to put full weight on their legs without problems.

## HUMAN HISTOLOGY

The ultimate test for HA is how it functions in the body. One stem from a patient dying of a non-hip-related cause was available for histologic analysis, six months after revision surgery. Clinical performance had been very satisfying despite prolonged use of immunosuppressive drugs (cyclosporin and corticosteroids). The explant x-ray confirms the good osseointegration.

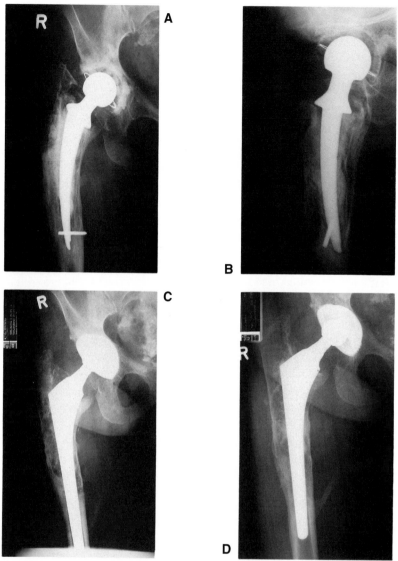

**FIG. 7.** Restoration of bone stock after revision of infectious cemented implant. **(A)**: preoperative condition, extensive bone loss and perforation of lateral wall; **(B)**: lateral view of same; **(C)**: three months after revision and bone grafting; **(D)**: four years postoperative, stable position and improvement in bone quality.

**TABLE 7.** *Average Engh's radiologic score in revision arthroplasty*

| Follow-up | 3 m | 6 m | 1 yr | 2 yr | 3 yr | 4 yr | 5 yr |
|---|---|---|---|---|---|---|---|
| Fixation score | 5.1 | 8.0 | 8.7 | 9.6 | 10.0 | 10.0 | 10.0 |
| Stability score | 8.6 | 7.9 | 5.5 | 3.7 | 4.9 | 8.3 | 8.3 |
| Total score | 13.7 | 15.9 | 14.2 | 13.3 | 14.9 | 18.3 | 18.3 |

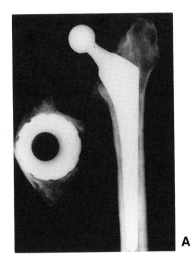

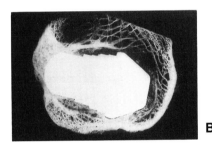

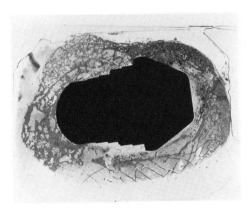

**FIG. 8.** Human histology of HA-coated retrieval six months after revisional arthroplasty. **(A)**: explant radiograph; **(B)**: microradiograph showing extensive new bone formation between previous demarcation line and femoral component surface; **(C)**: histology showing good new bone formation and extensive bone contact between HA-coated implant and femoral bone.

Radiologic cross-sections show that bone has regenerated from the old de-marcation line (of the previous loose stem) towards the complete HA–implant surface (Fig. 8). There is no fibrous tissue interposition and the HA coating is intact. The majority of the stem surface is surrounded by healthy bone, proving that osseointegration takes place within the first months after surgery. This case is discussed more in detail in the chapter on human retrieval analysis by Dr. Bauer, as well as in other literature (4).

## DISCUSSION

It is clear from both clinical and radiologic data, that HA-coated total hip replacement is a very satisfying procedure in revision arthroplasty. It meets the patient's need for pain relief early after surgery as well as the surgeon's desire to recover good bone stock. Although it is understandable that the clinical results are somewhat inferior to those of primary surgery, the absolute level of performance of HA-coated hips in revision arthroplasty is astonishing. At two years, the percentage of clinically significant pain problems is 6%.

Two years after surgery the average HHS is 91, and continues to improve slowly. At some of the shorter follow-up intervals, first -time revisions appear to do somewhat better. However, there is not much difference in overall results between first-time and multirevisions. Multirevision cases take much more time for ultimate recovery, but here , in particular, we can see that restoration of bone stock facilitates restoration of musculature. After two years the HHS for multirevisions is 89, indicating a good clinical result. Points are lost in these cases not by pain but by residual limp or impairment of range of motion.

In the entire group, limp is 12% more frequent at the two-year interval in comparison with primary arthroplasties, and range of motion is usually some-what more limited. The majority of patients, however, are able to flex their hips past 90 degrees, which is acceptable for most activities of daily living. These problems are caused by soft-tissue damage and are more dependent on the number and kind of previous surgeries. With time, strength and motion gradually increase to very satisfactory levels. Because pain is no longer experienced, patient satisfaction with the procedure is high. Because patients are able to ambulate freely and put maximal weight on their legs, muscle quality is much improved, and this also facilitates restoration of bone stock. Many patients are aware of this process and favor the strength provided by their HA-coated hips over their previous implants even when still functional.

To understand why so many hips perform properly even under difficult conditions, we must examine the x-rays. Bone regeneration, even without extensive bone grafting, is already clear on many x-rays at the two-year follow-up. In addition, Engh's radiologic scores point to very reliable bony ongrowth fixation of implants. At the two-year interval all femoral stems have confirmed bony ongrowth. There are no cases with radiologic loosening of cup or stem at five years. There were, however, two acetabular cups with early "settling" and breakage of the bone-graft fixation screws. The position of these components remained stable at later follow-up, although clear signs of bony fixation were not observed in these cases. Still, the involved patients were symptom-free. Longer follow-up is needed to further elucidate these cases. We must realize that in revision surgery bone loss sometimes can be so extreme that there are no ideal solutions. The best we can do is try to reconstruct the bony architecture and fix the implants as well as possible. If necessary, additional surgery could be performed at a later stage, to further reconstruct the hip.

Most current problems with mechanical loosening can be solved. Infectious loosening will remain a problem if we are unable to treat the concurrent infection effectively. Two failures in this series were caused by recurrent sepsis in infected loose arthroplasties. Although patients were ultimately satisfied with a Girdlestone resection condition, this clearly is not an ideal situation. Still, even under these adverse conditions the use of HA-coated implants has greatly extended the possibilities for reconstruction of difficult hips.

Current results using HA-coated devices in revision arthroplasty, in conjunction with bone grafting where appropriate, compare favorably with results from the literature on the same topic (5–12). Average HHS for HA-coated devices are higher and the incidence of mechanical loosening is lower.

## CONCLUSION

Although only 50 cases up to five years, this series proves the great potential of HA coatings, especially in difficult circumstances. In general, the experience with HA-coated implants in revision surgery is still limited. The clinical results are very satisfying, however, and the radiologically visible restoration of bone stock offers a good perspective for future implant performance and endurance. Clinical, radiologic, and histologic evidence all point to the excellent osseointegration properties of HA, even under clinically adverse conditions of revision arthroplasty.

## REFERENCES

1. Geesink RGT, Groot K de, Klein CPAT. Chemical implant fixation using hydroxylapatite coatings. *Clinical Orthopaedics* 1987; 225:147-70.
2. Stephenson PK, Freeman MAR, Revell PA, et al. The effect of hydroxyapatite coating on ingrowth of bone into cavities in an implant. *Journal of Arthroplasty* 1991; 66:51-8.
3. Søballe K, Hansen ES, Brockstedt-Rasmussen H, et al. Gap healing enhanced by hydroxyapatite coatings in dogs. *Clinical Orthopaedics* 1991;272:300-07.
4. Bauer TW, Geesink RGT, Zimmerman R, McMahon JT. Hydroxylapatite-coated hip stems: histologic analysis of autopsy retrievals. *Journal of Bone and Joint Surgery* 1991;73A:1439-52.
5. Goodman SB, Schurman DJ. Outcome of infected total hip arthroplasty: *Journal of Arthroplasty* 1988;3:97-102.
6. Harris WH, Krushell RJ, Galante JO. Results of cementless revisions of total hip arthroplasties using the Harris-Galante prosthesis. *Clinical Orthopaedics* 1988;235:120-6.
7. Hedley AK, Gruen TA, Ruoff DP. Revision of failed total hip arthroplasties with uncemented porous-coated anatomic components. *Clinical Orthopaedics* 1988;235:75-90.
8. Kavanagh BF, Fitzgerald Jr, Robert H. Multiple revisions for failed total hip arthroplasty not associated with infection. *Journal of Bone and Joint Surgery* 1987;69A:1144-9.

9.  Marti RK, Schuller HM, Besselaar PP, et al. Results of revision hip arthroplasty with cement: a five to fourteen-year follow-up study. *Journal of Bone and Joint Surgery* 1990;72A: 346-54.
10. Retpen JB, Varmarken JE, Rock ND, Jensen S. Unsatisfactory results after repeated revision of hip arthroplasty. *Acta Orthopaedica Scandinavica* 1992;63:120-7.
11. Rubash HE, Harris WH. Revision of nonseptic, loose, cemented femoral components using modern cementing techniques. *Journal of Arthroplasty* 1989;3:241-8.
12. Stromberg CN, Herberts P, Palmertz B. Cemented revision hip arthroplasty. *Acta Orthopaedica Scandinavica* 1992;62:111-19.

*Hydroxylapatite Coatings in Orthopaedic Surgery,*
edited by R. G. T. Geesink and M. T. Manley.
Raven Press, Ltd., New York, © 1993.

# Hydroxylapatite Coating of Custom Cementless Femoral Components

William L. Bargar, M.D., and Jeffery K. Taylor, M.D.

We have been designing and implanting custom cementless femoral stems since 1985. Our rationale was simple. Because of the extremely wide variation of the morphology of the proximal femur (both internally and externally) in the "normal" population, we believed that the only way to optimize the fit and biomechanics in each patient was to customize the implant. We took advantage of the methodology developed by Techmedica (Camarillo, CA) that utilizes CT as well as radiographic input and CAD/CAM manufacturing techniques, which improved accuracy and shortened manufacturing time to make this clinically practical.

Since 1985 we have implanted more than 300 stems. During this time our design rules have evolved, starting with a rectangular cross-section proximally and a long bowed fluted stem distally. We later shortened the stem and changed to a modified rhomboidal cross-section with beveled faces to increase metaphyseal fill (Fig. 1A,B). The ingrowth surfaces consisted of three mechanically attached proximal pads on the anterior, posterior, and medial metaphyseal surfaces.

In 1989, we first began to see a few isolated pad separations from the implant (Fig. 2A,B). Some of these were detected only incidentally on follow-up radiographs in asymptomatic patients. Others, however, occurred after strenuous activity by some patients, after which they became symptomatic with weight-bearing thigh pain. From 1989 to the present we have documented a 5% incidence of this complication. Almost half of these patients have required revision.

These pad separations were quite distressing to us, and we quickly set about researching ways to solve the problem. A review of the literature showed that almost all porous coatings have reported failures and either bead shedding, delamination, or pad separation. We began to investigate two solutions: diffusion bonding of the pads to the substrate or elimination of the pads entirely in favor of hydroxylapatite (HA). Diffusion bonding of these pads was difficult, because the fixturing required was different for each custom implant. Ultimately Techmedica solved this problem, but we became convinced that no matter how a porous surface is bonded to the substrate, there will be some incidence of failure. We also were intrigued by the added benefit of HA as a

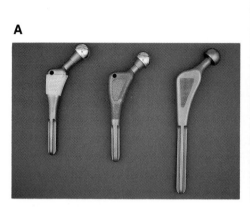

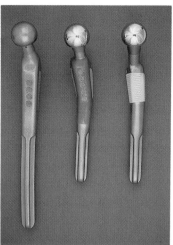

**FIG. 1** AP **(A)** lateral **(B)** views showing evolution of prostheses.

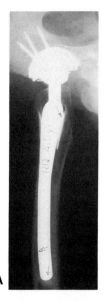

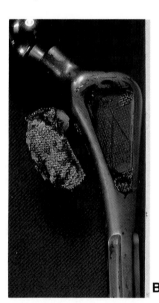

**FIG. 2** **(A)**: Lateral radiograph showing separation of the posterior ingrowth pad.**(B)**Post-operative photograph showing separation of the pad from the implant.

bioactive coating. As authors of other chapters have described, HA seems to induce osteoid to form adjacent to it and bonds directly to the bone. This is in contrast to a purely passive, porous metal surface that requires the bone to grow up to the surface and then into it to develop a mechanical interlock. Because retrieval studies had shown only spotty ingrowth into porous systems, and because all porous systems have reported coating failures, we chose to eliminate the porous coating entirely in favor of a bioactive HA coating. On the basis of early reports from other investigators in Europe and the United States, we recognized the need for high purity and crystallinity with uniform coatings of less than 70 μm.

Beginning in December 1989, we began using an HA coating (Bio-Interfaces, San Diego, CA) on a grooved, textured surface (Fig. 1). The groove geometry was specified by Bio-Interfaces on the basis of their experience with dental implants. Since then we have implanted almost 100 HA-coated stems, 26 of which have more than a two- year follow-up and are the subject of the clinical study reported here.

Simultaneously we recognized that long-term (more than one year) animal data were lacking to document HA's performance on femoral stems. Therefore, we began a canine study comparing implants with proximal porous pads versus HA-coated proximal grooves. This experience serves as the basis for the canine study reviewed below.

## CANINE STUDY

### Materials and Methods

Twelve skeletally mature male mongrel dogs underwent staged bilateral uncemented total hip replacement at 56 weeks and six weeks before harvest with MUTT canine total hips with titanium heads (Techmedica). Six of the dogs received bilateral stems with AP porous mesh (PC) ingrowth pads and six received bilateral stems with proximal circumferential 50 μm HA coating (Bio-Interfaces) applied to grooves on the metaphyseal segment. At harvest, AP and lateral x-rays, joint cultures, and synovial specimens were taken and femurs were frozen at -70°F before analysis.

Implants were evaluated for radiographic evidence of ingrowth. Gruen zones were marked, and the area and location of osteolytic lesions around the implant were noted and digitized.

A modification of a previously reported technique (6) was used to measure global and interfacial micromotion. Axial loads (0-450 N) were applied to the implant head, and torsional loads ($\pm$ 6 Nm) were cycled in internal and external rotation to the implant body. Data were collected at the level of the lesser trochanter through an array of three ball probes and six LVDTs. Implant-bone micromotion was calculated for the midpoint of the implant, the center of each implant face, and the stem tip.

After mechanical testing, specimens were embedded and sectioned at levels above and through the ingrowth/ongrowth regions and at the stem tip. Contact microradiographs, Scanning Electron Microscopy (SEM), and light histology were performed to evaluate bone apposition, HA status, osteolysis, and bone histology.

## Results

After initial recovery, all dogs ambulated normally. At harvest, all hips were located. No infections were noted. One dog (PC) was removed from the study because of a late femur fracture, leaving 11 dogs at the conclusion (n= PC-5, HA-6). Another dog required late reoperation to revise a broken modular head-neck component. Four reoperations were required to reduce acute dislocations. All femoral heads (Ti) were burnished, and although this had not been our initial intention we found that this acted as a generator of particulate debris within the joint space and may have contributed to the osteolysis we encountered in 56 -week specimens, in which all synovial specimens showed dark staining.

All HA and eight of ten PC implants appeared to be ingrown, with two PC implants being equivocal. There were no radiographic signs of loosening in any specimens. No osteolysis was seen at six weeks in any specimen. At 56 weeks, three of the six HA cases and all of the PC cases had some degree of osteolysis. With HA, osteolysis was minimal and was confined to the proximo-lateral shoulder of the implant. Three HA cases had no perceptible osteolysis. In the PC cases, osteolysis extended around the noningrowth surfaces of the implant, with cavitary lesions in the cancellous regions and endosteal scalloping of the diaphyseal cortex. Mean combined osteolytic area on AP and lateral x-rays was 7.2 mm$^2$ for HA and 143.5 mm$^2$ for PC ($p<0.01$).

Micromotion under both torsional and axial loading regimens was analyzed to compare differences in implant stability relative to time of implantation and type of fixation. Proximal torsional micromotion was significantly lower for HA stems at both six weeks ($p<.04$) and 56 weeks ($p<.05$). Both HA and PC stems demonstrated significant decrease in torsional micromotion at 56 weeks compared to six weeks (HA $p<.03$, PC $p<.04$). Similar differences seen with mean axial micromotion were not significant except for a small decrease in micromotion for HA stems from six to 56 weeks ($p<.04$)(Table 1).

TABLE 1. Mean micromotion

| Axial motion | 6 wks | 56 wks | p value |
|---|---|---|---|
| HA | 3.7 µm | 2.55 µm | <0.04 |
| PC | 5.6 µm | 4.8 µm | 0.38 |
| p value | 0.12 | 0.19 | |
| Torsion motion | | | |
| HA | 146 µm | 61 µm | <0.03 |
| PC | 922 µm | 191 µm | <0.04 |
| p value | <.04 | <.05 | |

Preliminary evaluation of six and 56-week specimens showed increasing bone ingrowth and apposition over time for the PC and HA specimens, respectively. The HA coating appeared to be unchanged in thickness between six and 56 weeks.

## Discussion

Despite adequate ingrowth or ongrowth in both groups, it appears that the HA group is significantly more stable in rotation. The increased wear of the titanium heads gave us an opportunity to evaluate the effect of circumferential HA coating versus porous pads in sealing the joint space from particulate debris and decreasing osteolysis adjacent to the stems. Osteolysis was more frequently seen in the PC group. When it was evident in the HA group it was proximal to the HA coating. Histology showed that these areas were filled with metallic particles. Because no burnishing of the stems was seen, we concluded that these particles came from the titanium heads.

HA coating was found to be missing in areas where the implant was proud and the coating exposed to the soft tissue or joint fluid. This was observed only in the one-year hips.

## CLINICAL STUDY

### Materials and Methods

Beginning in 1986, all patients who were thought to be candidates for cementless femoral components received a Techmedica custom femoral component. More than 300 of these components have been implanted in both primary and revision settings. One hundred consecutive primary cases and 100 revision cases that received a porous-coated custom stem with mesh pads have been followed for a minimum of two years (range two to six years). Beginning in December 1989, all custom cementless femoral components have been circumferentially proximally HA-coated over a groove-textured surface with no porous pads. Twenty-six cases have been followed for a minimum of two years (16 primaries and 10 revisions).

The design methodology has not changed significantly since 1986. A CT scan is obtained according to a standard protocol. Plain radiographs with magnification markers are also obtained. The CT images are digitally processed and aligned to create a three-dimensional model of the proximal femur with a standard coordinate system. Dimensional and shape parameters are extracted from the CT-based model, along with the plain radiographs, and are entered into a CAD/CAM system. This program designs the implant according to certain design rules.

The basic design rules have evolved over the years. The initial rectangular proximal cross-section with rounded corners has evolved into a modified rhomboidal cross-section, as shown in Fig. 1. Early implants were collarless but collars were subsequently added for revision cases. The distal stem has always had a cruciform shape in cross-section and an anterior bow matching the patient's own anatomic bow. The stem length for primary cases was initially quite long, extending to the isthmus. We subsequently established a rule that the stem length should be determined by extending down the canal until it had parallel endosteal contact for a distance of three stem diameters. Endosteal reaming was minimal early in the series, so that stems were longer. Later, in an attempt to improve AP fill distally in the oval-shaped canals, reaming was allowed to increase by 1 - 2 mm. This also enabled us to shorten the stem, since the endosteal region with parallel walls moves proximally with progressive reaming. Therefore, early in the series, implant lengths from osteotomy level to tip were approximately 165 mm on average; later, they decreased to 130 mm on average. The stem length on revision cases followed the same rule but was extended to bypass osteolytic defects or potential stress risers by three stem diameters. The bodies of the revision implants were also extended above the collar to make up for the proximo-medial segmental bone defects that were usually present. Version of the head-neck segment of the devices was also customized. Initially, 10° was chosen unless abnormal version of the proximal femur was detected; later, the position of the head was determined so that on an axial view of the CT model, a line drawn from the prosthetic head through the stem axis made a 25° angle with the posterior condylar line at the knee. This head position was achieved by altering the angle of version (anteversion or retroversion) and the take-off point from the body as needed. All implants were designed within a strain envelope to avoid implant breakage under physiologic loads.

An engineering drawing of the implant, along with transparencies at the appropriate magnification of the radiographs and photos of cut sections of the CT model was sent to the surgeon for review and approval. Consultation between the surgeon and design engineer resulted in modifications of almost half of the initial designs. The implant and a custom broach were manufactured and shipped to the hospital three weeks from the date of approval.

With the switch to HA coating, implants were manufactured by Techmedica with grooves on the anterior, posterior, and medial surfaces, and were bead-blasted circumferentially over the proximal 3 - 4 cm. The implant was then shipped to Bio-Interfaces for application of the HA coating before shipment to the hospital. This added an additional week to the manufacturing time.

### Results: Primary PC Stems

The first 106 custom primary stems, all with porous pads, have been followed two to six years (average 36 months). Of these, six have been lost to follow-up, leaving 100 stems for review.

At last follow-up the average total Harris hip score (HSS) was 93 (range 60 -100) with 76% excellent (score 90-100), 19% good (score 75-90), 5% fair (score 60-75), and 0% poor (score < 60). The fair and poor scores were mostly due to loss of points for function secondary to multiple-system disease. The mean Harris pain score (HPS -- maximum is 44 for no pain) was 41 (range 20- 40). There were 65% with no pain, 23% with slight pain, and 10% with mild pain. Analyzing thigh pain separately, 81% had no thigh pain, 12% slight, 7% mild, and 2% moderate, and none had severe thigh pain.

There were five revisions in the first 106 primary stems, two for failure of ingrowth and three for pad separation. There were no infections. In addition, there were four reoperations for osteolysis. All of these occurred in the first 26 cases in which a titanium modular head (28 mm diameter) was used. All of these cases had well-fixed stems at the time of reoperation, and only the head and liner were changed. Other complications included 1% dislocations, 5% femoral cracks, and 13% subsidence more than 3 mm. There were no cases of osteolysis in stems with chrome-cobalt heads.

Radiographic analysis showed that lucent zones of 1-2 mm were common over the smooth noningrowth surface of the stems. Ingrowth was judged to be present into at least one pad (no radiolucent zone over ingrowth pad and no progressive subsidence) in 83%, 5% showed no ingrowth and 12% were indeterminate owing to lack of tangential views of the ingrowth pads. Despite the large stems, stress shielding was rarely seen and was limited to the proximal two Gruen zones (1 and 7). Pedestal formation was seen in 15%. Failure of ingrowth and progressive subsidence correlated with pedestal formation, but the converse was not true.

## Results: Revision PC Stems

One hundred revision stems with porous pads have been followed for two to five years (average 46 months). Of these, 11 have died or are lost to follow-up and eight have been revised (see below) leaving 81 available for review. At final follow-up the average total HHS was 83 and the mean HPS was 38. Eighty-eight percent had minimal or no thigh pain.

There were eight revisions: three for failure of ingrowth, three for pad separation, one for infection, and one for unexplained pain. There were no reoperations for osteolysis. There were two infections, one of which was a recurrence after two stage-revision. There were three dislocations, 15 femoral cracks, 10 cases of subsidence over 3 mm, and six cases had ingrowth pad separation (three revised). There were no cases of osteolysis.

Radiographic analysis showed that lucent zones of 1-2 mm were common over the smooth noningrowth portions of the stem. Radiographic signs of ingrowth into at least one pad were seen in 73%, 15% had signs of no ingrowth, and 12% were indeterminate owing to nontangential views of the ingrowth pads. No stress shielding was appreciated and filling in of prior bone defects was common. Collars were added to revision stems later in the series and this virtually eliminated subsidence.

## HA Versus PC Stems

A study of HA-coated grooved femoral stems without porous pads was begun in December 1989. Since then, 26 stems have follow-up of more than two years (16 primary and 10 revision). These 26 stems were compared with the previous 26 stems (also 16 primary and 10 revision) at the same follow-up period.

Comparing the average HPS and HHS at three months, six months, one year, and two years for both primary and revision stems, there was no statistically significant difference, but this may be a result of the small sample sizes. Radiographic analysis showed that all HA primary stems had signs of bone attachment, whereas 81% of PC primary stems had signs of ingrowth into all three pad areas, 12% had ingrowth into one or two pad areas, and 7% were indeterminate. HA revision stems had 70% with signs of bone attachment and 30% were indeterminate. None had definite signs of failure of ingrowth. PC revision stems had only 30% with definite signs of ingrowth into all three pads, 30% with one or two pads ingrown, 10% with definite absence of ingrowth, and 30% were indeterminate. Radiolucent zones over the noncoated areas were less common in the HA groups.

There were no revisions in either group. Although no pad separations occurred in this PC group, the overall PC series described above had a 5% incidence of pad separation, half of which required revision.

## CONCLUSIONS

On the basis of our canine study and our initial clinical experience with HA-coated stems, we remain committed to their use. Although initial reports of off-the-shelf stems with HA coating are excellent (4), we do not believe that HA is a substitute for poor fit. Therefore, to optimize the results we will continue to use HA-coated custom-made implants when indicated.

The ultimate fate of HA on femoral stems is still unknown. Bauer et al. (1) have observed what appears to be remodeling of HA to bone on retrieved implants. There is concern, however, about possible long-term failure with cracking off of HA, thereby losing fixation and creating particulate debris that may also be abrasive to the titanium alloy stems.

Some authors recommend HA coating over a porous surface (2, 3, 5). This makes some sense, because canine studies indicate that the main advantage of HA is improved speed of bone attachment rather than improved strength of fixation as compared with porous coatings alone. These authors also believe that HA on porous coatings represents a "belt-and-suspenders" approach: even if the HA cracks off or dissolves, there will still be ingrowth to the porous coating. Our canine results, however, indicate drastically improved rotational stability of HA on grooves as compared to stems with porous pads. It would be of interest to compare circumferential HA-coated grooves to circumferential porous coating with and without HA. This awaits further study.

We chose to eliminate a porous coating because of our experience with pad separation. All porous coatings, however, have reported some incidence of failure (e.g., bead shedding, delamination). We are also concerned about HA coating of porous surfaces. In this situation there would be two interfaces subject to failure, HA-porous and porous-substrate. In addition, the porous coatings are more compliant than the base metal, which could lead to increased cracking off of HA on this more compliant surface.

In the future we plan to investigate an optimal groove design and orientation, one in which, regardless of the long-term fate of HA, the bone interdigitation with the grooves will provide both axial and rotational stability of the prosthesis.

## REFERENCES

1. Bauer TW, et al. Hydroxylapatite-coated femoral stems. Histological analysis of components retrieved at autopsy. *Journal of Bone and Joint Surgery* 1991, 73-A: 1439-52.
2. Collier JP, et al. Macroscopic and microscopic evidence of prosthetic fixation with porous-coated materials. *Clinical Orthopaedics* 1988, 235:173-80.
3. Collier JP et al. Results of implant retrieval from postmortem specimens in patients with well-functioning, long-term total hip replacement. *Clinical Orthopaedics* 1992, 274: 97- 112.
4. Geesink RGT, deGroot K., Klein CPAT. Chemical implant fixation using hydroxylapatite coatings. *Clinical Orthopaedics* 1987, 225: 147-70.
5. Hynes,DW, Freedman EL. The radiographic resolution of beads from porous-coated joint prostheses. *Journal of Arthroplasty* 1990, 5: 117-22.
6. Hayes DEF. Global: Interfacial micromotion of cementless femoral stems, *Orthopedic Research Society,* 1992.

Hydroxylapatite Coatings in Orthopaedic Surgery,
edited by R. G. T. Geesink and M. T. Manley.
Raven Press, Ltd., New York, © 1993.

# Early Clinical Results of Hydroxylapatite-Coated Total Knee Replacements

## Jan Verhaar, M.D., Ph.D.

It has been suggested that the evolution of knee arthroplasty has come to an impasse (1). After Charnley, Insall, and Marmor, many new designs have not clinically outperformed their predecessors. Poor implant design and polyethylene wear have recently been cited as contributors to high failure rates (1-3).

High rates of aseptic loosening have been reported with both the uncemented Kinemax® (4) and PCA® knee prostheses (5). After an average follow-up of 14 months, 20% of the Kinemax prostheses had been revised. PCA survival rates, defined as the point at which revision was recommended, were 77% at six years.

These figures contrast significantly with the 94% survival of the Total Condylar Knee reported by Ranawat and Boachie-Adjei (6) and the cumulative survival rate of 94% for the posterior stabilized prosthesis at 13 years, as reported by Stern and Insall (7). These successful implant designs had several features in common. The tibial and femoral component geometries were conforming, the patellar components were all-polyethylene, and the components were all fixed with polymethylmethacrylate.

Based on his study of polyethylene wear encountered in PCA and Synatomic® knee implants, Engh et al. concluded that five distinct design variables may contribute to accelerated wear (3). These are: a) thin polyethylene, b) screw holes in the tibial plate, c) high contact stresses due to reduced congruency, d) heat-pressed polyethylene and e) third-body wear debris. One or two of these variables may not, in themselves, be enough to induce excessive wear. However, a combination of more than one undesirable design feature may lead to the generation of polyethylene wear debris. This might explain why the PCA total knee prosthesis, in particular, has gotten a bad reputation with respect to polyethylene wear (3, 8-10).

The disappointing results seen with the PCA prosthesis and others have elicited editorial warnings regarding future innovations (1, 2). Although the editorials point out that the individual orthopaedic surgeon can improve his results through careful patient selection and improved surgical technique, the long-term material and design considerations cannot be ignored. Today, orthopedists are faced with a younger patient population presenting with incapacitating knee pain due to osteoarthritic changes. Although survival rates for total knee replacement (TKR) are encouraging, the probability of a good or excellent result after ten years has been reported at 60% (11). Moreover, the experience with total knee arthroplasty (TKA) in younger patients is mostly limited to rheumatoid arthritis. The largest series of TKAs for osteoarthritis in patients 55 years of age or younger, was published by Stern et al. (12) and was limited to 57 patients with a mean follow-up of six years. TKA may be a predictable and durable procedure in the elderly; however, with younger, more active patients, many questions remain unanswered.

The use of cement in TKA has been debated. Many authors have described reliable long-term results of TKR without radiographic evidence of "cement-disease" (12). There are, however, some theoretical advantages of cementless fixation over cement fixation. They include less bone loss during implantation, elimination of third-body wear caused by polymethylmethacrylate, better stress transfer and bone remodeling, safer implantation after previous bacterial arthritis, better restoration of bone stock, better loading of bone grafts, and easier removal of the implants without further bone loss at revision (13).

The goal of every artificial joint replacement should be to create an intrinsically stable joint. The stresses on the bone at the interface should be as low as possible. Because press-fit prostheses are not intrinsically stable, additional fixation has been necessary. This fixation has been traditionally achieved either through the use of polymethylmethacrylate or the use of porous surfaces (14).

Recently, Geesink reported that hydroxylapatite (HA) applied to the surface of metal implants creates an intimate bond between the bone, coating, and metal (15). The clinical results of human hip implantation with a follow-up of six years, as reported by Geesink, shows great similarity with cemented total hip results. This has never before been realized with any other cementless total hip system, including porous designs (16). HA seems to encourage bone to grow towards the prosthesis, filling gaps of between 1 and 2mm. This is a significant contribution, because bone cutting in TKA is not always as accurate as desired (17). In addition, with HA-coated implants, the entire coating area is available for bone apposition, whereas with porous surfaces, only 30% of the surface is available for bone ingrowth. Freeman and Tennant calculated that only 1% of the total surface area of porous coating is occupied by bone (14). This might explain why the histologic retrieval analysis of porous-coated tibial components have shown only limited bone ingrowth (18).

Based on the good, early results of HA-coated total hip replacements, we started a study in 1989 to determine the clinical and radiographic results of HA-coated femoral and tibial components in TKA. What follows is our preliminary experiences with HA-coated total knee prostheses. As such, our findings should not be interpreted as a plea for widespread clinical use of these implants in the very near future.

## MATERIALS AND METHODS

The study was conducted in the Netherlands at the Academic Hospital of Maastricht. Only patients younger than 70 years with a diagnosis of osteoarthritis of the knee were admitted to the study. Patients exhibiting a fixed flexion deformity of more than 20° and a varus or valgus malalignment of more than 15° were excluded.

The prosthesis used was an Osteonics Omnifit cobalt-chromium total knee (Osteonics, Allendale, New Jersey) (Fig. 1). The HA coating thickness was a uniform 50 μm and was applied to the stem via a plasma-spray process. The region of the coating is shown in Fig. 2. Only three of the five regions of the femoral component were HA-coated. The keel of the tibial component was not HA-coated. Six proportional sizes for both the femur and tibia were available. All patellae were resurfaced with an all-polyethylene patellar component which was secured in place with bone cement containing gentamycine (Gentapalacos ). Screw fixation was available in the tibial component. At the time of the operation, good quality bone and a good potential for implant stability were prerequisites for the use of HA. After the operation, full weight-bearing was permitted commencing on day seven.

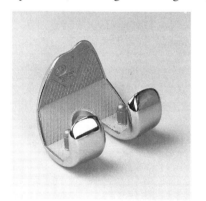 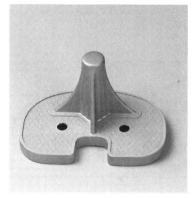

**FIG. 1.** The HA-coated Omnifit femoral and tibial components.

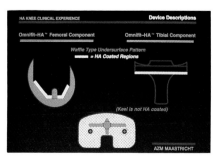

**FIG. 2.** Schematic illustration of the HA coating. Only the distal three areas of the femoral component were HA-coated. The tibial plate was HA-coated, but the keel remained uncoated.

In a two-year period, 24 patients (20 females and four males) with 26 TKRs were included in this study. The mean age of these patients was 61.4 years (range, 50 - 70 years). The average weight was 79.5 kg (range, 59 - 102 kg) and the average length was 167 cm (range, 150 - 190 cm). The right knee was resurfaced in 17 cases and the left knee in nine cases. Two patellae were non-resurfaced.

The average follow-up in this study was 12 months; the longest was for two years. All patients were seen at six weeks, three months, six months and one year. Yearly follow-up was continued. No patients were lost to follow-up.

No infection occurred. With the exception of a case of postoperative bleeding which resulted in stiffness of the knee and required manipulation under general anaesthesia, no major complications occurred. One patient has been reoperated on because of persistent patellar complaints. This patient had a previous hemipatellectomy and did not receive a patellar replacement at the time of surgery due to tightness of the extensor mechanism. The reoperation was a patellectomy without further complication and with good results.

The pre- and postoperative clinical investigation was conducted using the Hospital for Special Surgery (HSS) Knee Rating Scale in conjunction with the Knee Society Rating Scale. Radiographic studies were performed at each follow-up.

## CLINICAL RESULTS

Table 1 shows the pain at rest ratings based on the criteria of the HSS Scale.

**TABLE 1.** *Pain at rest*

| Rating | Pre- Op n = 26 | 6 Months n = 24 | 12 Months n = 18 | 24 Months n = 4 |
|---|---|---|---|---|
| None/Mild | 38 | 88 | 94 | 100 |
| Moderate | 50 | 12 | 6 | 0 |
| Severe | 12 | 0 | 0 | 0 |
| Total | 100 | 100 | 100 | 100 |

*The numbers are in percentages.*

Table 2 shows the pain on walking ratings based on the criteria of the HSS Scale.

**TABLE 2.** *Pain on walking*

| Rating | Preop n = 26 | 6 Months n = 24 | 12 Months n = 18 | 24 Months n = 4 |
|---|---|---|---|---|
| None/Mild | 8 | 79 | 89 | 100 |
| Moderate | 34 | 13 | 11 | 0 |
| Severe | 58 | 8 | 0 | 0 |
| Total | 100 | 100 | 100 | 100 |

*The numbers are in percentages.*

Table 3 shows the walking and standing ratings based on the criteria of the HSS Scale.

**TABLE 3.** *Walking and standing ability*

| Rating | Preop n = 26 | 6 Months n = 24 | 12 Months n = 18 | 24 Months n = 4 |
|---|---|---|---|---|
| Unlimited Range | 0 | 25 | 39 | 50 |
| Walking Five to Ten Blocks / Standing Intermittent | 8 | 33 | 44 | 50 |
| Walking One to Five Blocks / Standing 1/2 Hour | 92 | 42 | 17 | 0 |
| Walk Less Than One Block | 0 | 0 | 0 | 0 |
| Unable to Walk | 0 | 0 | 0 | 0 |
| Total | 100 | 100 | 100 | 100 |

The numbers are percentages.

Table 4 shows the mean HSS score and the mean Knee Society Score.

**TABLE 4.** *Mean total knee scores*

Mean HSS Knee Score

| | |
|---|---|
| • 3 months: | 77 |
| • 6 months: | 77 |
| • 12 months: | 82 |
| • 24 months: | 91 |

Mean Knee Society Score

| | Pain/Motion | Function |
|---|---|---|
| • 3 months: | 75 | 67 |
| • 6 months: | 75 | 74 |
| • 12 months: | 81 | 79 |
| • 24 months: | 91 | 88 |

The overall scores presented are comparable to the early results found with other cemented and uncemented studies. The time needed for full recovery seemed longer than that for cemented knee arthroplasties, but this could not be confirmed. We did not have a control group with patients identical in age and diagnosis.

## RADIOGRAPHIC RESULTS

With *in vivo* HA-coated total hip femoral components, subcortical cancellous bone formation along with diaphyseal subperiosteal cortical thickening has been described. We saw none of this with any of the HA-coated knee implants. With respect to the femoral components of the total knee, we noticed good bone contact with the distal (HA-coated) zones, and, as time progressed, we noticed a radiolucency and sclerotic line beneath the anterior and posterior zones (Fig. 3). This radiolucency was not accompanied by any bone reaction around the femoral pegs. The interpretation of these findings is difficult. The reactions might be caused by micromotion or some form of stress shielding due to a very good binding of the bone to the distal part of the femoral component.

The tibial components showed some condensation in the central area of the tibial plate, but with longer follow-up radiolucencies starting at the sides of the plates were seen in some cases (Fig. 4). Reactive lines around the stem of the tibia were also noted on many x-rays. However, there was no radiolucency around the stem. These findings are suggestive of some form of fibrous tissue interface, but in the central part of the tibial plate, no radiolucency has been noticed that might indicate bony ingrowth.

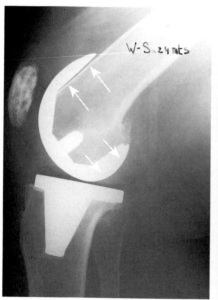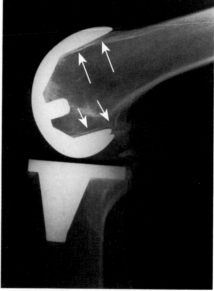

**FIG. 3.** Two lateral radiographs of HA-coated femoral components after a follow-up of two years. There is a good contact between the femur and the distal part of the femoral component. There is no contact between the bone and uncoated anterior and posterior part of the femoral component.

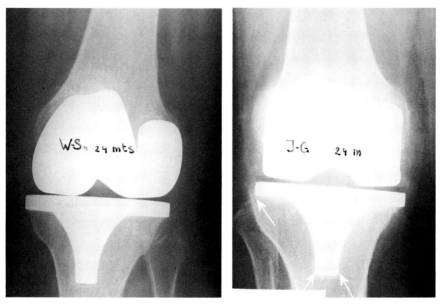

**FIG. 4.**   An AP radiograph of two HA-coated Omnifit knees, showing line formation around the stem and some radiolucencies at the sides of the tibial plate.

## CONCLUSIONS AND FUTURE PERSPECTIVES

These very early results may already lead to some conclusions. The clinical and radiographic results prove that HA-coated total knees do better than press-fit uncoated prostheses (4). Although the clinical results are rewarding, we are not fully convinced that we achieved bony ingrowth in all of our femoral and tibial components. Although Søballe et al. has shown that an unstable HA-coated implant has a more sure attachment to bone than an unstable non-HA-coated implant (19), we believe that long-term predictable results can only be achieved with bony ingrowth fixation.

We concluded from our observations that full HA coating of the femoral component may better distribute the stresses at the bone / implant interface than the partial HA coating we used in this series. Although bone loss in the distal anterior femur after TKA has been reported (20), the clinical relevance appears to be limited. Full coating might prevent the radiolucency seen at the anterior and posterior sides of the femoral component. The tibial components did not unequivocally show bony ingrowth, however additional follow-up is needed to accurately assess bone remodeling around the components. We also believe further biomechanical research is required to create an optimal stable implant for the proximal tibia. New keel designs, longer stems, or improved interfaces might lead to implants that provide much better intrinsic stability, which we consider a prerequisite for bony ingrowth (21, 22).

## REFERENCES

1.  Bauer GC. What price progress? - failed innovations of the knee prosthesis. *Acta Orthopaedica Scandinavica* 1992; 63: 245-6.
2.  Goodfellow J. Knee prostheses - one step forward, two steps back. *Journal of Bone and Joint Surgery (Br)* 1992; 74-B: 1-2.
3.  Engh GA, Dwyer KA, Hanes CK. Polyethylene wear of metal backed tibial components in total and unicompartmental knee prostheses. *Journal of Bone and Joint Surgery (Br)* 1992; 74-B: 9-17.
4.  Nafei A, Nielsen S, Kristensen O, Hvid I. The press-fit Kinemax knee arthroplasty. *Journal of Bone and Joint Surgery (Br)* 1992; 74-B: 243-6.
5.  Moran CG, Pinder IM, Lees TA, Midwinter MJ. Survivorship analysis of the uncemented porous-coated anatomic knee replacement. *Journal of Bone and Joint Surgery (Am)* 1991; 73-A: 848-57.
6.  Ranawat CS, Boachie-Adjei O. Survivorship analysis and results of total condylar knee arthroplasty. *Clinical Orthopaedics* 1988; 226: 6-13.
7.  Stern SH, Insall JN. Posterior stabilized prosthesis. *Journal of Bone and Joint Surgery (Am)* 1992; 74-A: 980-6.
8.  Jones SMG, Pinder IM, Moran CG, Malcolm AJ. Polyethylene wear in uncemented knee replacements. *Journal of Bone and Joint Surgery (Br)* 1992; 74-B: 18-22.
9.  Nolan JF, Bucknill TM. Aggressive granulomatosis from polyethylene failure in an uncemented knee replacement. *Journal of Bone and Joint Surgery (Br)* 1992; 74-B: 23-7.
10. Tulp NJA. Polyethylene delamination in the PCA total knee. *Acta Orthopaedica Scandinavica* 1992; 63: 263-6.
11. Nelissen RGHH, Brand R, Rozing P. Survivorship analysis in total condylar knee arthroplasty. *Journal of Bone and Joint Surgery (Am)* 1992; 74-A: 383-9.
12. Stern SH, Bowen MK, Insall JN, Scuderi GR. Cemented total knee arthroplasty for gonarthrosis in patients 55 years old or younger. *Clinical Orthopaedics* 1990; 260: 124-9.
13. Rackmann S, Mintzer CM, Walker PS, Ewald FC. Uncemented press-fit total knee arthroplasty. *Journal of Arthroplasty* 1990; 5: 302-14.
14. Freeman, MAR, Tennant R. The scientific basis of cement versus cementless fixation. *Clinical Orthopaedics* 1992; 276: 19-25.
15. Geesink RGT. Hydroxylapatite-coated hip implants. *Thesis*. Rijksuniversiteit Limburg te Maastricht, Maastricht, the Netherlands, 1988.
16. Geesink RGT. Hydroxylapatite-coated total hip prostheses. Two-year clinical and roentgenographic results of 100 cases. *Clinical Orthopaedics* 1990; 261: 39-58.
17. Toksvig-Larsen S, Ryd L. Surface flatness after bone cutting. *Acta Orthopaedica Scandinavica* 1991; 62: 15-18.
18. Cook SD, Barrack RL, Thomas KA, Haddad RJ. Quantative analysis of tissue growth into human porous total hip components. *Journal of Arthroplasty* 1988; 3: 249-54.
19. Søballe K, Brockstedt-Rasmussen H, Hansen ES, Bünger C. Hydroxylapatite coating modifies implant membrane fromation. *Acta Orthopaedica Scandinavica* 1992; 63: 128-40.
20. Mintzer CM, Robertson DD, Rackemann S, Ewald FC, Scott RD, Spector M. Bone loss in the distal anterior femur after total knee arthroplasty. *Clinical Orthopaedics* 1990; 260: 135-43.
21. Volz RG, Nisbet JK, Lee RW, McMurtry MG. The mechanical stability of various noncemented tibial components. *Clinical Orthopaedics* 1988; 226: 38-42.
22  Yoshii I, Whiteside LA, Milliano MT, White SE. The effect of central stem and stem length on micromovement of the tibial tray. *Journal of Arthroplasty* 1992; supplement; 7: 433-8.

*Hydroxylapatite Coatings in Orthopaedic Surgery,*
edited by R. G. T. Geesink and M. T. Manley.
Raven Press, Ltd., New York, © 1993.

# The Histology of HA-Coated Implants

Thomas W. Bauer, M.D., Ph.D.

Many animal studies, as well as early experience with human implants have suggested that calcium phosphate ceramics are biocompatible and may have desirable properties for weight-bearing orthopedic implants. Our understanding of the interface between bone and hydroxylapatite (HA) is incomplete, however, and it is appropriate to speculate about the potential consequences of HA degradation *in vivo.* The purpose of this study is to use experience with prospective animal studies as well as human clinical and autopsy retrievals to review our understanding of the bone/HA/implant interface. Several different mechanisms whereby HA coatings might disappear from the implant surface will be suggested, and we will speculate about the long term consequences of HA coatings on total joint implants.

## BACKGROUND

A thorough discussion of the chemistry and physical properties of calcium phosphate ceramics is beyond the scope of this study, but previous investigators have demonstrated the importance of the calcium and phosphate content as well as the density and crystallinity of ceramics in determining the extent of bone apposition and ceramic solubility (20). There is some evidence of partial conversion of various calcium phosphate compounds to more stable apatites *in vivo*, but non-hydroxylapatite calcium phosphates (eg. tricalcium phosphate, tetracalcium phosphate, etc.) tend to be more soluble than HA at neutral pH.

Precise chemical and crystallographic characterization has not always been complete, but previous studies have demonstrated the osteoconductive properties of calcium phosphates, especially hydroxylapatite. Porous and non-porous blocks of HA (16, 17, 21, 25, 26), and coatings of HA on metal substrates (6, 9, 10, 13-15) have shown early bone apposition with histologic features of excellent biocompatibility. Bone apposition appears to be well advanced as early as three weeks (4, 15), and in some animal studies, HA has shown greater than 90% apposition at 96 weeks (15). Most authors have shown no evidence of fibrous membranes or delamination (15), and have shown attachment strengths equivalent to, or stronger than, porous coatings (7, 9).

In previous studies we evaluated the extent and distribution of bone apposition to HA coatings from five femoral stems (1) and acetabular components (3) retrieved at autopsy from patients who died of causes unrelated to the implants. In this study, we will use examples from previous animal studies, human autopsy retrievals, and more than 30 clinically retrieved human HA-coated implants to illustrate the bone/HA interface and to propose several different potential mechanisms whereby HA coatings may be removed from the implant.

## MATERIALS AND METHODS

For animal studies, we have used a model in which cortico-medullary plugs are inserted into the distal femur of rabbits. Although not weight-bearing, the surface of the implant is exposed to both the cortical and medullary bone environment, rather than cortex alone. Plugs are left *in vivo* variable lengths of time, and different specimens are used for mechanical testing (push out tests), or histology (Fig 1). Our histologic preparation methods are similar for both animal test specimens and human retrievals:

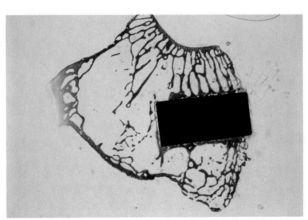

**FIG. 1.** Low magnification photomicrograph of a rabbit distal femur containing a corticomedullary plug. Bone apposition is extensive in this 4 week specimen, and there is no evidence of a fibrous membrane.

1) **Fixation**: After retrieval, each implant with surrounding bone is fixed in either 10% neutral buffered formalin or 70% ethanol. Recent studies have suggested that during formalin fixation, crystals of phosphate-containing salts may precipitate from the buffer onto the surface of exposed HA coatings (19). While not influencing the light microscopic appearance of implants surrounded by bone, this phenomenon may alter the ratios of calcium and phosphate

detected by energy dispersive x-ray spectroscopy. No such precipitation occurs in ethanol. Furthermore, direct dissolution of calcium phosphate coatings may occur during incubation in inadequately buffered formalin with a low pH. For these reasons, we currently recommend using 70% ethanol as the primary fixative rather than formalin. Depending on the amount of adjacent bone, fixation times vary from two days to more than one week. Large specimens, such as human autopsy retrievals are often rough cut into segments several cms in length before fixation.

2) **Embedding**: After fixation, the specimens are washed in water, dehydrated in a graded series of alcohols and embedded in Spurr plastic. After the plastic has polymerized, additional rough cuts are made and the resulting 1-2 mm thick blocks are radiographed, then ground using varying grits of sandpaper with Buehler grinding and polishing equipment. Final sections range from 35-60 μm in thickness and are stained with Cole's hematoxylin and eosin.

3) **Quantitation**: Several different methods can be used to visualize the final histologic sections. Back-scatter electron microscopy can provide images of the tissue as well as data concerning calcium and phosphate ratios, but does not reveal optimum cellular detail. We have also found it difficult to recognize and interpret histologic processing and sectioning artifacts by SEM, and find it especially difficult to distinguish *in vivo* delamination from artifactual cracks. We have found light microscopy, however, to provide good detail of the interface between bone and HA, as well as satisfactory resolution of cellular detail. EDX can also be performed on rough cut sections before, or after preparation for light microscopy. Interactive image analysis and light microscopy are used to measure the extent of bone apposition (expressed as percent of total surface available), trabecular bone areas, and HA thickness.

## RESULTS

### A) Animal Studies:

The corticomedullary plug model described above has proven to be a useful screening test to compare bone apposition and shear strength of different surface treatments. The results of our animal studies, like those of many other investigators, have confirmed the biocompatibility of HA coatings and the excellent bone apposition that occurs within the first several weeks *in vivo* (Fig. 2). We have also shown equivalent bone apposition and shear strength of HA coatings applied to either titanium or chrome-cobalt alloy substrates (2).

### B) Human Retrieval Studies:

Six HA-coated femoral components (1), and five HA-coated acetabular components (3) retrieved at autopsy have been histologically analyzed. Low magnification views of sections through the femoral (Fig. 3) and acetabular (Fig. 4, 5) components suggest that bone apposition is good, with struts of bone extending from the cortical endosteum to the implant surface. These struts

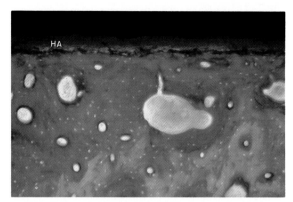

**FIG. 2.** Higher magnification photomicrograph of an HA-coated corticomedullary plug. Direct bone apposition to the HA coating is evident.

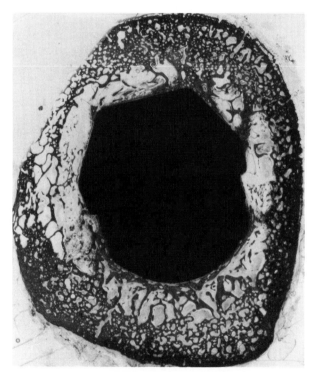

**FIG. 3.** Cross section of an HA-coated implant and proximal femur retrieved at autopsy nine months after total hip arthroplasty. Obtained just distal to the lesser trochanter, this section illustrates the bone remodeling occurring near the distal extent of the hydroxylapatite coating. Although somewhat difficult to visualize at this magnification, bone apposition is extensive, especially along medial and anterior aspects and at the "corners." Cortical porosity is also somewhat increased. (Reprinted with permission from Collier JP, Bauer TW et al, CORR 274:97-112, 1992).

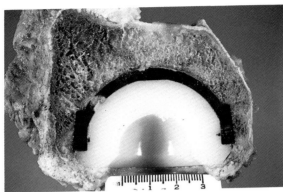

**FIG. 4.** Gross photograph illustrating the rough-cut acetabular component from a 9 month autopsy specimen. No fibrous membranes or areas of osteolysis are apparent and there is good bone apposition, especially to the rim. An incompletely bridged screw hole is also evident in the photograph.

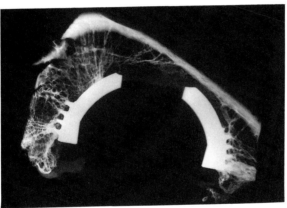

**FIG. 5.** Specimen radiograph of acetabular component retrieved at autopsy from a 37 year old woman 2 years after arthroplasty. Bone apposition is most prominent around the rim of this HA-coated screw cup, especially at the "peaks" of the threads. "Spot welds" of apposition to the dome are also apparent.

appear most prominent along the medial and anterior aspects of the femoral stem, areas where we would expect load to be transmitted from implant to cortex. There are also areas of cancellous condensation near the normalization steps and the corners of the implant, as if responding to torsional forces. There is increased proximal femoral cortical porosity present as well, suggesting a component of proximal stress shielding.

Higher magnifications reveal several features of bone apposition. First, HA can be identified over most of the surface of each implant, at each section level. Where present, the HA is of relatively uniform thickness. Bone apposition is also present over much of the implant surface (Figs. 6, 7). There are areas,

# THE HISTOLOGY OF HA-COATED IMPLANTS

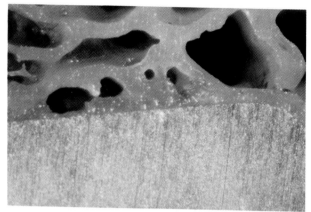

**FIG. 6.** Macrophotograph showing trabecular bone directly against the surface of an Omnifit-HA femoral component retrieved at autopsy 6 months after insertion. The bone appears somewhat translucent in this illustration, and appears to be in direct contact with the implant.

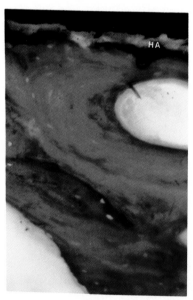

**FIG. 7.** Higher magnification photomicrograph of bone apposition to an HA-coated femoral stem retrieved at 9 months. The superficial aspect of the HA stains relatively darkly, probably representing adsorbed proteins, while the HA in direct contact with the substrate has a more transluscent appearance in this photograph. (Hematoxylin and eosin).

however, of apparent resorption of both bone and HA, and these areas are sometimes accompanied by osteoclasts (Fig. 8). In the regions of bone and HA resorption, small granules of HA are often present next to the stem, usually within histiocytes (Fig. 9). Small particles of metal may also be present. In rare areas, especially along the medial aspect of the stem, HA appears to have completely disappeared and bone is present immediately adjacent to the titanium substrate.

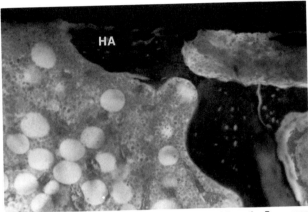

**FIG. 8.** Photomicrograph of a portion of a femoral stem retrieved at 4.5 months. Bone resorption appears to have occurred, and a remodeling canal is associated with resorption of both bone and the HA coating, but no fibrous membrane is present.

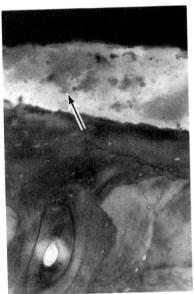

**FIG. 9.** Photomicrograph of an area of recent bone and HA resorption. Small granules of HA are present, primarily within histiocytes (arrow). Rare particles of metal also appear to be present, although it is unclear whether these are from the implant or are the result of sectioning artifact.

For the femoral stems, bone apposition and HA preservation are most prominent in regions of probable load transmission, especially the medial aspect of the implant. In areas where we would expect less load transmission (eg. posteriorly near the greater trochanter), there appears to be relatively less bone apposition, and somewhat greater loss of HA. The acetabular cups show similar findings, with bone and HA present in areas of expected load transfer (eg. the "peaks" of screw and knurled surfaces of the rim), and there appears to be non-random bone and HA resorption in areas of reduced load transfer (eg. the "valleys" between screw threads of the rim) (Fig. 10).

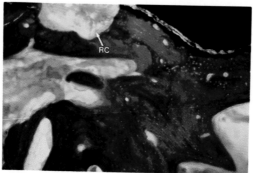

**FIG. 10.** Photomicrograph of the rim of an HA-coated dual geometry acetabular component. Bone apposition and preservation of HA appear most prominent at the "peaks" of the knurled surface, while bone and HA resorption are more prominent in the "valleys" (arrow), perhaps illustrating the influence of transmitted load on bone remodeling.

### C) Clinical Retrievals:

Besides autopsy retrievals described above, we have evaluated more than 30 HA-coated implants that have been clinically retrieved at the time of revision arthroplasty. Most of these have been revised because of post-operative fractures or infection. While those removed within several weeks of surgery are explanted without difficulty, implants that have been *in situ* for longer periods of time are often extremely difficult to extract, requiring the use of osteotomes to disrupt the bone-implant interface. The analysis of these retrieved implants is difficult, because the interface is nearly always compromised, and the extent of artifacts induced by implant removal cannot be determined with certainty. Some of these implants are completely surrounded by an intact coating of HA with a variable amount of adherent bone. Other implants, however, show apparent loss of HA coating (Fig. 11), sometimes as early as several weeks *in vivo*. Because the adjacent bone is not available for study, we can only speculate on the mechanism of HA loss (see next page).

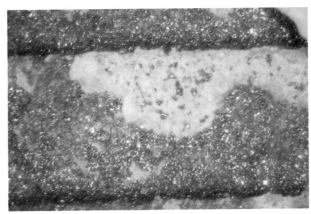

**FIG. 11.** Photograph of the surface of an HA-coated femoral component retrieved at the time of revision for a postoperative fracture approximately one week after arthroplasty. Areas of HA are absent from the implant surface. Adjacent bone was not available for study, so it is unclear whether this HA loss is due to delamination, dissolution, abrasion, or (less likely) osteoclastic resorption.

## DISCUSSION

Based on the above observations as well as previous animal studies, we have hypothesized that there are several mechanisms whereby HA coatings can be lost from the surface of the implant. The non-random distribution of bone and HA loss, as well as the frequent presence of osteoclasts, suggests that bone remodeling in response to changing loads may be one mechanism of HA loss (1, 3).

It has long been recognized that all bone remodels, and that bone in areas of changing mechanical loads may remodel relatively rapidly. The control of remodeling by load and local growth factors is incompletely understood, and represents an area of intense current investigation (27). It appears that once a remodeling unit has been activated, osteoclast precursors bind to the surface of a bony trabeculum, differentiate into multinucleated osteoclasts, and begin to resorb bone. Osteoclasts secrete hydrogen ions into the extracellular space, and by concentrating these ions close to the cell surface, create a local pH of approximately 4.8 (11). This acid environment dissolves endogenous bone mineral, while enzymes dissolve the organic component of bone matrix. Complex feedback mechanisms, possibly involving growth factors such as TGF-beta eventually inhibit osteoclast function. Under appropriate systemic and local homeostasis, osteoclasts are replaced by osteoblasts which gradually restore normal bone volume.

It is clear that many factors influence the extent and orientation of the new bone that is formed during the course of remodeling. These factors include: 1) the overall calcium and phosphate metabolism of the organism, controlled in part by systemic hormones, 2) local metabolic factors, such as the recruitment of osteoclasts by cytokines during inflammation, 3) the local availability of adequate raw materials (such as calcium and phosphate ions), 4) the location within the bone (eg. subperiosteal, cortical, or trabecular), and 5) the mechanical load being transmitted at that specific site. The mechanisms whereby all of these factors interact to influence the extent and orientation of new bone are unclear, and represent areas of productive research. While many factors could be involved in regulating bone resorption and apposition to HA-coated implants, the pattern of bone resorption and deposition suggests to us that normal bone remodeling in response to changing mechanical loads may be involved. Other authors have also suggested the cell-mediated consumption of calcium phosphate coatings by osteoclasts (19, 23).

Experience with animal studies as well as human clinical retrievals suggests that osteoclastic resorption is only one mechanism of HA loss. Other potential mechanisms include: 1) delamination, 2) dissolution, and 3) abrasion.

## Delamination

Bonding of the plasma-spray coating to the substrate is extremely important, and is influenced by many factors, including the temperature of the applied ceramic, and the texture of the implant. The adherence of the coating to the metal appears to be mostly mechanical, and is enhanced by a limited extent of surface roughness. Using high resolution electron spectroscopic imaging, however, Filiaggi and co-workers have mapped the distribution of calcium and phosphate ions over a titanium alloy substrate and have suggested phosphate diffusion into the metal as deep as 25 µm, possibly along grain boundaries (12). This suggests that under some conditions an actual chemical interaction may contribute to the mechanical bond between plasma spray coatings and titanium substrates.

While presenting a significant theoretical problem, in our studies we have confirmed *in vivo* delamination in only two specimens. One was a canine stem that was HA-coated in approximately 1983, and retrieved after 4.5 years. This femoral stem was functioning very well, but a loose acetabular component prompted removal. Histologic analysis revealed areas in which the HA coating had separated from the metal substrate and had become completely surrounded by lamellar bone. Bone was present between the HA, and the implant, in part in direct apposition to the underlying metal implant (Fig. 12). No histiocytic reaction was present and there was no foreign body giant cell reaction. Instead, the presence of numerous cement lines adjacent to the delaminated HA suggest very gradual consumption by remodeling.

The second example of delamination was a human clinical retrieval in which the HA coating had been applied to a textured, previously plasma-sprayed, titanium substrate. In this case the HA appears to have separated from the "peaks" of the textured substrate. Again, small plates of bone were present surrounding the delaminated HA, without evidence of a histiocytic or foreign body giant cell reaction. We have not recognized delamination in any of the Omnifit-HA autopsy stems analyzed to date.

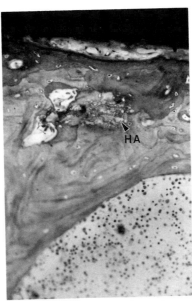

**FIG.12.** Photomicrograph of an HA-coated canine femoral component retrieved at 4.5 years. In this specimen a portion of the HA coating appears to have delaminated *in vivo* and is surrounded by lamellar bone. Bone is present between the delaminated HA and the implant surface. There is no evidence of a fibrous membrane or a proliferative histiocytic response to the delaminated HA, and no metal wear debris is present.

## Dissolution

It is well-recognized that non-HA calcium phosphates have a higher solubility at neutral pH than pure HA. Composites of HA and TCP used for bone graft substitutes or coatings, for example, show more rapid dissolution than coatings of nearly pure HA. While some conversion of other calcium phosphates to apatites probably occurs *in vivo*, it is likely that some of the loss of ceramic coatings seen in clinically retrieved specimens may represent dissolution. Plasma-spray coatings might be thought of as granules of highly crystalline HA bonded together by a matrix of less crystalline HA and other calcium phosphates. Components of the coating that are not densely crystalline HA are likely to preferentially dissolve. As this occurs, the more dense HA crystals appear to be released from the coating and are phatocytized by local histiocytes. Once intracellular, these particles may be seen within phagolysosomes where eventual consumption is likely.

Although not necessarily of clinical significance, it would appear that coatings containing a high content of dense, crystalline HA are likely to undergo less rapid dissolution, than coatings of either lower crystallinity or higher content of non-HA calcium phosphates. Experience with HA coatings from different manufacturers suggests to us that there may be marked differences in the composition and density of coatings produced by different manufacturers or by different application processes. These differences will certainly influence the longevity of the coatings, although at the present time we do not know the clinical significance of rapid, versus very slow, HA loss.

## Abrasion

It is reasonable to suspect that if an HA-coated implant is never stable, then the coating may become damaged by simple abrasion. We have received several such cases, one of which, for example, was placed next to a large segment of bone graft that failed to become incorporated. The loss of HA in this case is unlikely to represent osteoclastic resorption or dissolution, but simply abrasion.

## Consequences of Particulate HA

As illustrated above, the focal disintegration of HA is often accompanied by particles of calcium phosphate that become phagocytosed by histiocytes. Does this debris induce osteolysis, as is commonly believed for polyethylene wear debris? Certainly this is an area of concern, but the absence of radiographic evidence of osteolysis in the available clinical series of HA-coated femoral components (8, 13) suggests that distal femoral osteolysis induced by HA may not be a clinically significant problem. Furthermore although histiocytes can be identified to contain HA debris, these cells do not appear to proliferate into the large sheets of histiocytes commonly seen in membranes around cemented, or uncemented non-HA coated implants, and the lysosomes within the histiocytes are likely to eventually completely digest the calcium phosphate crystals (unlike polyethylene). Finally, solid blocks of HA, and particles of HA, have been available for several years for maxillofacial augmentation and for filling bone defects. The calcium phosphates in these applications may also undergo slow resorption, yet we are unaware of any cases of osteolysis known to be induced by these materials. Therefore, at the present time we view HA debris as ultimately biodegradable, and not, therefore, as likely to induce osteolysis as non-degradable wear debris.

Could particulate HA accelerate polyethylene wear by acting as a third body? Three body wear may be a major component in accelerated polyethylene wear. Many different types of particles can make their way into the joint space, including particles of bone cement or barium sulfate, loose metal beads or metal wires, fragments of bone, and particles of HA. Ultrahigh molecular weight polyethylene (UHMWPE) itself may also contain dense inclusions. Although we have no direct evidence of HA particles embedded in polyethylene of retrieved acetabular cups, it is logical to suspect that if these ceramic granules obtained access to the joint space, then like the erosive arthropathy induced by precipitation of endogenous hydroxylapatite crystals into joint fluid ("Milwaukee shoulder", "apatite-deposition arthritis") (22, 23), accelerated polyethylene wear would be a likely consequence.

## SUMMARY

The biocompatibility and osteoconductive properties of HA coatings appear to be beyond reasonable question. The longevity of these coatings *in vivo*, however, is unclear. We speculate that there are several different mechanisms whereby calcium-phosphate coatings could be lost from the implant surface. Three of these mechanisms (delamination, dissolution, and abrasion) can be influenced by manufacturing, application, and surgical techniques. The fourth mechanism, ie. consumption by osteoclasts during bone remodeling, can be influenced by coating density, but is unlikely to be easily overcome by manufacturing methods. Instead, it would appear that the biologically-controlled loss of HA coatings is a likely consequence of skeletal remodeling. If so, then it follows that simply coating an implant with HA will not necessarily lead to permanent bone apposition. Instead, the factors that influence load transfer from implant to bone, including the macroscopic and microscopic geometry, the flexibility of the underlying implant, and the state of the host bone will ultimately determine the extent and distribution of bone apposition.

## REFERENCES

1.  Bauer TW, Geesink RGT, Zimmerman R, McMahon JT. Hydroxyapatite-coated femoral stems. Histological analysis of components retrieved at autopsy. *Journal of Bone and Joint Surgery.* 1991;73-A:1439-52.

2.  Bauer TW, Friedman RT, Garg K, Draugh R. Effects of substrate metal composition on bone apposition to hydroxyllapatite. *Laboratory Investigations.* 1992;66:3A.

3.  Bauer TW, Stulberg BN, Ming J, Geesink RGT. Uncemented acetabular components. Histologic analysis of retrieved hydroxylapatite-coated and porous implants. *Journal of Arthroplasty.* 1992 (In press).

4.  Bloebaum RD, Merrell M, Gustke K, Simmons M. Retrieval analysis of a hydroxyapatite-coated hip prosthesis. *Clinical Orthopedics and Related Research.* 1991;267:97-102.

5.  Collier JP, Bauer TW, Bloebaum RD, Bobyn JD, Cook SD, Galante JO, Harris WH, Head WC, Jasty MJ, Mayor MB, Sumner DR, Whiteside LA. Results of implant retrieval from postmortem specimens in patients with well-functioning, long-term total hip replacement. *Clinical Orthopedics and Related Research.* 1992;274:97-112.

6.  Cook SD, Thomas KA, Kay JF, Jarcho M. Hydroxylapatite-coated titanium for orthopedic implant applications. *Clinical Orthopedics and Related Research.* 1988;232:225-43.

7.  Cook SD, Thomas KA, Dalton JE, Volkman TK, Whitecloud TS, Kay JF. Hydroxylapatite coating of porous implants improves bone ingrowth and interface attachment strength. *Journal of Biomedical Materials Research.* 1992 ;26:989-1001

8.  D'Antonio JA, Capello WN, Crothers OD, Jaffe WL, Manley MT. Early clinical experience with hydroxylapatite-coated femoral implants. *Journal of Bone and Joint Surgery.* 1992;74-A:995-1008.

9.  de Groot K, Geesink, RGT, Klein, CPAT, Wang TF. Plasma sprayed coatings of hydroxylapatite. *Journal of Biomedical Materials Research.* 1987;21:1375-81.

10. Ducheyne P, Hench LL, Kagan A, Martens M, Burssens A, Mulier JC. The effect of hydroxylapatite impregnation on skeletal bonding of porous coated implants. *Journal of Biomedical Materials Research.* 1980;14:225-37.

11. Fallon MD. Alternatives in the pH of osteoclast resorbing fluid reflects changes in bone degradative activity. *Calcified Tissue International.* 1984;36:458.

12. Filiaggi MJ, Coombs NA, Pilliar RM. Characterization of the interface in the plasma-sprayed HA coating/Ti-6Al-4V implant system. *Journal of Biomedical Materials Research.* 1991; 25:1211-29.

13. Geesink RGT, de Groot K, Klein CPAT. Chemical implant fixation using hydroxylapatite coatings. *Clinical Orthopedics and Related Research.* 1987;225:147-70.
14. Geesink RGT, de Groot K, Klein CPAT. Bonding of bone to apatite-coated implants. *Journal of Bone and Joint Surgery.* January 1988;70B(1):17-22.
15. Hayashi, K, Uenoyama K, Matsuguchi N, Sugioka Y. Quantitative analysis of *in vivo* tissue responses to titanium-oxide- and hydroxyapatite-coated titanium alloy. *Journal of Biomedical Materials Research.* 1992;25:515-23.
16. Holmes RE, Hagler HK. Porous hydroxyl-apatite as a bone graft substitute in mandibular contour augmentation. A histometric study. *Journal of Oral Maxillofacial Surgery.* 1987;45:421-9.
17. Jarcho M. Calcium phosphate ceramics as hard tissue prosthetics. *Clinical Orthopedics and Related Research.* 1981;157:259-78.
18. Kawaguchi H, Ogawa T, Shirakawa M, Okamoto H, Akisaka T. *Journal of Periodontal Research.* 1992;27:48-54.
19. Kieswetter K, Bauer TW, Brown SA, Van Lente F, Merritt K. Effects of histological processing on hydroxyapatite coatings. *Transactions of the Society of Biomaterials.* 1992;15:65.
20. Klein CPAT, Driessen AA, de Groot K, van den Hooff A. Biodegradation behavior of various calcium phosphate materials in bone tissue. *Journal of Biomedical Materials Research.* 1983;17:769-784.
21. Krajewski A, Ravaglioli A, Mongiorgi R, Moroni A. Mineralization and calcium fixation within a porous apatite ceramic material after implantation in the femur of rabbits. *Journal of Biomedical Materials Research.* 1988;22:445-457.
22. McMarty DJ, Halverson PB, Carrera GF, Brewer BJ, Kozin F. "Milwaukee Shoulder" - association of microspheroids containing hydroxyapatite crystals, active collagenase, and neutral protease with rotator cuff defects. *Arthritis and Rheumatology.* 1987;30:651-60.
23. Mueller-Mai CM, Voigt C, Gross U. Incorporation and degradation of hydroxyapatite implants of different surface roughness and surface structure in bone. *Scanning Microscopy.* 1990;4:613-624.
24. Ohira T, Ishikawa K. Hydroxyapatite deposition in osteoarthritic articular cartilage of the proximal femoral head. *Arthritis and Rheumatology.* 1987;30:651-60.
25. Oonishi H. Orthopaedic applications of hydroxyapatite. *Biomaterials.* 1991;12:171-8.
26. Uchida A, Nade SML, McCartney ER, Ching W. The use of ceramics for bone replacement. A comparative study of three different porous ceramics. *Journal of Bone and Joint Surgery.* 1984;66B:269-75.
27. Vaes G. Cellular biology and biochemical mechanism of bone resorption. A review of recent developments on the formation, activation, and mode of action of osteo-clasts. *Clinical Orthopedics and Related Research.* 1988; 231:239-71.

# Subject Index

# Subject Index